Understanding Clinical Governance and Quality Assurance

D0995421

By the same author:

*Quality Assurance**

* Also by Palgrave Macmillan

Understanding Clinical Governance and Quality Assurance

Making It Happen

Diana Sale

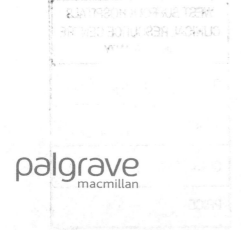

palgrave
macmillan

First published 2005 by
PALGRAVE MACMILLAN
Houndmills, Basingstoke, Hampshire RG21 6XS and
175 Fifth Avenue, New York, N.Y. 10010
Companies and representatives throughout the world

PALGRAVE MACMILLAN is the global academic imprint of the Palgrave
Macmillan division of St. Martin's Press LLC and of Palgrave Macmillan Ltd.
Macmillan® is a registered trademark in the United States, United Kingdom
and other countries. Palgrave is a registered trademark in the European
Union and other countries.

ISBN–13: 978 0–3333–98510–6 paperback
ISBN–10: 0–333–98510–9 paperback

This book is printed on paper suitable for recycling and made from fully
managed and sustained forest sources.

A catalogue record for this book is available from the British Library.

Library of Congress Cataloging-in-Publication Data

   p. cm.
   Includes bibliographical references and index.
   ISBN 0–333–00000–0
   1.

10   9   8   7   6   5   4   3   2   1
14   13   12   11   10   09   08   07   06   05

Printed and bound in China

This book is dedicated to my family: my husband Mike with thanks for so many happy years together; my lovely daughters Joanna and Caroline; and the very latest addition to the family, Harry, a five-month-old bundle of absolute perfection – definitely three-star quality!

Contents

List of Figures and Tables

Figures

Tables

Foreword

I was delighted to be asked to write the foreword to this comprehensive book that explains clinical governance and quality assurance. Although clinical governance and quality assurance are now a welcomed and accepted part of the routine delivery of healthcare, concerns continue about implementing clinical governance amongst some managers and healthcare professionals. This book will be of value to everyone involved in the practicalities of clinical governance and assuring the quality of care for patients. It is valuable reading for those undertaking a variety of academic courses with quality assurance as an element of their studies.

Diana Sale has successfully supported private and public sector healthcare organisations to set up systems of quality assurance and clinical governance both here in the UK, in Ireland and in Portugal. In this book she draws upon this experience to give a clear account of the theory behind quality assurance and clinical governance and expands on the practical skills that are essential to the successful implementation and maintenance of clinical governance systems.

The seven pillars of clinical governance are described in detail and each pillar concludes with a checklist of suggested action to turn theory into practice, with the result that clinical governance is a reality and not a paper exercise. Essentially this is a practical book which is underpinned by theory and is motivated by the need to support a system of clinical governance that will ensure patients receive the highest possible quality of care, based on high standards, safety, and improved patient services. The book also includes relevant theories, concepts and methodoligies that have been applied successfully over the years, including Deming, Crosby and Juran's work on total quality management, Donabedian's approach to setting and monitoring standards and Maxwell's Six Dimensions. The book also covers the practical skills to support an effective system of clinical governance which include project management, managing change, mentoring, managing poor performance, leadership, facilitating skills, working with groups, preparing a strategy, process mapping, risk management, and workforce planning.

Clinical governance is driving the national agenda to improve healthcare, and this readable and comprehensive book will support staff in delivering the best quality of care for patients.

Sir Ian Carruthers OBE
Chief Executive, Dorset and Somerset Strategic Health Authority

Preface

Clinical governance has been at the top of the agenda for the NHS since 1999, with the aim of setting in place systems that assure good-quality care for patients and their carers and families. This book is about making the principles, philosophies and methodologies of quality assurance a reality, and that requires the people who deliver and manage care to have the skills and knowledge to meet the clinical governance agenda.

Clinical governance is a quality assurance framework within which to assure the quality of patient care and services in a trust or healthcare organisation. It is not different to quality assurance, but is an approach to assuring the quality of care. Clinical governance consolidates the quality agenda by 'closing the loop' through the monitoring of standards by national organisations which include the Healthcare Commission (England and Wales), previously known as the Commission for Healthcare Audit and Inspection (CHAI); the Clinical Standards Board for Scotland; the National Patient Safety Agency for England. The NHS Performance Framework, and the National Patient and User Surveys.

In the past, quality assurance was often seen as someone else's responsibility – perhaps a team of people in a healthcare organisation with the management of quality assurance as their remit – but clinical governance is not someone else's responsibility. It is not a 'spectator sport'; it includes everyone involved in the delivery of healthcare services both in the public and in the private and voluntary sectors. It is everyone's responsibility, a team approach that requires knowledge and skills to ensure that patients receive good quality care and services every time, all the time. Like any successful team it requires strong, effective leadership and skilful, knowledgeable, well-trained clinical and non-clinical team members who work together to deliver the quality agenda.

Today most staff working in NHS trusts, and other healthcare organisations have a clear idea of what clinical governance is all about and the role that they are expected to play in the system. However, I have written this book because I believe that there are other skills and knowledge which support an effective system of clinical governance. This includes a good working knowledge of clinical governance and quality assurance, its history, and the tools which have been used effectively, tried and tested and whose valid methodology and approach is still applicable today. Certain chapters may be more relevant or may appeal more to people in their quest for meeting the clinical governance agenda depending on their different backgrounds, remits and interests.

However, the primary leadership is for nurses and therapists at all levels of their careers, for managers both in the NHS and the private and voluntary sectors, and for students undertaking leadership courses at degree or masters level such as Leadership London, Clinical Leadership, the Royal College of Nursing Leadership Programme and Leading an Empowered Organisation (LEO). Also, as reference for the MBA and Health Management programmes as supplementary text. There are other skills that are very useful, if not essential, in today's health service, such as the management of change, project management, working with groups and effective facilitation. There is information in several chapters to support project managers in the numerous current projects and others that are proposed in the government's plans to modernise the NHS and in the private and voluntary sectors to support the desire continuously to improve the quality of care for their patients.

Some chapters are more relevant to directors of nursing and heads of service, such as the chapters on strategy and the management of change. Others support a much wider readership, offering guidance on how to work effectively with groups together with information on being an effective facilitator, while the chapters on the seven pillars of clinical governance may be of interest to non-executive directors of NHS trusts and governors and trustees in the private and voluntary sector to support their responsibilities in assuring clinical and corporate governance.

There are three sections to the book. First is the background to the history of quality assurance leading up to the time that this book was written. The appendix sets out some of the key events, legislation, reorganisations and people that have influenced the development of the measurement of quality of care from the first century AD up to the present day. Chapter one addresses the question 'What is quality assurance and how did it evolve?' I have included potted histories of some of the gurus of quality assurance such as Donabedian, Maxwell, Oakland, Crosby, Koch, Juran and Deming to mention just a few. The work of Deming is of particular relevance to the private sector as it forms the basis of the continuous quality assurance programmes in private hospitals all over the UK.

Chapter 2 describes the backgorund to clinical governance, and the national agencies and bodies that drive the clinical governance agenda. Then Chapters 3 to 9 expand on each of the seven pillars of clinical governance and look at how to make the key elements work in practice. For example, in Chapter 3, Patient and Public Involvement, there is information about how to assess patient satisfaction and methods of involving patients in evaluating and planning their care and services. This section concludes with a 'making it happen' checklist. In other words, if the organisation has implemented all the items on the checklist then this element of clinical governance is likely to be in place. This format is repeated for each of the seven pillars of clinical governance. Pillar five, which is about education, training and continuing professional development, includes a very informative contribution on practice development and quality improvement by Brendan McCormack, Director of Nursing Research, and Helen Chambers, Quality Manager, who both work in the Practice Development Unit at the Royal Hospital in Belfast.

Chapter 10 brings the previous chapters together as a strategy or plan that gives structure to the process of clinical governance. It is said that 'if you don't know where you are going then there is little chance that you will arrive there'. A strategy pinpoints exactly where you want to be, how you will get there and when you will arrive. Writing a strategy is a skill to be learned, and this chapter sets out some useful guidelines and advice on how to write one. This is supported by an excellent example of a clinical governance strategy provided by Barbara Merricks, who is the Director of Primary and Community Services and the Lead Director for Clinical Governance for North Dorset Primary Care Trust. As the process of clinical governance develops, it is essential to know 'when we have arrived', and this is achieved through measurement at a variety of levels across the organisation, but also at organisational and national levels in the form of benchmarking and the measurement of performance indicators by measuring how well the organisation is doing against external targets and indicators.

Essence of Care is a benchmarking tool, and Carole Annetts describes how she led the Essence of Care project for South West Primary Care Trust and North Dorset Primary Care Trust. This chapter also gives an overview of organisational approaches to quality assurance, including Total Quality Management, quality circles and quality improvement processes, which concludes the first section of this book.

The second section of the book takes the form of a review of some of the most commonly used 'off-the-shelf' tools for measuring the quality of care and an overview of the process of setting and monitoring standards.

There are other skills that I believe are essential to support continuous quality improvement, including the management of change, project management and good facilitation skills to lead and support staff in the process of change required to ensure a robust system of clinical governance. The final and third part of the book is about some of these skills and includes worked examples of project plans, work plans and change management.

The last chapter is called clinical governance – the tools for the job which include some of the skills that lead to successful meetings: supporting listening skills, coping with and resolving conflict, facilitating brainstorming sessions, forcefield analysis, and so on. In fact, these are the skills which turn a clinical governance strategy into reality through supporting change in the culture of the organisation and improved approaches to the management and delivery of care for patients.

This book is not intended as an academic text but to give information on supporting and maintaining a successful system of clinical governance in an

NHS trust or a private or voluntary sector healthcare organisation. It is about supporting the people who deliver and manage care with the skills and knowledge to meet the clinical governance agenda.

Diana N. T. Sale

Acknowledgements

I should like to take this opportunity to thank Jo Ley-Sale for helping me with the production of this book, ensuring that it was produced in an efficient and timely fashion, and Caroline Sale who undertook an enormous amount of research to support the book. Once a book is written there is always that moment of doubt about the content – is it accurate, up to date, interesting and readable? My sincere thanks go to Pam Homer, Director of Nursing at Joseph Weld Hospice, and Bob Oreschnick of Healthcare Consulting for wading their way through the draft manuscript and offering sound advice and positive encouragement.

I am very grateful for three contributions to this book: Barbara Merricks, Director of Primary and Community Services and Lead Director of Clinical Governance for North Dorset Primary Care Trust (PCT) and her excellent clinical governance strategy; Carole Annetts, a project manager for North Dorset PCT and South and West Dorset PCT and her account of the PCTs' innovative approach to the use of Essence of Care, and to Brendan McCormack, the Director of Nursing Research, and his colleague Helen Chambers, a quality manager on a Practice Development Unit, at the Royal Hospitals Trust in Belfast. Their valuable contribution is about the role of practice development in clinical governance.

Thanks are due to the publishers Appleton-Century-Crofts for extracts from *The Nursing Audit* by Phaneuf and *Quality Patient Care Scale* by Wandelt and Ager. Permission was kindly granted by Newcastle-upon-Tyne Polytechnic Products Ltd to reproduce extracts from Monitor, the Juran Institute for extracts from their work on Total Quality Management, Philip Crosby for extracts from his work on the Quality Improvement Process, and the Deming Institute for extracts from Deming's work on Total Quality Management

Every effort has been made to trace all the copyright holders of text used in this book. If any have been inadvertently overlooked, the publishers will be pleased to make the necessary arrangements at the first opportunity.

Diana N. T. Sale

Quality Assurance: What Is It, and How Did It Evolve?

1

Chapter Contents:

- defining quality assurance
- levels of evaluation of the quality of care
- evaluation of the quality of care
- quality assurance concepts, theories and principles.

This chapter defines quality assurance and describes its origins. The appendix sets out a chronological overview of some of the significant milestones in the history of quality assurance from the first century right up to the present day. It includes key events, people and legislation that have brought us to clinical governance and a systematic approach to quality assured healthcare.

Defining Quality Assurance

There are many definitions of the term 'quality assurance' written by people who have researched the subject thoroughly. A definition that is both appropriate and easily understood is that given by Williamson (1979): 'Quality assurance is the measurement of the actual level of the service provided plus the efforts to modify when necessary the provision of these services in the light of the results of the measurement.'

Another definition, according to Schmadl (1979), is that the 'purpose of quality assurance is to assure the consumer of nursing of a specified degree of excellence through continuous measurement and evaluation'. Øvretveit (1992) describes quality as 'all activities undertaken to predict and prevent poor quality'. An alternative definition is from the British Standards Institution (BSI, 1990): 'A management system designed to give maximum confidence that a given acceptable level of quality of service is being achieved with a minimum of total expenditure.' The word 'quality' is defined by *The Concise Oxford Dictionary* as 'degree of excellence' and the word 'assurance' as 'formal guarantee; positive declaration'. So, from these definitions, 'quality assurance' may be interpreted as a formal guarantee of a degree of excellence.

Levels of Evaluation of the Quality of Care

There are various levels at which evaluation of the quality of care may take place (see Figure 1.1):

■ national level
■ Strategic Health Authority, NHS trust or other health organisation (board level)
■ local level – wards, departments, GP practices, clinics, units.

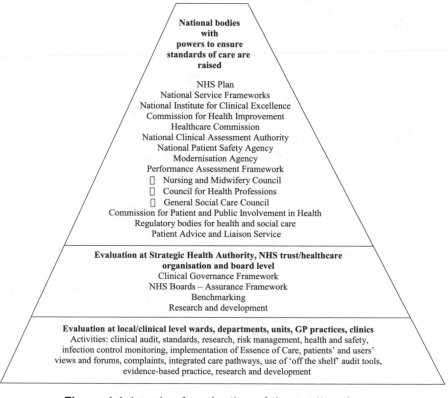

National bodies
with
powers to ensure
standards of care are
raised

NHS Plan
National Service Frameworks
National Institute for Clinical Excellence
Commission for Health Improvement
Healthcare Commission
National Clinical Assessment Authority
National Patient Safety Agency
Modernisation Agency
Performance Assessment Framework
☐ Nursing and Midwifery Council
☐ Council for Health Professions
☐ General Social Care Council
Commission for Patient and Public Involvement in Health
Regulatory bodies for health and social care
Patient Advice and Liaison Service

Evaluation at Strategic Health Authority, NHS trust/healthcare organisation and board level
Clinical Governance Framework
NHS Boards – Assurance Framework
Benchmarking
Research and development

Evaluation at local/clinical level wards, departments, units, GP practices, clinics
Activities: clinical audit, standards, research, risk management, health and safety, infection control monitoring, implementation of Essence of Care, patients' and users' views and forums, complaints, integrated care pathways, use of 'off the shelf' audit tools, evidence-based practice, research and development

Figure 1.1 Levels of evaluation of the quality of care

National Level

NHS Plan

The Government's NHS Plan is the blueprint for health services for the next ten years. *The NHS Plan: A Plan for Investment; A Plan for Reform* (DoH, 2000b) underpins the Government's reforms set out in *The New NHS, Modern, Dependable* (DoH, 1997):

The NHS Plan – which was published in July 2000 is a radical action plan which sets out measures to put patients and people at the heart of the health service and promises a 6.3 per cent increase in funding over five years to 2004.

Within the NHS Plan the Government set out the arrangements for performance review and promises:

- more power and information for patients
- more hospitals and beds
- much shorter waiting times for hospital and doctor appointments
- cleaner wards, and better food and facilities in hospitals
- improved care for older people
- tougher standards for NHS organisations and better rewards for the best.

The priorities of the NHS Plan are to:

- target the diseases which are the biggest killers, such as cancer and heart disease
- pinpoint the changes that are most urgently needed to improve people's health and wellbeing and deliver the modern, fair and convenient service that people want.

The targets set out in the NHS Plan end in 2005 and will be replaced by national standards (DoH, 2004; see also Chapter 11 – Benchmarking).

The NHS Plan outlines the role of the Modernisation Board and the Modernisation Agency. Ten task-forces were set up to drive the agenda for coronary heart disease, cancer, mental health, older people, children, waiting times and access to services. The remaining four concentrated on the NHS workforce, quality, reducing inequalities and promoting public health and investment in facilities and information technology (DoH, 2000b).

The plan outlines an approach that ensures that health services are driven by continuous quality improvement for all aspects of the service provided, which includes clinical care, support services, management processes, the quality of life and the patient experiences of healthcare. The Plan states that healthcare organisations must have systems that allow for review and reform of policy, procedures and the delivery of care thus ensuring that care is constantly improved; a culture that supports learning from mistakes leading to a reduction in errors, supported by clinical supervision and ongoing learning and development of all staff – in other words, clinical and corporate governance.

Also at this level is the Audit Commission looking at 'best value' in the delivery of services, which is now incorporated into the Healthcare Commission.

National Service Frameworks

National Service Frameworks (NSFs) form one of a range of measures to raise quality and decrease variations in services. They were introduced in *The New NHS, Modern, Dependable* (DoH, 1997) and *A First Class Service: Quality in the New NHS* (DoH, 1998) and re-emphasised in *The NHS Plan* (DoH, 2000b) as drivers in delivering the Modernisation Agenda. The NSFs set national standards and define service models for a defined service or care group, put in place strategies to support implementation and establish performance milestones against which progress within an agreed timescale can be measured.

NSFs establish standards and define service needs for specific groups of patients and there is only one new framework a year. Each NSF is developed with the assistance of an external reference group which includes health professionals and representatives of users and carers, health service managers, partner agencies and other advocates to establish clear, evidence-based NSFs for major care areas and disease groups. This approach ensures greater consistency for patients in the availability and quality of services right across the NHS. The Government uses NSFs as a way of being clearer with patients about what they can expect from their health service. The first NSFs began with mental health and coronary heart disease, with their priority status reflected in the guidance given on the development of health improvement programmes. The rolling programme of NSFs was established in 1998 and to date there are NSFs for:

- mental health (1999)
- coronary heart disease (2000)
- national cancer plan (2000)
- older people (2001)
- diabetes (2001)
- renal services (2002)
- children's services
- long-term conditions focusing on neurological conditions (in the future).

With each NSF the best evidence of clinical cost-effectiveness is taken, together with the views of users, to establish principles for the pattern and level of services required. These then establish a clear set of priorities against which local action can be framed:

The selection of the future topics will be informed through:

- demonstrative relevance to the Government's agenda for health improvement and tackling health inequalities, set out in The New NHS, Our Healthier Nation and wider policies on social exclusion
- an important health issue – in terms of mortality, morbidity, disability or resource use

- an area of public concern
- evidence of a shortfall between actual and acceptance practice, with real opportunities for improvement
- an area where care for a patient may be provided in more than one setting (for example, hospital, GP surgery or at home) and by more than one organisation (for example, NHS and/or local authority/voluntary sector)
- an area where local services need to be recognised or restructured to ensure service improvements, and
- a problem, which requires new, innovative approaches.

The programme also informs the Chief Medical Officer's Annual report (DoH, 1998, para. 2.43).

At the top of the pyramid are the national bodies with powers to ensure that standards of care are raised and these include the National Institute for Clinical Excellence, Commission for Health Improvement (CHI) now incorporated into the Healthcare Commission, the National Clinical Assessment Authority, the National Patient Safety Agency, the Modernisation Agency, the NHS Performance Assessment Framework, Commission for Patient and Public Involvement in Health and the Patient Advice and Liaison Service.

National Institute for Clinical Excellence (NICE)

NICE was formed in April 1999. It is a Special Health Authority and part of the NHS. According to its website:

> It is the independent organisation responsible for providing national guidance on treatments and care for those using the NHS in England and Wales. Its guidance is for healthcare professionals and patients and their carers, to help them make decisions about treatment and healthcare. NICE guidelines and recommendations are prepared by independent groups that include professionals working in the NHS and people who are familiar with the issues affecting patients and carers. NICE produces guidance in three areas of health:
>
> - the use of new and existing medicines and other treatments within the NHS in England and Wales – technology appraisals
> - the appropriate treatment and care of patients with specific diseases and conditions within the NHS in England and Wales – clinical guidelines, and
> - whether interventional procedures used for diagnosis or treatment are safe enough and work well enough for routine use – interventional procedures.

NICE also funds four enquiries that undertake research into the way patients are treated to identify ways of improving the quality of care. These investigations are known as Confidential Enquiries.

NICE makes recommendations about whether interventional procedures used for diagnosis or treatment are safe enough and work well enough for routine use. Responsibility for interventional procedures was transferred to NICE in April 2002, following a recommendation made in the Kennedy Report that aims to produce an NHS centred on patient's needs in which systems are in place to ensure safe care and to maintain and improve the quality of care. (www.nice.org.co.uk)

There are numerous sources of evidence to support best practice and inform the clinician in the setting of their standards so the question is – Why is a single statement of best practice from NICE of benefit to clinicians and patients? Andrew Dillon (Lugon and Secker-Walker, 2001) suggests the following benefits:

- there is consistent definition of best practice
- there is economy of effort from a single, thorough appraisal of the evidence
- health professionals and patients can be informed simultaneously
- there is equitable access to clinical services
- there is consistent use of resources.

NICE was established to provide guidance to health professionals and patients in England and Wales on the clinical cost and effectiveness of selected technologies and other health interventions. Technology appraisals include

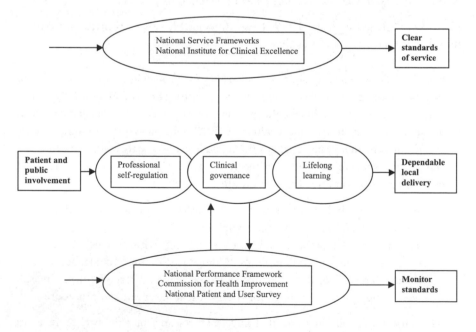

Figure 1.2 The Quality Framework
Source: DoH, 1997

those for medical devices, pharmaceuticals, equipment, diagnostic procedures, clinical procedures and some aspects of health promotion. Topics are selected for NICE by the Department of Health in England and by the National Assembly for Wales following consultation with stakeholders from outside and inside the NHS against a framework of the National Service Frameworks (NSFs) and the priorities set for the NHS. The Institute works in conjunction with the Commission for Health Improvement (CHI) now known as the Healthcare Commission, the Health Development Agency (HAD) and the NHS Research and Development (R&D) Programme. NICE also works closely with the agencies in Scotland that are similar to those in England and Wales, as mentioned above. These include the Scottish Intercollegiate Guidelines Network (SIGN) and the Health Technology Assessment Board for Scotland (HTB). It also funds clinical audit at national level and provides funds for effective practice publications. The Institute is part of the modernisation of the NHS in England and Wales as set out in the government's framework *A First Class Service* (DoH, 1998) and *The New NHS, Modern, Dependable* (DoH, 1997).

Commission for Health Improvement (CHI)

The Commission for Health Improvement was set up 'to provide independent assessment of local systems to assure and improve quality in the NHS, with the power for rapid intervention to address serious service problems. It also has the function of providing advice and guidance to the Health Service' (DoH, 2001).

The CHI is a non-departmental public body (CHI, 2002). It was established under the 1999 Health Act as part of the Government's reforms to help improve patient care. It has statutory powers and is accountable to the Government for its work, but operates independently. Its main functions are:

- to provide independent scrutiny of local clinical governance arrangements to support, promote and deliver high-quality services. CHI is carrying out a rolling programme of reviews of clinical governance arrangements in every NHS organisation
- to carry out studies that monitor and review the implementation of National Service Frameworks, National Institute of Clinical Excellence (NICE) guidance and other key NHS policy priorities
- to provide national leadership to develop and disseminate clinical governance principles and to identify and share good practice.

CHI has adopted six key principles that underpin its work:

- the patient's experience is at the heart of CHI's work
- CHI is independent, rigorous and fair

■ CHI's approach is developmental and supports the NHS in continuous improvement
■ CHI's work is based on best available evidence and focuses on improvement
■ CHI is open and accessible
■ CHI applies the same standards of continuous improvement to itself that it expects of others.

The five principle aims of CHI's clinical governance reviews are:

■ to provide the public and people using the NHS services with objective and fair assessments of NHS organisations' progress towards introducing effective clinical governance
■ to help the NHS achieve evidence and continuous improvements in the quality of patient care
■ to help the NHS reduce unacceptable variations in the quality of clinical services
■ to identify and disseminate good practice in clinical governance
■ to increase understanding of clinical governance and the factors that determine its effectiveness.

Since April 2000, the CHI have undertaken reviews of NHS trusts to monitor the quality of clinical services at local level, against national standards, and intervene as necessary to deal with problems of poor quality. The CHI has a rolling programme across NHS organisations, which involves teams of auditors who visit and check that clinical governance is in place. The CHI visits each organisation at least once every four years, targets those that are not meeting the required standard and arranges to visit these trusts more frequently. The CHI works with the NHS to help improve the standards in poorly performing trusts and also highlights good practice that they encounter during their visits. The CHI has the power to investigate any service where concerns have been raised or there is clear evidence of serious failure of the management of a trust.

The Government announced in 2002, subject to primary legislation, that a new single commission was to be set up to inspect both the public and private healthcare sectors (NHS Executive, 2002). The CHI has been succeeded by the Commission for Healthcare Audit and Inspection (CHAI) with more responsibilities (see under Healthcare Commission). It has incorporated the Office for Information on Healthcare Performance and manages the national patient and NHS staff surveys. In April 2004 it re-established itself as the Healthcare Commission. See also Chapter 11 – Star Ratings.

Healthcare Commission

The Healthcare Commission is a new organisation established in April 2004 and is the public name of the Commission for Healthcare Audit and Inspection

(CHAI).This new organisation covers England and Wales and brings together the CHI, the National Care Standards Commission (NCSC) – inspection and licensing of private and voluntary healthcare – and the Audit Commission who undertake national 'Value for Money' studies in healthcare.

In future it is expected that the Mental Health Act Commission will merge into the Healthcare Commission, once further legislation has been completed. The Healthcare Commission, pilot for mental health reviews with the Commission for Social Care Inspection is planned for 2005. The merging of existing organisations is as a result of the following:

- greater patient involvement in healthcare and an increased choice about their treatment, which demands better information on healthcare so that informed decisions can be made
- NHS budgets are largely devolved to PCTs, increasing the diversity in the provision of healthcare through the private sector and foundation trusts which demand reliable and meaningful information on healthcare
- the publication of the consultation document, *Standards for Better Health – Health Care Standards for Services under the NHS* (DoH, 2004). The Healthcare Commission is responsible for developing criteria against which to assess compliance with these standards. The Welsh Assembly Government is undertaking a similar programme of work
- increased funding for the NHS and the need for monitoring outcomes, how the money is used, value for money and the return on investments
- continuing issues of equity and access. The inspection by multiple agencies is widely seen as excessive and one of the key roles of the Healthcare Commission is to co-ordinate and reduce the workload involved in the inspection process.

The Healthcare Commission will continue reviews and investigations but there will be three significant differences:

- the reviews will reflect national standards (the pilot reviews against standards are planned for the end of 2004/beginning of 2005 and will include standards in medicine management, the children's National Service Framework and public health)
- the Commission will move away from the whole system approach of clinical governance reviews to one that is targeted on issues that emerge from the screening process and local intelligence
- the reviews will cover NHS trusts and the private and voluntary sector.

The Healthcare Commission will also conduct and publish surveys of NHS patients and staff and again this will be confined to England. The result is a more cohesive approach to inspection, publishing reports and dissemination of good practice. As part of the complaints reforms (DoH, 2003) the Healthcare Commission will have responsibility for following up complaints that have not been resolved locally through the local resolution process (see Chapter 6 – Complaints).

Standards for Better Health

Standards for Better Health (DoH, 2004) is a consultation document published in February 2004 which ended in May 2004. This document proposes the establishment of two sets of standards covering NHS healthcare in England:

> The Health and Social Care (Community Health and Standards) Act 2003 confers powers on the Secretary for State to publish statements of standards in relation to the provision of health care by and for English NHS bodies and cross border Special Health Authorities. Standards for Better Health, health care standards under the NHS February 2004.

The consultation document states:

> The publication of the standards provides the opportunity to draw several strands of the performance regime together in a redesigned format and we are currently considering how best to co-ordinate these, which include:
>
> ■ agreed healthcare standards and inspection criteria, and a defined method which the Healthcare Commission (CHAI) will use to review trusts
> ■ a redesigned performance ratings system from the Healthcare Commission, (CHAI) incorporating the Healthcare standards
> ■ a national Public Service Agreements (PSA) targets for 2005–8, and
> ■ a new Planning and Priorities Framework (PPF) for 2005–8.
>
> The establishment of these standards will set the framework for decentralising the management of the health service in line with our policy to shift the balance of power from central government to the NHS.

A set of 24 core standards will establish a level of quality of care which can be expected by all NHS patients, regardless of where they are treated. These standards are coming into effect from the end of 2004.

The second set of standards proposed are ten developmental standards, designed to enable the overall quality of health care to rise to a higher standard in the long term as additional resources invested in the NHS take effect.

Criteria with which to measure the standards will be developed and subsequently monitored by the Healthcare Commission. The standards have been divided into the following domains:

- safety
- clinical and cost effectiveness
- governance
- patient focus
- accessible and responsive care
- care environment and amenities
- public health.

For more information, see Chapter 6.

National Clinical Assessment Authority (NCAA)

The NCCA was established as a Special Health Authority in April 2001 with a remit to provide support to the NHS when the performance of an individual doctor is giving cause for concern. The NCCA works closely with the General Medical Council and the Healthcare Commission as part of a framework to protect patients and improve the quality of care. The publication of the report *An Organisation With a Memory* (DoH, 2000a) drew attention to the absence of a systematic approach to identifying serious lapses in standards of care and of an analysis of the events, learning from these and introducing systems of change to prevent them recurring.

National Patient Safety Agency

This agency was set up in July 2001 following the publication of *Building a Safer NHS* (NHS Confederation, 2001). The role of the National Patient Safety Agency is to run a national reporting system for the recording of adverse healthcare events. See also Chapter 4 – Risk Management.

Modernisation Agency

The Modernisation Agency, created in April 2001, is part of the Department of Health and was set up to help healthcare staff redesign local health services in line with good practice (DoH, 2000b).

The agency provides a problem-solving service to the NHS which includes the following:

- it helps to diagnose problems and support possible solutions. The agency has a key role in conjunction with the Strategic Health Authorities in the assessment of an NHS organisation for eligibility to access the NHS Plan Performance Fund and how the fund may be used
- it provides practical tools and training skills
- it secures patient and carer involvement

- it co-creates solutions which means that the agency adapts and modifies innovation and best practice from one trust so it can be used by another trust
- it identifies good practice, for example the NHS Beacons Learning Handbook which lists services that have been innovative in meeting specific health care needs across all sectors. The Beacons Learning Handbook can be obtained through the Beacon website at www.nhs.uk/beacon.

The agency works closely with organisations on a national and international basis, for example the Royal Colleges, the European Quality Forum and the academic institutions. The following teams carry out the work of the Modernisation Agency:

- the National Patient's Access Team – this team helps NHS organisations meet the NHS Plan maximum-waiting-time targets. See also Chapter 11 – Benchmarking
- the National Clinical Governance Support Team which is a multidisciplinary team that helps NHS organisations to develop and implement systems of clinical governance
- the National Primary Care Development Team which supports all aspects of primary care development such as medicines management programmes, and the healthy communities collaborative which includes social care and primary care collaboratives
- the Changing Workforce Programme whose role is to address issues such as expanding the breadth or depth of a job, design new roles to meet patient needs and improve access to treatment and care
- the Leadership Centre whose role is to bring together the different leadership initiatives and support the NHS University. See Chapter 6 for more information on leadership.

NHS Performance Assessment Framework

This is a mechanism by which NHS organisations monitor the delivery of health services against the Government's plans for improvement and is discussed in detail in Chapter 11 – Performance Indicators.

Commission for Patient and Public Involvement in Health (CPPIH)

Community Health Councils were abolished in 2003 and the Commission for Patient and Public Involvement in Health (CPPIH) was set up with responsibility to make appointments to Patient Forums. This organisation sets national standards and provides training and monitoring of the Patient's Advice and Liaison Service (PALS), Patient Forums and the Independent Complaints Advocacy Services (ICAS).

Patient Advice and Liaison Service (PALS)

In the discussion document *Involving Patients and the Public in Healthcare* (DoH, 2001b), a series of proposals were made to improve public involvement in the NHS. These included:

- patient's forums to be set up in every NHS Trust and PCT in England, as an independent body of patients and people from the local community. This forum is empowered to inspect all aspects of the work of a trust including that of the service provided by the GPs and the NHS work provided by the private sector. One member of the forum is elected to serve on the trust board
- the role of PALS is to provide information to patients about health and local health services, both NHS and voluntary services and support groups. PALS are in a position to alert trusts and PCTs to gaps in service provision and possible or potential problems. They also support patients with concerns, problems and complaints helping them through the process to resolve issues as quickly as possible.

Other national standards include the National Minimum Standards for Care Homes for older people, and the standards for younger adults and adult placements. Examples of other organisations offering evaluation of the quality of care at this level include the Health Quality Service Accreditation and the Bristol University Hospital Accreditation Programme. At this level the organisation is measured against pre-set standards or criteria set by an organisation outside the trust or healthcare organisation. There are also national standards set by the Royal Colleges and professional organisations such as the Chartered Society of Physiotherapists and any British Standards, formally BS 5750 now ISO 9000, and regulatory bodies for health and social care which include:

- the Royal Colleges
- the Nursing and Midwifery Council
- the Council for Health Professions
- the General Social Care Council.

Trust or Organisational Level

The next level is that of the Chief Executive and the board of the NHS trust or healthcare organisation. This level is responsible for ensuring that the provision of services meet the requirements set out at national level. Since the publication of *A First Class Service* (DoH, 1998) and the accompanying legislation, the Chief Executive is now required to be accountable for the quality of patient care in the same way that he/she already guarantees financial probity in the handling of public money by the trust. In 1999 the Government published *Clinical Governance: Quality in the New NHS* (DoH, 1999), which states that trusts must demonstrate that they have mechanisms in place through which they can account for this responsibility and take action on the outcomes of these processes in their organisation. To meet this requirement each trust has set up a clinical governance committee. This committee provides regular reports about progress towards clinical governance and/or reports to highlight problems or deficiencies, including complaints, clinical negligence, incidents and poor performance, to the Chief Executive and the trust board who take appropriate action.

Local/Clinical Level

The next level is the base of the pyramid and the most important level – the clinical area, ward, department, unit, clinic, GP practice, and so on. Here the quality assurance activities may be varied and numerous, including research,

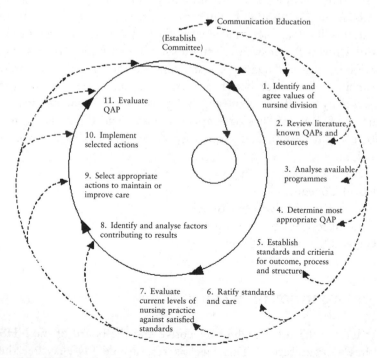

Figure 1.3 Steps in implementing a quality assurance programme (QAP)
Source: Lang, 1976

clinical audit, integrated care pathways, setting and monitoring of standards, comparing standards against national standards, benchmarking, evidence-based practice, systems of patient/client feedback, implementation of National Service Frameworks and NICE directives and guidelines, continuing professional development and lifelong learning, reflective practice, risk management, health and safety, infection control, and so on.

Evaluation of the Quality of Care

All these levels require an evaluation of the quality of patient care and the service provided. There are a variety of conceptual models of evaluation that have been published and may be used by anyone, from any background, as a model of evaluation. Lang's framework for change (Lang, 1976) as set out in Figure 1.3 has eleven steps and has been used successfully as a model for quality assurance.

The model can also be adapted, as shown in Figure 1.4, for use by a quality assurance committee, or the ward sister or charge nurse, head of department or professionals in their particular clinical area.

The Quality Assurance Cycle

The quality assurance cycle as set out in Figure 1.4 is used as a systematic approach to assuring the quality of care:

- *identifying values*: the first step of the quality cycle is to get together with colleagues in your ward or department and write a philosophy of care, discussing your personal beliefs about patient care, the national-level directives that are driving the provision of health care, the profession's code of conduct, any specific departmental guidelines or standards, beliefs about the uniqueness of individuals and their human rights, the philosophy of care of the trust or organisation and society's values. This does not have to be a long, detailed account but a simple summary of the beliefs held by the group
- *setting objectives*: the next step is to set some objectives – what is hoped to be achieved by measuring the quality of care. This should include the measurable effect of care given to patients and the performance of the staff involved in the delivery of patient care or service
- *describing patient care in measurable terms*: before the quality of care can be measured, it must be described in terms of the process of the delivery of care or service. To this end, it is necessary to identify standards and criteria. On reviewing the literature, it is evident that a number of tools have been

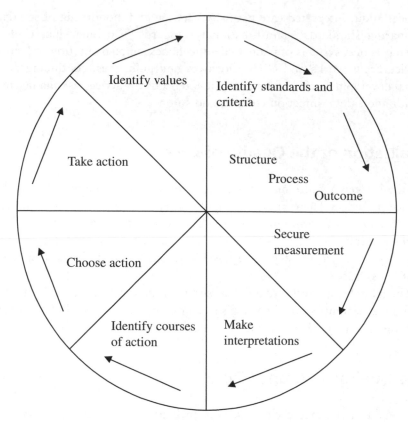

Figure 1.4 A quality assurance cycle adapted from Lang's cycle as in Figure 1.3

developed and are in use all over the country. Many approaches are based on criteria and standards, and can be categorised into a structure, process and outcome framework. Some authors of these tools favour the measurement of process while others favour outcome

- *securing measurement*: to measure the quality of care, the appropriate tool must be selected. The tools are essentially data collection systems using retrospective and concurrent audit; that is, systems for collecting information which, when collated, will give an indication of the quality of patient care for a particular ward or department

- *evaluating the results*: evaluation of the results involves comparing 'what is' with 'what should be' and then identifying what needs to be done to achieve an acceptable standard of care or service

- *taking action – completing the cycle*: taking action is achieved by developing a plan to ensure that care is given, or the service is provided, according to the agreed standard. If this last vital step is not taken, then there has been little point in the exercise, and there will be no improvement of patient care. Where standards are found to be low, or where there is poor quality of care, action must be planned and taken to change practice, and the cycle starts again.

Quality measured is not always quality assured, as shown in Figure 1.5. When the gaps have been identified and actions drawn up and implemented and the resulting change leads to the standard being achieved, then the loop has been closed and only then is quality is assured.

Quality Assurance Concepts, Theories and Principles

Within the world of quality assurance there are some key people whose work has influenced the development of quality assurance over the last 40 years, both in the United Kingdom and abroad. It is said that the quality revolution in industry started in Japan in the 1950s inspired by the writings of Deming and Juran (Macdonald and Piggott 1990). Some of these people include:

- W. Edwards Deming
- Joseph Juran

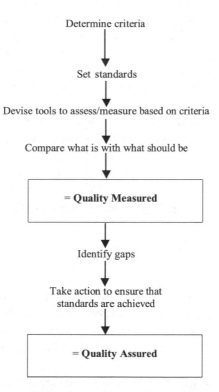

Figure 1.5 Quality measured, quality assured

- J. Drew
- Philip B. Crosby
- John Oakland
- T. J. Peters and R. H. Waterman
- Robert Maxwell
- Avedis Donabedian
- Dr John Øvretveit
- Hugh Koch
- Karoru Ishikawa

W. Edwards Deming

One of quality assurance's gurus from the USA who died in 1994, he is considered to be the founding father of the quality movement. In his early work, Deming recommended uniformity as the path to quality and promoted the idea of a 'quality culture' through motivating and developing people (Deming, 1986).

Today Deming's work is the primary resource used as the basis of quality assurance systems in the private healthcare sector across the UK. Deming, a statistician, is widely acknowledged as the initiator of the use of statistical quality control measures that were used extensively by Japanese industry in the 1940s. His early work was based on statistics and founded on his experience of sampling techniques used during the period he worked for the US Government in the Department of Agriculture and the Bureau of Census. Deming drew on the work of his tutor, Walter Shewhart (1931), and the need to focus on problems and variations in production processes, which should be identified and systematically reduced to: 'a predictable degree of uniformity and dependability, at a low cost and suited to the market' (Deming, 1982).

He divided the need to identify the cause of problems and variations into:

- 'special causes' which can be assigned to individual equipment, machinery or operators
- 'common causes' which include faulty raw materials which are shared by several operations and as such are the responsibility of management.

He believed in the use of statistical process control (SPC) charts as the key method for identifying special and common causes and assisting with the diagnosis of quality problems. His aim was to remove outliers, which are quality problems relating specifically to the cause of failure of an individual or piece of equipment.

Deming had a quantitative approach to identifying and solving problems. He was critical of companies that looked for chance variation which, he believed, occurred in the absence of statistical methods. He recommended the use of measurement of performance through statistical methods in all areas and not simply conformance to product specifications. His philosophy was that productivity improves as variability decreases and, as everything varies, then to control quality successfully a statistical method is required.

Deming advocated worker participation in decision-making and was critical of management, holding them responsible for 94 per cent of quality problems because he felt that management should help their workers to work 'smarter, not harder'. He was also critical of 'motivational programmes' because he believed that 'doing one's best' was just not good enough. Workers must know what to do and have the resources with which to do the job. He raised concerns about inspection as a method of quality control when it is used in isolation, as this approach neither improves nor guarantees quality. In 1982 he was influenced by the work of Juran and Feiganbaun when they worked together in Japan and from this came Deming's systematic approach to problem-solving which is the 'plan, do, check, action' (PDCA) cycle as shown in Figure 1.6. The cycle is continuous; once the cycle has been systematically completed, it just starts again and again and again ...

This approach is now commonplace; it has been reinterpreted in other methodologies such as the EPDCA cycle in Oakland's work and is central to the application of the ISO 9001: 2000 standard.

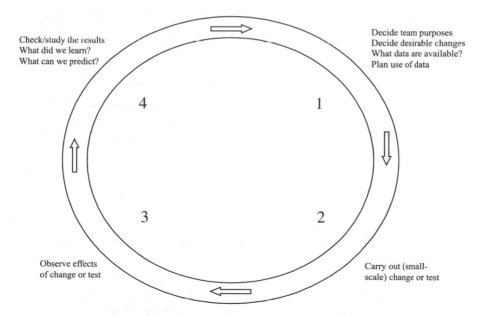

Figure 1.6 The Deming/Shewhart or PDCA cycle

Deming also believed in a systematic, methodical approach to quality initiatives and the need for continuous quality improvement action. He set out seven fundamental beliefs which the called the Seven Deadly Sins (Deming, 1986):

- lack of constancy
- short-term profit focus
- performance appraisals
- job-hopping
- use of visible figures only
- excessive medical costs
- excessive costs of liability.

Deming has four principal methods:

- the PDCA cycle
- statistical process control
- the 14 principles for transformation (see Chapter 11 – Total Quality Management)
- the seven-point action plan (see Chapter 11 – Total Quality Management).

Dr Joseph M. Juran

Joseph Juran came from the USA and had an engineering background. He started his career as an engineer in 1924 and later worked as an executive, civil servant, academic, arbitrator, director and management consultant. In the early 1950s he was invited to Japan where he lectured on quality. He is best known for the broad management aspects of quality, the important role of communication, the co-ordination of functions and the 'human' element. He stated that an understanding of the human element associated with the job would help to solve technical problems and that such an understanding might be the prerequisite of a solution. He focused on quality management from the top of an organisation and identified eight success factors which would indicate that an organisation had improved quality (Juran, 1988). In these organisations top managers had:

- personally led the quality process
- adopted quality improvement plans, and roles and responsibilities were clearly identified
- included all those affected
- trained management staff in quality planning, control and improvement
- trained the workforce to participate in quality improvement
- included quality improvement in strategic planning

■ applied quality improvement to business planning and operational processes
■ used modern quality methodology instead of empirical quality planning.

Juran (1998) organised quality management into three parts called a quality trilogy:

■ *quality planning*: determining who the customers are and their needs, and developing processes which result in products which respond to these needs
■ *quality control*: evaluation of the product performance and comparing this to product goals and then acting on the difference
■ *quality improvement*: identification of improvement projects and establishing the project teams with resources, training and motivation to diagnose the cause of the problems, identify solutions and establish mechanisms to monitor and maintain progress.

J. Drew

Drew undertook a survey of 21 hospitals to establish what quality assurance techniques were being used. It was established that there were 42 different techniques being used and that they fell into the following categories:

■ comments from patients and others
■ special rounds of patient units
■ checks and tests of procedures
■ patient and other records
■ others, for example inspection teams of outside agencies, nurses, consultants, infection control nurse, and so on.

The survey highlighted that each hospital was using at least one quality assurance tool, but that there was a lack of co-ordination and information-sharing between hospitals in the same area. Drew stressed the need for the sharing of techniques in order to establish a uniform and complete system of quality control. Since then, nurses all over the world have evaluated the care given to their patients to a greater or lesser degree (Drew, 1964).

Philip B. Crosby

Crosby, one of America's quality gurus, has a background in quality control. He is a graduate of the Western Reserve University and, following military service, he went into quality control in manufacturing. He combines the preventative focus of quality assurance with the Deming and Juran systematic and disciplined approach, while taking account of prevailing staff attitudes. He is a significant contributor to quality assurance and, although his work has been developed in industry, many of the principles he proposed have relevance to and influence over health care.

Crosby (1979) defined quality management as: 'A systematic way of guaranteeing that organised activities happen the way they are planned. It is a management discipline concerned with preventing problems from occurring by creating the attitudes and controls that make prevention possible.' Crosby also highlights 'customer requirements' as the cornerstone of quality. He maintains that quality is 'no more and no less than conformance to customer requirements'. His best-selling book, *Quality is Free*, was first published in 1979. His approach is known as the quality improvement process (QIP). He sets out three questions which are essential to answer (Crosby, 1988):

- what is the definition of quality?
- how is it achieved?
- how can it be measured?

See Chapter 11 for Crosby's Quality Improvement Process.

J. S. Oakland

John Oakland is a British guru of quality assurance and the author of *Total Quality Management* (1989). He is Executive Chairman of Oakland Consulting plc and prior to this was Professor of Total Quality Management and head of the European Centre for Total Quality Management at the University of Bradford Management Centre in the UK. He stresses the importance of the customer/supplier interface, which he describes as a "quality chain', with the customer and the supplier forming the vital links. He concludes that the chain can be broken at any point if an individual or other essential piece of equipment does not meet requirements (Oakland, 1989). He examines the management of quality through two central concepts (Oakland, 1986):

- *quality of design*: 'a measure of how well the product or service is designed to meet its purpose'
- *conformance to design*: the extent to which the product or service actually achieves the quality of design; the need to build statistical process control into the production process.

See Chapter 11 for Oakland's Total Quality Management.

T. J. Peters and R. H. Waterman

Peters and Waterman published *In Search of Excellence: Lessons from America's Best-Run Companies*. Creating quality requires an organisation continually to strive for excellence. There are seven key variables in the organisation to focus on (the Mckinsey 7-S Framework:

- strategy
- structure
- people
- management
- style
- systems
- procedures guiding concepts and shared values, and the skills contained within the organisation (Peters and Waterman, 1982).

Robert Maxwell

In 1984 Robert Maxwell, while leading the King Edward's Hospital Fund for London, published a paper in the *BMJ* entitled 'Quality Assessment in Health' (Maxwell, 1984). He went on to say: 'Concern about the quality of care must be as old as medicine itself. But an honest concern about quality, however genuine is not the same as a methodological assessment based on reliable, evidence' (Maxwell, 1984). Maxwell's six dimensions arise from his belief that quality of care cannot be measured in a single dimension. Each of the six dimensions needs to be recognised separately; each requires different measures and different skills (Maxwell, 1984).

Maxwell's six dimensions

1. *Acceptability*
   - how humanely and considerately is this treatment/service delivered?
   - what does the patient think of it?
   - how would I feel if it were my nearest and dearest?
   - what is the setting like?
   - are privacy and confidentiality safeguarded?
2. *Effectiveness (for individual patients)*
   - is the treatment given the best available in a technical sense, according to those best equipped to judge?
   - what is their evidence?
   - what is the overall result of the treatment?

3. *Efficiency and economy*
- is the output maximised for a given input or conversely is the input minimised for a given level of output?
- how does the unit cost compare with the unit cost elsewhere for the same treatment/service?

4. *Access*
- can people get this treatment/service when they need it?
- are there any identifiable barriers to the service for example, distance, inability to pay, waiting lists and waiting times, or straightforward breakdowns in supply?

5. *Equity (fairness)*
- is this patient or group of patients being fairly treated relative to others?
- are there any identifiable failings in equity. For example, are some people being dealt with less favourably or less appropriately in their own eyes than others?

6. *Relevance to need (for the whole community)*
- is the overall pattern and balance of the services the best that could be achieved, taking account of the needs and wants of the population as a whole?

To expand on this he used the accident and emergency department services as an example:

- *access*: it is possible to assess access to this service in terms of ambulance response times and waiting times in the department
- *relevance to need*: this would require further work in the form of review and analysis of the different roles within the department such as the service for major trauma, minor injuries and primary care
- *effectiveness*: technical effectiveness might include the adequacy of equipment and staffing in the department, the incidence of complications, and some form of follow up assessment
- *social acceptability*: this could include the environment within the department and include privacy, and standards of communication between the patient and the GP
- *efficiency and economy*: this would look at workload and unit cost comparisons with other accident and emergency departments.

By using these six dimensions it is possible to assess the quality of the department as a whole rather than in a fragmented way. Maxwell also stressed the need to keep the approach and system simple, while providing a framework within which the quality of care could be studied, discussed, protected and improved. He believed that this would take 'encouragement, experiment, and sharing of ideas and require a mixture of assessment methods including standard data analysis, sampling and follow up, professional peer review, consumer opinion tailored to an understanding of the multidimensional nature of quality itself' (Maxwell, 1984).

Avedis Donabedian

In 1990 Avedis Donabedian, a retired professor of public health in the USA, wrote an article entitled 'The Seven Pillars of Quality'. In this article he describes the seven attributes of healthcare that define its quality:

1. Efficacy: The ability of care at its best to improve health.
2. Effectiveness: the degree to which attainable health improvements are realised.
3. Efficiency: the ability to obtain the greatest health improvement at the lowest cost.
4. Optimality: the most advantageous balancing of costs and benefits.
5. Acceptability: conformity to patient preferences regarding accessibility, the patient-practitioner relation, the amenities, the effects of care, and the cost of care.
6. Legitimacy: concerning all of the above.
7. Equity: fairness in the distribution of care and its effects on health.

Consequently, health care professionals must take into account patient preferences in assessing and assuring quality. When the two sets of preferences disagree the physician faces the challenge of reconciling them.

Donabedian's concept that quality of care has several dimensions was developed into the seven headings outlined above. He stated that quality of care was judged by conforming to a set of standards, which came from three sources:

- the science of health care that determines efficacy
- the individual values and expectations that determine acceptability
- social values and expectations that determine legitimacy.

This develops the argument that quality cannot be judged by healthcare professionals alone but must include the patient's views and preferences as well as those of society in general. He also develops the debate around the pursuit of each of the several attributes of quality which can be mutually reinforcing, but also that the pursuit of one attribute may be in conflict with another so that a balance has to be achieved. The most common conflicts arise when the preferences of society are at variance with the preference of individuals. For example, as a society we may see the care offered in our acute trusts as more of a priority than that of patients with mental health problems.

Dr John Øvretveit

Dr John Øvretveit has carried out consultancy research into health and commercial service organisation in the UK and abroad. He is Professor of Health Policy and Management at the Nordic School of Public Health in Gothenburg, Sweden, and at the Faculty of Medicine at Bergen University, Norway. He is an expert in Total Quality Management.

Hugh Koch

Hugh Koch is a Management Consultant in Health Care Associates at the Health Service Management Centre at the University of Birmingham. He is a British expert in Total Quality Management and is discussed in more detail in Chapter 11 – Total Quality Management.

Karoru Ishikawa

Best known for pioneering the quality circle approach to quality assurance in Japan in the 1960s (Ishikawa 1976, 1985). In Japan this approach incorporated the education of workers in statistical quality control and included:

- Pareto charts
- cause and effect diagrams
- stratification
- check sheets
- histograms
- scatter diagrams
- Shewhart's control charts and graphs.

This differs from the approach used in the UK in the 1980s which is outlined in Chapter 6 – Total Quality Management.

As demonstrated in this quick walk through some of the theories, philosophies and methodologies of quality assurance, it is clear that the concept of clinical governance is not new but is a whole-system approach that supports a quality assured service and takes account of the key elements that support corporate, clinical and self governance, as set out in Figure 1.7.

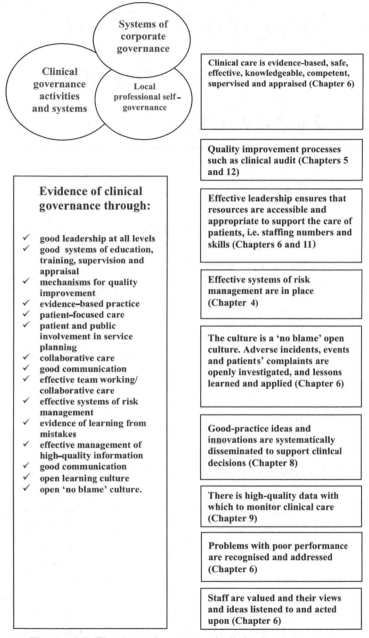

Figure 1.7 The key elements of clinical governance

Most important is the cultural change that supports learning from mistakes, lifelong learning and working as an effective team with the patient as the focus of the service. All the criteria identified in this flow chart are explored in detail in the chapters that follow.

The Seven Pillars of Clinical Governance: An Overview

2

Chapter Contents:

- clinical governance background information
- what is clinical governance?
- the purpose of clinical governance
- the key elements of clinical governance.

Clinical governance is about assuring sustainable continuous quality assurance improvement, which can only be achieved by the determined and conscious efforts of the clinical and non clinical staff who have the appropriate support of their organisation to deliver best practice. To obtain improvements in quality systems there needs to be in place appropriate support to facilitate individuals and organisations in the pursuit of clinical excellence.
(NHS Executive 1999)

Clinical Governance Background Information

In the 1990s and the early 2000s there were a series of situations and notable failings in the care of patients, for example the Kent and Canterbury cervical smear tests inquiry and the failings of the breast-screening service in Exeter, both of which led to the unnecessary deaths of an excessive number of women under the care of the NHS. Then there was the notorious GP, Dr Shipman, who murdered a large number of his patients. The public inquiry into heart surgery at the Bristol Royal Infirmary covered a period of ten years from 1980 to 1990 and identified over thirty children under the age of one year who died unnecessarily, and many more were injured. The NHS was described as 'having no system of monitoring quality, no reliable data and no agreement about what constituted quality' (Bristol Royal Infirmary Enquiry, 2001).

These incidents and many others cast a shadow of doubt about the overall standards of patient care in the NHS. A report on standards in public life (Nolan Report, 1995) and a report on controls assurance (Cadbury Report,

1992) resulted in a framework for corporate governance for the public and private sectors (DoH, 1994).

Since the inception of the NHS in 1948, the ethos has been that 'the patient comes first' and high standards of conduct are expected of those who work in the NHS. Accountability, probity and openness are three key values in public services, and the aim of corporate governance is to ensure that these values are at the heart of the NHS.

The Cadbury Report recommended that the board of directors of all listed companies in the UK should report on the effectiveness of the internal control systems of the company. In the NHS this translates into Strategic Health Authorities (SHAs) and trust boards who must be assured that risks are assessed and managed. To confirm to the general public that this is the case, a statement to this effect accompanies the annual report, and the annual accounts confirm that the board of directors believe the systems to be in place.

The chief executives of the SHAs and the trusts must now sign two assurance statements, one for controls assurance and one for clinical governance, on behalf of the board to confirm probity, accountability and quality assurance across their healthcare organisation. Both these statements are subject to external audit, one for finance and one for the quality of clinical care.

What is Clinical Governance?

Clinical governance is a systematic approach to managing quality assurance and quality control. It is, therefore, essential that the development of an effective and dynamic approach to clinical governance be based on a sound understanding of the principles of quality assurance, its history, how it can be applied, the methodology, approach and the use of tools that support the measurement of quality and the management of change, in the light of measurement, to ensure continuous quality improvement. Clinical governance is a systematic approach to assuring the quality of patient care. A system of clinical governance includes corporate, clinical and self-governance. These elements are intrinsically linked, as shown in Figure 1.7. The three key elements include:

- corporate governance, or the system of governance, is the mechanism of leadership, decision-making, information-sharing and accountability in a trust or healthcare organisation
- clinical governance is delivered through an integrated system of organisational and professional responsibility, which is the shared responsibility of clinical professionals and the organisation. This includes the formal and informal processes of setting standards, measurement and action to improve care

■ self-governance or local professional governance relates to the individual and collective systems of professional self-management (standards of professional practice, professional conduct, education and training, professional development and the identification and resolution of poor practice), collaboration, ownership of clinical issues and accountability for clinical outcome.

In the Government's paper *A First Class Service: Improving Quality in the New NHS* (DoH, 1998), clinical governance is defined as 'A framework through which NHS organisations are accountable for continuously improving the quality of their services and safeguarding high standards of care by creating an environment in which excellence in clinical care will flourish.' Within this document the government sets out the Quality Framework.

Clinical governance is a system designed to improve patient care as the Government's White Paper (DoH, 1998) emphasises the importance of involving patients and the public not only in the gathering of their views about care and services received but also through their contributions to NHS policy and planning decisions. Patient involvement was further reinforced by the publication of the NHS Plan (DoH, 2000): 'Patients and citizens will have a greater say in the NHS, and the provision of services and the needs of different groups and individuals within society ... Patients and citizens will have a greater say in the NHS, and the provision of services will be centred in patient need.'

Since April 1999 trusts have had a legal duty to put in place systems for monitoring and assuring the quality of care provided for their patients: 'It is the duty of each Health Authority, Primary Care Trust and NHS Trust to put and keep in place arrangements for the purpose of monitoring and improving the quality of healthcare which is provided to individuals' (Health Care Act 1999, section 18).

On an annual basis the chief executive of a trust signs a report on the quality of clinical care, which in turn is agreed by the trust board, all the members of which are accountable for the quality of patient care. In order to do this, there must be regular reporting systems of information and performance indicators in place. To support this, trusts have developed systems of clinical governance led by a clinical governance head, which is either the medical director or the director of nursing and a clinical governance committee. The clinical governance committee is a subcommittee of the board and is chaired by a non-executive director. Some trusts have a clinical governance committee, which has a joint remit of clinical and corporate governance. In this situation the clinical governance committee has replaced the audit committee, which previously had the remit for financial accountability and probity of the trust. As the non-executive chairman of the clinical governance and risk subcommittee for North Dorset PCT, which has responsibility for community hospitals and services, primary care and also mental health services across two PCTs, I believe it is better that the audit committee retains specific responsibility for financial probity and all that this entails. The clinical governance and risk agenda is very large and the subcommittee already meets on a monthly basis so the added responsibilities of the audit committee would render the agenda too large to manage.

Through clinical governance the government requires the development of evidence-based guidelines to set standards of care, and monitoring by health care commissioners to ensure that such guidelines are implemented by clinicians to provide clinically effective and economically efficient care (DoH, 1999). In 1998 the Government published a consultation paper which outlined its policy for ensuring quality in the NHS. The paper suggested that standards would be set by the National Institute for Clinical Excellence (NICE) and the National Service Frameworks, and delivered through clinical excellence, lifelong learning and professional self-regulation. To fulfil this objective, the Government introduced a wide range of policies to modernise and improve the NHS and in particular set up two important organisations: the National Institute for Clinical Excellence (NICE) and the Commission for Health Improvement (CHI). Details about these organisations and changes that have occurred since 1999 may be found in Chapter 1.

The Purpose of Clinical Governance

The purpose of clinical governance is to ensure that patients receive the best quality of care that the NHS can provide. This includes the organisation's systems and processes for monitoring and improving services including:

- patient and public involvement
- risk management
- clinical audit
- clinical effectiveness programmes
- staffing and staff management
- education, training and continuing personal and professional development
- the use of information to support clinical governance and healthcare delivery.

Clinical governance is a quality framework not dissimilar to the European Foundation for Quality Management (EFQM) framework, which can be used to co-ordinate disparate quality initiatives and the process of change. This systematic approach allows trusts to use different tools to track and resolve problems such as integrated care pathways (see Chapter 8).

The Key Elements of Clinical Governance

There are fifteen key elements, which have been subdivided into the seven pillars of clinical governance. This chapter and Chapters 3 to 9 discuss and expand on each of the key elements and establish how each one can be achieved. The fifteen key elements of clinical governance may be summarised as:

- quality improvement processes, such as clinical audit, are in place and integrated with the quality programme for the organisation as a whole
- leadership skills are developed at clinical team level
- evidence-based practice is in day-to-day use with the infrastructure to support it
- good practice, ideas and innovations, which have been evaluated, are systematically disseminated within and outside the organisation
- clinical-risk-reduction programmes of a high standard are in place
- adverse events are detected and openly investigated; lessons learned are promptly applied
- lessons for clinical practice are systematically learned from complaints made by patients
- problems of poor clinical performance are recognised at an early stage and dealt with to prevent harm to patients
- all professional development programmes reflect the principles of clinical governance
- the quality of data collected to monitor clinical care is of a high standard
- there is monitoring of all clinical staff to ensure that they meet professional requirements for updating or reregistration, for example CME (Continuing Medical Education) and PREP (Post-Registration Education Requirements)
- a forum discusses all clinical practice and agrees/reviews new practices
- the culture is open and participative
- there is an ethos of teamwork between all staff
- the patient is a partner in care.

The key elements have been further organised into the Healthcare Commission's seven pillars of clinical governance:

- patient and public involvement
- risk management
- clinical audit
- staffing and staff management
- education, training and continuing personal and professional development
- clinical effectiveness programmes
- use of clinical information to support clinical governance and healthcare delivery.

Pillar One – Patient and Public Involvement

3

Chapter Contents:

- the patient as a partner in care
- tools for assessing patient satisfaction
- methods for involving patients.

This first pillar describes how patients are involved in decisions concerning their care and treatment and how they and patient organisations can influence the way that NHS services are provided.

The Government set out the anticipated benefits and its expectation for patient involvement in clinical governance in the paper *Clinical Governance: Quality in the New NHS* (NHS Executive, 1999
). Within this document there are some key expectations of benefits of change:

- an organisation-wide strategy for involving patients, users, carers and the public, including strategic plans for communication with them
- a designated senior individual to oversee a strategy for patients', users' and carers' involvement in clinical governance
- user representatives on clinical governance committees or groups
- use of involvement methodologies, for example patient panels and focus groups
- training and education for all individuals on effective patient, user, carer and public involvement.

This can be achieved through a variety of approaches. The most common of these is a system of clear, well-written patient information leaflets that are distributed across the trust, either by the staff, when talking to patients and their carers, or displayed on well-organised racks in wards, departments and GPs' surgeries. The use of written information is most effective when presented to the patient at the same time as the doctor, nurse or therapist is discussing his/her care or treatment.

Each trust should have a planned timetable for patient-satisfaction surveys, which will include the traditional completion of a questionnaire post-care or a suggestion box, or more innovative approaches; for example, if there has been a series of similar complaints about a service, it may be appropriate to visit the patients and their carers at home to discuss the issue and then compare the findings prior to establishing a way of learning from the problem and implementing policy and procedure to prevent the issue from recurring. Other areas of patient and public involvement include:

- input or feedback from patients and the wider public. The trust is also required to inform the public as a whole about what the organisation is doing and how well it is performing
- patient surveys
- public meetings
- Community Health Council liaison
- Patient Advocacy and Liaison Service partnerships
- client care focus groups
- patient support groups
- patients' suggestions mechanisms
- stakeholders' suggestions mechanisms
- complaints
- patient literature and notices
- patient's charter and patients' rights leaflet.

The choice of methods will depend on a number of factors such as the purpose of the initiative, the skills of the staff using the approach, the types of patients involved and the preferences of the patients and their carers with regard to the different methods.

Tools for Assessing Patient Satisfaction with Services

Patient-satisfaction surveys have been around for a long time. As early as 1957, in the USA, Abdellah and Levine set out a system to establish patients' views. Work by Raphael led to the development of the King's Fund questionnaire, which was modified by Raphael in 1969. The use of questionnaires that ask patients about the quality of their care is often criticised, as critics suggest that patients are reluctant to be negative about the nursing care they receive, particularly if they are an in-patient at the time or scheduled to be readmitted (Nehring and Geach, 1973).

Current Department of Health policy expects health services to be responsive to the needs of patients, their carers and the general public, as set out in the policy documents *The New NHS, Modern, Dependable* (DoH, 1997) and

A *First Class Service* (DoH, 1998). In these documents it is quite explicit that there is an expectation that patients and the public must be involved in a range of activities across the NHS and that their input should be seen as integral to the working of the health service. *The NHS Plan* (DoH, 2000) stated:

> to shape its services around the needs of different groups and individuals within society' highlights the Government's desire to focus the provision of health services on patient's needs ... patients and citizens will have a greater say in the NHS, and the provision of services will be centred on patients' needs.

It is clear that patient experiences are a very important part of quality assurance and play an essential part in clinical governance. The patients' and the public's views on both the process and outcomes of care are essential for a clear understanding of how they live and cope with illness, how they access services they require and what difficulties they encounter, what was good about the treatment they received and any bad effects of the treatment. They also answer questions about the standard of care and how well or badly the care was delivered; whether the care was well co-ordinated by health and social services both in hospital and at home; how accessible, efficient and effective the delivery of care was in hospital and at home; how much information they were given, and whether the quality of the information was sufficient to make decisions and judgements about their care. These are questions to which health professionals need answers if they are to assess the quality of care that is provided.

Methods for involving patients include:
- patient-satisfaction surveys and questionnaires
- consultation with patient representatives and groups
- patient councils and panels
- workshops and conferences
- case studies
- observational studies
- tracking patient care
- patient stories and diaries.

The choice of the method to be used to gather the views of patients and the general public will depend on the resources available, including the skills and expertise of the staff, and the time and money available. Patient surveys are most commonly used as they are possibly one of the simplest ways of gathering evidence about the patient's views. They include structured questionnaires and telephone surveys, which can be used to gain the views of a large number of people – the quantitative survey.

Questionnaires

The techniques for asking questions have been thoroughly researched and there are many different approaches. Payne (1951), Maccoby (1968), Gordon (1969) and Oppenheim (1979) all put forward excellent information and advice on the art of asking questions. Ward (1982) gives many examples of different approaches to patient surveys. From these findings and recommendations, the following points arise:

- questions should be phrased so they do not patronise the respondent, while at the same time being easily understood at all intellectual levels
- questions must be expressed simply and clearly, avoiding ambiguity
- questions should be asked one at a time. Two topics should not be included in one question, for example 'Was your discharge planned and negotiated with you?' The care may have been planned with the patient but not necessarily negotiated. Two separate questions should be asked, as the answers could be very different
- questions should be short
- the respondent should be given an opportunity to write his or her comments
- respondents tend to choose a middle answer if given a choice, so a simple 'yes' or 'no' will overcome this problem
- sometimes a respondent may show a bias by answering 'yes' to every question. To avoid this, a question can be asked where a positive answer is required and then later in the questionnaire the same or a similar question where a negative response is required. Including different forms of the same question can also check for inconsistency and misunderstandings.

These are only a few suggestions, but they may help you when you come to prepare a questionnaire to gather the views of patients and their carers. Other techniques include in-depth interviews and focus groups. Although these approaches involve smaller numbers of people, they have the added advantage of giving patients and carers the opportunity to raise issues and concerns that the professionals who designed the questionnaires and interviews had not thought of. Focus groups are small groups of service users who are invited to describe their experiences of a particular service. These techniques are also useful when gaining views from those who have sight problems, who are unable to read or for whom English is not their first language. This approach is a qualitative technique. In some instances it may be useful to combine the techniques outlined above, for example a questionnaire distributed to a large number of people followed by a structured interview with a few patients on issues raised in the questionnaires.

The results of patient surveys can be used to inform clinical governance activities, to monitor standards as part of clinical audit, to inform service strategy and service changes or developments and to review services.

Workshops and Conferences

Other techniques include workshops and conferences where patients are invited to participate and work alongside representatives from the health services and other stakeholders in order to gain their views on specific areas of a service. These events can be consultative, where the patients' views are collected but the patients are not involved in the decisions made as a result of the workshop, or collaborative, where the patients participate actively in the recommendations made at the workshop.

Case Studies, Observational Studies, Patient Stories, Diaries and Patient Tracking

The patients' experiences as they receive care, treatment and therapy can also be assessed through the use of case studies, observational studies, patient tracking, patient stories and diaries. Observational studies are used to record what happens to patients at a particular point in time, for example during an out-patient appointment or an episode of care such as a dressing or a surgical intervention. Patient tracking, however, involves what happens at different points in the patient's care. For example, the trackers will track the experience from the GP, through admission to the hospital, care in hospital and the discharge process and then back into the community. This information may also be recorded by the patient, who keeps a diary of his experience, in his own words, of the care as it happens. Some patients keep a record as a written diary; others use a tape recorder. They then share and discuss the experience with a health professional. This information is then used to measure the effectiveness of the service and make changes to improve it as a result of the analysis of the data. For more information on PALS, patient councils and patient forums and groups, see Chapter 1.

Patient Councils and Panels

Setting up a council or panel gives an organisation the opportunity to meet formally and on a regular basis with a group of service users. The Royal Colleges (Kelson, 1996) have put forward some criteria for setting up success-ful and effective patient liaison groups and councils which are as follows:

- an explicit remit for the group with clear terms of reference
- clear membership criteria for all members (including professionals, if relevant)
- regular attendance and finite terms of office
- a range of interests represented appropriate to the task of the group
- established links between the group and other initiatives within the organisation
- mechanisms within the organisation to ensure that the group's activities are disseminated and acted upon
- resources, training and administrative support for the group
- monitoring of the group's effectiveness and the organisation's responsiveness to it.

Consultation with Patient Representatives and Groups

There are a large number of patient organisations which are led by service users. Their remit is to provide up-to-date information to the general public, to offer support in the form of local groups and publications, and to influence policy makers and professionals, usually on specific problems such as Parkinson's disease (Wilson, 1999). These groups have access to their members and they can draw on their networks to provide people willing to talk about their experiences as a patient, which is a very valuable source of information.

An integrated care pathway (ICP) is an excellent approach to the concept of the patient as a partner in their care (see also Chapter 8). An ICP provides information to the patient about his/her condition and expected treatment. Patient ICPs are presented in the same format as the multidisciplinary ICP. The patients complete the ICP as part of their care by building the sequence of care, treatments, interventions and events into a diary. The information is discussed with the staff on a day-to-day basis which supports ongoing evaluation of the care the patients have received. On discharge the patients' ICPs are collected and collated as part of the audit of the ICP and the patients' perspective of their care and treatment are used as part of the audit.

Conclusion

This aspect of clinical governance is about valuing the patient and his/her carers. It is about ensuring that the patient's experience meets his/her needs, and includes the environment, which should be clean, comfortable, in good decorative order and risk-free. Dietary and all other care needs must be met. The benchmarking approach used in *Essence of Care* (DoH, 2001) is a valuable tool for ensuring that these essential elements of the quality of patient care are in place (see also Chapter 11 – Essence of Care). Confidentiality must be assured through the Caldicott Guardian arrangements demonstrated in a records management strategy, electronic data security and patient access to medical records. Most importantly, the patient must be well-informed about options, outcomes of treatment and interventions to empower him/her to make informed choices as a partner in his/her care.

Making It Happen

Patient and Public Involvement

The trust will need to:

- develop strategic plans and policies
- implement strategy, policy and procedure
- provide training for staff in:
  - ☐ patient/service user care (customer care)
  - ☐ communication skills
  - ☐ obtaining patient consent to treatment skills
  - ☐ knowledge about confidentiality issues, and
  - ☐ handling complaints
- support patients or service users with patients' advocates, support for carers, interpreters, translation services, signers and link workers
- monitor effectiveness of strategy, plans and policy.

Pillar Two – Risk Management 4

Chapter Contents:

- clinical-risk-reduction programmes
- risk management
- clinical negligence scheme for trusts
- controls assurance
- an organisation with a memory
- learning from mistakes.

Risk management is having systems to understand, monitor and minimise the risks to patients and learning from mistakes. Key elements include:

- clinical-risk-reduction programmes of a high standard are in place, adverse events are detected, and openly investigated, and lessons learned are promptly applied
- lessons for clinical practice are systematically learned from complaints made by patients
- problems of poor clinical performance are recognised at an early stage and dealt with to prevent harm to patients
- the culture is open and participative.

Clinical-risk-reduction Programmes

There are numerous books, articles and plenty of information on a variety of websites on the subject of risk management and controls assurance. Within the context of this book it is not possible to give a detailed account of risk management. What follows is an overview of risk management and controls assurance, which aims to give some baseline information in order to link risk management with clinical governance.

Wilson (1994) suggests that, 'risk in its simplest form is the potential for unwanted outcome', and Williams and Heins (1976), define risk as 'a variation in the outcomes that could occur over a specified period in a given situation'. Therefore risk may be seen as exposure to events, which may threaten or damage the organisation and its interests, for example when a patient is injured while in the care of an NHS Trust or healthcare organisation. This results in the patient and his/her carers making a formal complaint, which requires resources to respond to the complaint. If proven, then there is a resource requirement in the form of litigation and legal costs. These costs reduce the resources available for patient care, and staff involved are demoralised, sometimes resulting in sickness as a result of stress. Patients question the quality of care that the organisation provides and its reputation is adversely affected. This sequence of events has far-reaching consequences and the solution is to prevent it happening in the first place.

Clinical Risk

Clinical risk is defined by Wilson and Tingle (1999), as 'a clinical error to be at variance from intended treatment, care, therapeutic intervention or diagnostic result; there may be an untoward outcome or not'. However, clinical risk cannot be seen as applying to one profession in isolation, as patient care is reliant on a team of people including clinical and non-clinical staff. For example, hospital-acquired infection may be the result not only of the poor hand-washing techniques of staff caring for patients, but also of poor standards of ward cleanliness. If the hand hygiene of clinical staff is addressed but the ward remains dirty and dusty, then patients will continue to acquire infections. The management of risk has to be a holistic approach both to manage the current risk and to prevent risk in the future.

Risk Management

Risk management is the systematic identification, assessment and reduction of risks to patients and staff through:

- the provision of appropriate, effective and efficient levels of patient care
- the prevention and avoidance of untoward incidents and events
- the learning of lessons and the changing of behaviour or practices as a result of near misses, incidents and adverse outcomes
- the communication and documentation of care in a comprehensive, objective, consistent and accurate way.

Risk management is described by the Department of Health (DoH, 1994) as 'concerned with harnessing the information and expertise of individuals within the organisation and translating that with their help into positive action which will reduce loss of life, financial loss, loss of staff availability, loss of the availability of buildings or equipment and loss of reputation'.

Clinical risk management can be seen as having three component parts:

- identifying risk
- analysing risk
- controlling risk.

The identification of risk is through the analysis of data collected about accidents, incidents, near misses and the results of systematic reviews of services. The aim is to get a better understanding of the issues and identify ways of controlling the risk. The principle of clinical risk management is to improve the quality of healthcare and patient care in order to minimise risk and protect the patient. Risk management is essentially a framework for safe practice. Clinical governance provides a framework within which to improve and assure the quality of care and services for patients.

The three components of clinical risk management can be developed into a risk management cycle similar to the quality assurance cycle and the audit cycle. See Figure 4.1.

The cycle starts with the identification of the risk which is the process through which a trust or healthcare organisation becomes aware of the risks within its environment which could potentially put patients and staff at risk, and result in litigation, loss of reputation, and so on. NHS Trusts have reporting systems through which they identify risks. This is a system that

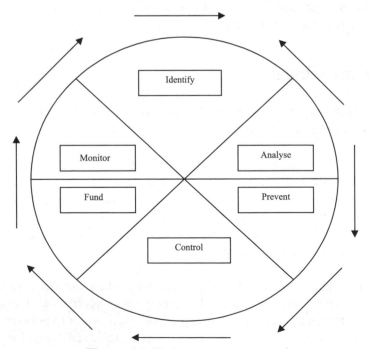

Figure 4.1 Risk management cycle

allows staff to report potential or actual incidents, accidents and near misses. Every report received is reviewed and the details added to the system, which is usually electronic. Effective management of the incidents, accidents and near misses is achieved through early identification, and positive action taken to manage the risk.

This is followed by an analysis of the risk and existing controls. Risk analysis is the process of establishing the potential severity of loss associated with the identified risk and the likelihood of this occurring. An effective claims management system and a well-run approach to responding and managing complaints are an essential part of a risk management system. These systems will generate information with which to manage risks and prevent them from occurring. Part of clinical governance is to focus on and tackle adverse healthcare events (DoH, 1999). Many very similar events will have occurred before either in the same organisation or in another trust. Part of the analysis is to identify patterns and trends both locally and nationally and to take action to prevent the adverse event from occurring. The trust or healthcare organisation must have systems for the identification of the controls which are in place to prevent the adverse incident.

Prevention is achieved by taking the actions and additional measures required to control the risk and by having physical and systems controls in place to reduce the risk through:

- comprehensive risk-assessment processes
- current, up-to-date, evidence-based policies, procedures, protocols pathways and clinical guidelines to support staff to deliver care that results in desired outcomes
- contingency and disaster planning which is important for reducing the effects of major internal incidents such as loss of electrical power or other utilities
- risk management training and education.

The next part of the cycle is to fund the residual risk, which is when an organisation manages and accepts an identified risk and the potential losses associated with the risk and makes plans to cover any financial consequences of the anticipated losses. These include risks that cannot be reduced, transferred or avoided and the setting-up of funds for use in the event of such an adverse incident. Some of these risks can be transferred through a system such as the Clinical Negligence Scheme for Trusts (CNST, 2002) (see below), which is administered by the National Health Service Litigation Authority (NHSLA), and is one of the two schemes providing reimbursement to healthcare trusts in relation to clinical negligence claims. The other scheme is the Existing Liabilities Scheme (ELS), which deals with cases arising from incidents that occurred before 1 April 1995 and is managed by the NHSLA and their solicitors. The

Welsh Risk Pool (WRP) is a similar system to the CNST but covers both clinical and non-clinical claims.

The final part of the cycle is to monitor as part of a continuous quality improvement. This is an ongoing evaluation of the effectiveness of the techniques used to identify, analyse and manage risks that have occurred or have been prevented from occurring in the trust or healthcare organisation. Effective risk management is achieved through an open and blame-free culture that supports staff in reporting mistakes and untoward or adverse incidents, followed up with processes that support learning from mistakes, and ongoing training and development to prevent a recurrence.

Clinical Negligence Scheme for Trusts

In 1995 the CNST was designed to help trusts to meet the cost of clinical negligence claims, in order to protect them against the costly consequences of clinical negligence payments. The CNST is administered by the National Health Service Litigation Authority (CNST, 1997) and is one of the systems for providing reimbursement to NHS trusts, in the case of negligence claims. The trust pays a premium based on the size of the hospital trust, the specialities and the claims history, and the premium is discounted for minimising and managing clinical risk. The level of this discount is linked to the trust's compliance with the CNST standards, which range from levels one to three. The higher the compliance with the standards, the greater the discount on the premium. These are national standards and the original CNST risk management standards include the following:

1. the board has a written risk management strategy that makes its commitment to managing clinical risk explicit
2. an executive director of the board is charged with responsibility for clinical risk management throughout the trust
3. the responsibility for management and co-ordination of clinical risk is clear
4. a clinical-incident reporting system is operated in all medical specialities and clinical support departments
5. there is a policy for rapid follow-up of major clinical incidents
6. an agreed system of managing complaints is in place
7. appropriate information is provided to patients on the risks and benefits of the proposed treatment or investigation, and the alternatives available, before a signature on a consent form is sought
8. a comprehensive system for the completion, use, storage and retrieval of medical records is in place. Record-keeping standards are monitored through the clinical audit process

9. there is an induction/orientation programme for all new clinical staff
10. a clinical risk management system is in place
11. there is a clear, documented system for management and communication throughout the key stages of maternity care.

Source: CNST risk management standards (reproduced from CNST Risk Management Standards and Procedures Manual of Guidance, April 1997)

The CNST's original standards are set out in a manual and each standard is developed into a series of statements which are categorised as level one (a basic or minimum level), level two (more difficult to achieve) or level three (the most difficult to achieve). When the trusts joined the scheme they were encouraged to be assessed but in many cases this did not happen and yet they continued to be members of the system. Of those that were assessed, only 50 per cent over the first two years were able to comply with the basic level. The CNST was set up to reduce financial risks but today it is a voluntary organisation, administered by the NHS Litigation Authority, that can support the clinical risk element of clinical governance.

At the time of writing there are another ten standards with a separate set for maternity services and these include (NHS Litigation Authority, 2002):

1. learning from experience
2. response to major critical incidents
3. advice and consent
4. health records
5. induction, training and competence
6. implementation of clinical risk management
7. clinical care
8. the management of care in Trusts providing mental health services
9. ambulance services
10. maternity care.

Trusts are assessed at least once every two years with regard to the first seven standards.

There is a similar scheme available from the Welsh Risk Pool in Wales, as set out below, and the Clinical Negligence and Other Risks Indemnity Scheme in Scotland.

The Welsh Risk Pool risk-management standards include 11 general standards:

1. risk profile
2. risk management strategy
3. incident reporting system
4. patient records

5. clinical audit
6. complaints
7. policies and procedures
8. communications
9. supervision of junior staff
10. assessing competence
11. health and safety, and related issues.

They also included one set of specialist standards for each of the following:

12A. mental health
12B. ambulance services
12C. operating theatres
12D. accident and emergency
12E. maternity
12F. community.

Controls Assurance

CNST standards have been instrumental in the management of clinical risk. However, there is a need for a holistic management of risk, which has been introduced through controls assurance, and is an integration of all risk management activities: clinical, non-clinical, health and safety.

In the health service circular, *Governance in the New NHS* (DoH, 1999), it states that 'Implementing and maintaining effective risk management and organisational controls is fundamental to ensuring the success of clinical governance, providing a solid foundation upon which to build an environment in which quality care can be provided and clinical excellence can flourish.' Figure 4.2 (DoH, 1999) illustrates the relationship between basic financial controls, non-clinical and non-financial controls, and those of clinical systems. The paper goes on to say that the 'common thread' linking clinical governance and wider controls assurance is risk management, which is defined as 'the culture, processes and structures that are directed towards the effective management of potential opportunities and adverse effects' (Standards Australia, 1999).

A holistic risk management approach includes both clinical and non-clinical aspects of risk. Trust boards of all organisations are now required to provide an annual assurance that there are robust systems in place across the organisation to manage risk (DoH, 2001). Griffiths (2000) outlines four stages in an integrated risk management system:

1. *policy and strategy – getting the framework right*: defining the types of risk relevant to the specific assessment concerned, and identifying what measurement scales will be used

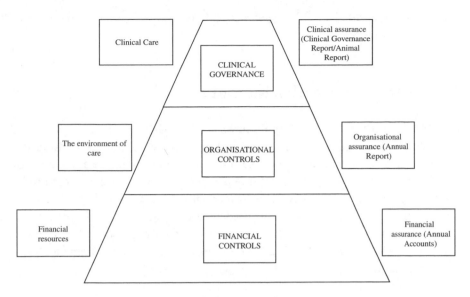

Figure 4.2 Controls assurance and clinical governance
Source: DoH, 1999b

2. *planning and assessment – producing the plan*: the plan incorporates the results of the setting of the context at the first stage and defines how risks will be identified, assessed, prioritised, recorded and managed. It is at this stage that an outline risk register is produced. This register will contain all risk information and a summary of responses to risks. The planning will establish the processes by which risk identification and assessment will take place at all levels of the organisation and the structures necessary to facilitate those processes

3. *implementation and change management*: the culture needs to be one that takes controls assurance seriously and the staff must be supported with resources, education and training to discharge their responsibilities under controls assurance

4. *monitoring and reviewing the system*: information from incidents, complaints, audits and inspections should be used to monitor the effectiveness of existing controls. The risk management core standards require a systematic analysis of incidents, complaints and claims so that practice can be reviewed and trends monitored.

The guidance issued by the NHS Executive (1999), sets out a number of targets for achievement by trusts over a five-year period. The targets are based around the achievement of controls assurance performance levels. Level one requires the framework outlined above to be in place. Level two builds on this and level three requires full convergence between clinical governance and controls assurance.

An Organisation with a Memory

In 1999 a report called *An Organisation with a Memory* (DoH, 2000) was produced by an expert committee chaired by Professor Liam Donaldson, the Chief Medical Officer. This report examined the number, nature and causes of avoidable failure in the NHS. It went on to identify what was considered to be the best approach to the early identification of problems including the collecion and analysis of data. The report made recommendations for improvement and the government responded to the report with a paper called *Building a Safer NHS for Patients*, (DoH, 2001) and in this report it recommended the following actions:

- the establishment of a mandatory, national reporting scheme for adverse health care events
- the setting up of a new National Patient Safety Agency (see also Chapter 1)
- the setting up of a new system for handling investigations and inquiries across the NHS
- the following four specific areas of risk to be targeted:
  - □ by December 2002 to reduce to zero the number of patients killed or paralysed by misadministration of spinal injections
  - □ by the end of 2005 to reduce by 25 per cent the number of instances of harm in obstetrics and gynaecology which lead to litigation
  - □ by the end of 2005 to reduce by 40 per cent the number of serious errors in the use of prescribed drugs
  - □ by March 2002 to reduce to zero the number of suicides by mental health patients as a consequence of hanging from non-collapsible beds or shower curtain rails on wards
- the development of a strategy for patient safety research to improve understanding of the underlying causes of why things go wrong.

Learning from Mistakes

When something does go wrong, staff still feel concerned about discussing what went wrong, often through fear of being made to look stupid or even the loss of their job. Some of them have had bad experiences in the past and witnessed colleagues being blamed for mistakes that were not entirely their responsibility, even being used as a scapegoat for another member of staff or the organisation. These people have learned to keep their head down and often find it difficult to unlearn this behaviour.

Adverse incidents occur for a variety of reasons including:

- poor communication between departments, organisations and staff
- lack of policy, procedure and guidelines or systems failure
- roles and responsibilities that are blurred and not clearly defined which leads to staff exceeding the scope of their competencies
- lack of training, knowledge and skills
- poor co-ordination of care
- a heavy workload, being short-staffed and, as a result, taking short cuts to meet the care needs of patients
- in some cases deliberate harm to patients, such as in the Beverly Allitt case where a nurse working in a paediatric ward was found to be responsible for the unexpected deaths of a number of children (Clothier, 1992).

When and wherever adverse incidents occur they must be reported and lessons learned so as to prevent the incident from recurring and putting other patients at risk. Therefore systems must include:

- *local reporting of incidents*: this must include a description of the nature of the incident, the severity of the outcome, the cause or reason for the incident and the action required to correct the situation. This report can be used to share and reflect with colleagues and, if necessary, to support changes in policy and practice in order to 'close the loop' and prevent the incident from occurring again
- *critical incident analysis*: this is the analysis of the information supplied by the people involved in the incident through reflection on what has happened in order to clarify and understand decisions that were made and then identify areas of practice that need to be improved or changed. This is essentially an educational tool which can be used to review the incident in report form for general discussion, for personal development and for individual learning
- *significant event auditing*: this takes the form of a team approach and includes clinical and non-clinical events linked with patient safety, clinical effectiveness and patient satisfaction. Both positive and negative aspects of care are discussed and areas of improvement identified and then acted upon
- *organisational cause analysis*: this is a systems approach to the investigation of errors and adverse incidents. The analysis includes a review of the following factors and issues to establish how patient safety was compromised:

☐ work environment factors
☐ patient factors
☐ staff factors
☐ communication issues
☐ organisational issues
☐ policy issues.

The analysis looks at the causes at different levels of the trust or healthcare organisation to identify the influences that are compromising patient safety followed by the drawing-up of an action plan to prevent events from recurring.

■ *root cause analysis*: an incident or a cluster of incidents leads to an investigation and a question is asked that leads to further questions, for example:

☐ an incident occurred – why did it happen?
☐ how did it happen?
☐ what was the reason for that?

One question leads to another, tracking the problem to establish the cause.

Conclusion

This aspect of clinical governance is about minimising the clinical risk to patients through systems that support the detection of adverse events and incidents which are promptly investigated, acted upon and lessons learned are disseminated across the trust or healthcare organisation.

It is vital to have systems in place that detect problems after the event but even more important for a trust to create an open and participative culture which ensures that problems of poor clinical performance are recognised and dealt with to prevent harm to patients.

Making It Happen

Risk Management

The trust will need to ensure:

■ strategic planning for the management of risk
■ integration of all risk management activities – clinical, non-clinical, health and safety
■ integration of risk management with audit and quality improvement programmes

- consideration of risk in decision-making
- involvement of patients, service users, carers and other health organisations, social services and so on, in risk management
- resources for risk management including budgets for risk management activities and specialist teams and support such as infection control, tissue viability, and so on
- processes for risk assessment and reporting incidents, near misses and investigations
- processes for risk management, including trigger events and protocols
- processes for the prevention and control of risk
- processes for the dissemination of lessons learnt from risk management activities
- training and education for staff in risk prevention and management.

Pillar Three – Clinical Audit

5

Chapter Contents:

- definition of clinical audit
- the audit cycle
- four main principles of clinical audit
- eleven steps to successful audit
- summary of guidelines for success.

Quality improvement processes, such as clinical audit, are in place and integrated with the quality programme for the organisation as a whole.

Clinical audit is the continual evaluation and measurement by health professionals of their work and the standards they are achieving. For some years clinical audit has been used within the health service and it has grown from its origins as medical audit to the system that we have today, which is a multidisciplinary, multiprofessional audit of clinical care.

Clinical Audit – Definition

Clinical audit is 'the systematic and critical analysis of the quality of clinical care, including the procedures for the diagnosis, treatment and care, the associated use of resources and the resulting outcome and quality of life for the patient' (NHS Executive 1996). It is a simple system which allows professionals to measure their performance, to recognise good practice and, if necessary, to make improvements. A clinical audit is not undertaken in isolation by one person but is developed with the help of colleagues and the support of management. Clinical audit is an essential part of the desire by every professional involved in patient care to deliver good quality of care.

The Audit Cycle

The audit cycle (see Figure 5.1) is a process not dissimilar from the quality assurance cycle process.

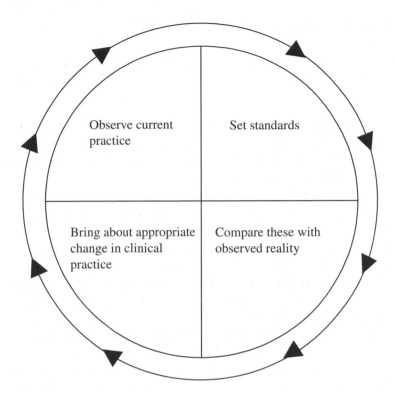

Figure 5.1 The audit cycle

1. *observe current practice*: the first part of the cycle is to observe current practice and make an assessment of its quality
2. *set standards of care:* the setting of standards is often seen as a difficult part of the cycle and is discussed in detail in Chapter 12
3. *compare expectations with reality*: having established what the standards are, there is a need to compare these with clinical practice. What is the reality? Where are the gaps? Is there a difference between the standards which were set and the standards that actually apply when patient care is delivered? Having monitored the standards and identified the gaps, then make comparisons. This will form the body of the clinical audit, which will be described in more detail further on in this chapter
4. *bring about appropriate change*: this is perhaps the most important part of the cycle. If necessary changes have been identified, then these must be agreed with your colleagues. Changes in practice need to be carefully reviewed to ensure that they will result in the improvement of patient care. Having set up and implemented the changes, then the changes must be monitored. Observe the effects and improvements and whether there are any problems associated with making the changes.

Four Main Principles of Clinical Audit

Essentially there are four main principles which apply to the development of clinical audit, and these are applicable to any clinical area and any professional group:

1. *defining the objectives*: it is important to remember that any effective care requires individuals to work as a team and depends on that team holding the same values and expectations to avoid the confusion created by people working to different objectives.

   The first step under this particular principle, therefore, is to identify the mission statement of the organisation and to write the philosophy of care for the particular area in which your team is working.

   Having identified the philosophy of care for a particular area, the next step is to identify the key objectives of the service. Many areas will already have been through this process while undertaking a 'setting of standards' exercise a few years ago, so this will just be a continuation of the work that has already been undertaken

2. *developing standards and ways to measure them*: many professionals have already written their standards, and audit may be seen as a link between standard-setting and more in-depth monitoring of quality and audit. As discussed previously, it is important to understand the language used, so that areas of quality are not muddled; when professionals talk about auditing standards instead of monitoring standards, it gives the impression that every standard needs to be audited in depth, which of course is not true

   The monitoring of standards should be seen as a 'snapshot' of activity, looking at whether or not standards are complied with and good-quality care is achieved. If there is an area within those standards that staff are having difficulty achieving, then this may be the area that is pulled out and developed for clinical audit. In other words, audit should be seen to be a 'detailed portrait' of the area of activity being monitored, and monitoring of standards should be seen as a simple 'snapshot'

3. *agreeing, implementing and monitoring change*: monitor the standards and identify current performance; compare what should be with what is. Identify the gaps and take action to ensure that the gap is closed and the audit cycle is completed. The clinical audit process will identify areas of excellence and also identify areas in need of improvement. At this point, in clinical audit, the ways of improving patient care must be discussed and agreed by the group

   Clinical audit is not something that is taken on by one person; it is achieved through a group of people. This means that the tasks and the workload should be shared among the group and that individual people should be made responsible for specific areas of work that have been identified.

Communication

Within the organisation there needs to be a clinical audit strategy which sets out the clinical audit objectives and a detailed work programme of audits to be carried out. This strategy, when communicated to all staff, will not only publicise the purpose and outcome of the audits to be undertaken, but it will prevent duplication of studies and allow the results of the audits to be shared to benefit patients across a whole healthcare organisation or trust. Communication should not be limited to those professionals involved in the audit but should be extended to patients and their relatives. Communication should also be aimed at management, at policy-makers and at those who are accountable for the resources, because without their support, the changes identified – with resource implications – may never take place.

The Eleven Steps to Successful Audit

Having outlined the four principles of audit, the next step is to put these principles into practice. The cycle of audit activity which results in a systematic improvement in clinical practice can be described in eleven steps (see Figure 5.2).

1. *win the support and commitment of colleagues*: the first part of this step is to obtain support from management, as discussed earlier in this chapter. Without their support, audit is likely to flounder because of a lack of resources. It is important to reiterate at this point that the involvement of management, through the presentation of clear objectives and the likely implications of the audit, will move the group closer to good communication with the managers. During this first step it is a good idea to establish whether there are any specific resources available for audit. These may be in the form of data collection clerks, information technology systems or other resources such as particular personnel with expertise or access to previous studies that are closely linked to the proposed audit.

   The research undertaken at the beginning of this study, which includes a review of the mission statement and the objectives of the organisation followed by the group's philosophy and objectives, will be key in demonstrating how the audit will fit in to the clinical governance strategy.

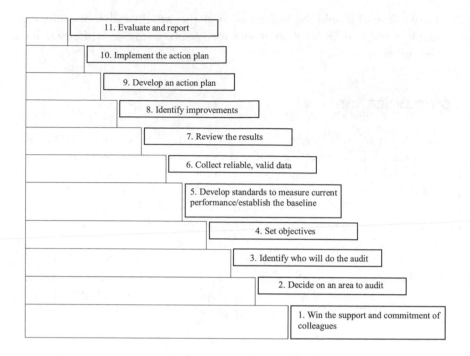

Figure 5.2 Eleven steps to audit

2. *decide on an area to audit*: if you already have standards, integrated care pathways and guidelines which are being monitored and have identified an area where it is felt that performance could be improved, then the selection of the area to audit quite logically follows on from this. If, on the other hand, there has been no such activity, standards/pathways/ guidelines have not been monitored and there are no particular areas that need to be audited, then the following questions might help with the decision:

- review areas of clinical care and ask, Why do staff do it that way? Then identify ways that it might be done and ask, Why don't staff do it this way?
- are there delays in the provision of care? If so, why do these delays occur and what can be done to improve the timing of provision of care?
- discuss with colleagues whether or not patients have unnecessary complications. If they do, what can be done about it? In what specific areas do these complications occur?
- discuss whether equipment is always used correctly and, if not, what can be done about it?
- are the most suitably qualified people delivering the care? Who is doing what? Who should be doing what?

- a key area to address is whether or not clinical practice is safe. If not, why not and how can it be improved?
- would a change in resources improve the quality of care? What resources are available at present, what resources are required and where are the gaps?

Clinical audit may be used to audit an integrated care pathway or some guideline where outcomes are not being achieved or areas of clinical care that are high volume, high risk or high cost. Audit may stem from a complaint or a critical incident or from outside pressures such as a National Service Framework, an area of care or concern raised by the Healthcare Commission Review or any other outside body

3. *identify who will do the audit*: the group to conduct the audit will probably arise quite naturally from the chosen area in which the audit is being undertaken, whether it be a ward, a department, a whole hospital or the patient's home or community. As mentioned above under the topic of resources, there may be key people available who will affect the choice or make up the group. There will be several groups of people working at various levels of the organisation. It may be important to involve some of the managers in the audit to ensure that both sides of the clinical audit are taken into account: that is, clinical care and the management of that care.

Having identified the scope of the audit, decide how much time should be spent on it. The staff who are involved in clinical audit already have a heavy professional workload and are working hard delivering patient care. Be realistic, therefore, about how much time can be given to delivering a successful audit. At this point it is also important to consider what the audit will require apart from time. For example, will it require:

- information technology support
- the development of data collection forms
- data input support
- secretarial support?

Clinical audit must be evidence-based, in other words based on recognised research evidence that is proven to be effective or on expert clinical judgement. This will involve a computer search to establish current literature and research findings. However, many audit topics deal with local issues for which the literature may provide evidence that is only of superficial relevance. If this is the case, then it is even more important to develop local standards and criteria through discussion with the relevant stakeholders.

An evidence base may also be provided through existing protocols, national initiatives, professional consensus, peer group consensus, national guidelines, professional journals, national and regional organisations, and so on

4. *set the objectives for the audit*: the objectives should be set and agreed by the audit group. Objectives must be measurable, achievable and in line with the strategy and objectives for the audit programme and the organisation as a whole, as set out in the business plan and the clinical governance strategy

5. *develop standards to measure current performance*: if there are no standards, or if existing standards have not been monitored, then this is the moment to agree, write and set the standards specifically for the audit that you have in mind. Every standard should be broken down into measurable elements that will indicate whether or not it is being met. These are known as audit indicators or audit criteria. The audit indicators are the foundations around which to collect data

Establishing the baseline or identifying the level of current practice may also be achieved though a comparison with other centres, through clinical judgement or through the assessment of current practice as a result of direct observation

6. *collect the data*: there are already numerous potential sources from which to gather relevant data without gathering new data, for example the patient or client record, the care plans developed by nurses and other professionals, and so on. If guidelines are being used to support care or as part of a pathway, this will be relevant data to collect. If your audit is part of the monitoring of a pathway, then the information from the recorded 'variances' may be the data to collect. The audit may require a review of complaints reports, so identify who is responsible for the complaints received from patients and relatives and then talk to them and establish whether there have been any complaints relating to the area of the selected audit. Another area that may be relevant to the audit is that of accident reports indicating numbers of incidents and near misses, all of which will be collected and collated by the clinical risk department.

There is an enormous amount of information to be gathered from the Korner-based data. These data give information on length of stay, cases per consultant and bed occupancy. If this information is relevant to the audit, make arrangements to gather it from the finance department or the information technology department or whichever department holds it. If in doubt as to where these data are held, then ask at the library; the staff will probably be able to tell you where you can obtain them.

The audit may require new sources of information to be developed. It is important to try to restrict this information to what is essential. If new data collection forms are required, make sure that they are clear and easy to understand and quick to complete.

It may be necessary to conduct interviews with patients, clients or other service users. If interviews are to be used for collecting data, then make sure that the key questions to be asked are written down in an unambiguous fashion, so that all the interviewers ask the same questions (see Chapter 5 for more information on structured interviews). This will facilitate the collection of the data. It may be necessary to create a special audit questionnaire. Remember that it is in these areas that there may be problems with confidentiality, so ensure that whatever is developed is in line with the trust's policy on confidentiality, the data protection act and Caldicott.

For the chosen topic to be audited decide which data are essential to the audit answer the following questions:

- what are the purposes of the data?
- what data items are required?
- what are the sources of the data?

The sample used must be large enough to meet the objectives of the audit but not so large that unnecessary time is spent collecting and collating data that are not required or have no purpose. The skills of a statistician may be helpful in making an accurate decision but experience and clinical judgement will tell you what is a reasonable sample size.

Pilot all aspects of data collection to ensure that the data collected are accurate, reliable, ethical and valid. Check that all data collection forms result in the collection of data that meet the purpose as intended, are unambiguous and straightforward to use

7. *review the results*: once all the required data have been collected, the next step is the data analysis. This can take a great deal of time and so it is essential to be sure that the data collected were required and necessary to meet the audit objectives. Taking each indicator in turn, quantify the degree to which the standards have been met and identify areas where the service delivered has not conformed to the standards set. This needs to be clearly documented as the group collate and analyse the data.

During this process the group may discover that one indicator has a significantly lower rate of achievement than the others, or that there is a pattern of failure emerging which indicates a need for a specific remedy. It is important to note the indicators and the way that the study is progressing and to discuss this at regular meetings of the whole group so that everyone is clear about how the study is going

8. *identify improvements*: through analysis of the data and peer group discussion: identify any necessary improvements

9. *develop an action plan*: this should identify how the group intends to rectify any problems that the audit has identified. This action plan should specify the following:

- improvement to be achieved
- actions that need to be taken

- resources (if any) that are needed
- how improvement can be measured
- timescales by which improvements should be achieved
- who is responsible

One method of exploring possible solutions is for the group to focus on one particular problem through brainstorming, (brainstorming is explored in more detail in Chapter 16) or by using a mock solution in a systematic way. It is essential that ideas be explored on paper or within the group prior to using them in direct patient care. If the outcome of the audit indicates a change in the delivery of patient care, it is essential that those changes be piloted and the results monitored prior to implementation on a larger scale

10. *implement the action plan*: once the action plan has been drawn up and people have been identified to co-ordinate certain aspects of the initiative, it is essential that the new strategy be put into effect. Any changes should reflect the results of the monitoring process and these may have to be modified again after a further period of evaluation. This should not necessarily be seen as the end result, as there may need to be further changes to ensure that the delivery of care has been improved

11. *evaluate and report*: once the group is confident that the standards are now firmly in place, that changes have been identified and that those changes when measured provide an assurance that the quality of care has been improved and can be sustained, then the audit report can be prepared for all those involved in the service and for management. A reaudit should be planned to check that patient care has improved.

Summary of guidelines for successful audit

- commitment:
  - ☐ commitment to the study
  - ☐ group of staff who are keen to be involved.
- scale of the study:
  - ☐ start with a small study
  - ☐ be clear about the scope of the study.
- key elements:
  - ☐ handling the data
  - ☐ acquiring the evidence base about current good practice
  - ☐ drawing up checklists
  - ☐ devising ways of communicating
  - ☐ developing resources
  - ☐ acquiring additional relevant skills required, such as critical appraisal of research, computer skills, and so on.

■ decisions to be made:
  ☐ how the audit is to be carried out
  ☐ what should be looked at
  ☐ how it should be studied
  ☐ what should be done with the results.
■ rules for success:
  ☐ look at topics that are relevant to the group's work
  ☐ ensure that professional groups maintain responsibility for their own practice
  ☐ be clear about policies, procedures and confidentiality
  ☐ ensure that the study is not too time-consuming
  ☐ ensure that the group is representative of the team delivering the particular area of care
  ☐ get the support of management
  ☐ make sure that you close the audit cycle and demonstrate improvements/changes for the improvement of patient care.

In the early days of medical and clinical audit it was unusual to include the patients in the process of clinical audit. As part of clinical governance it is essential to include the patients in clinical audit, either by giving feedback about care or at a strategic level where patients and their representatives select audit topics and are involved in the process of audit and the implementation of identified changes (Kelson, 1996). At a local level, Salford Community Health Council successfully introduced facilitated patient-led mental health services audits in adolescent psychiatry and adult forensic services (Casley et al. 1998).

Conclusion

Quality processes such as clinical audit, and this includes other initiatives such as integrated care pathways, standards, and so on, should not only be in place but should also be integrated with the quality programme for the organisation. They should not be seen as isolated and detached from the rest of the quality programme but as part of a complete system of clinical governance and quality assurance.

A quality assurance programme is a systematic approach which supports the review and improvement of the quality of a service given. This systematic approach can be developed using an established framework such as Lang's model (Lang, 1976), or frameworks such as Donabedian (1990) and Maxwell (1984), all discussed in Chapter 1. On their own these frameworks and individual quality processes are not enough to sustain long-lasting and continuous quality improvement, as they tend to be set up and led by individual groups or departments. Often these individual initiatives identify problems that need to be resolved and require an organisational approach to planning and managing the change required to implement and sustain improvement. See Chapter 13 for more information on the management of change. A systematic approach through clinical governance can address these issues.

Making It Happen

Clinical Audit

The trust or healthcare organisation must ensure that there is:

- strategic planning for clinical audit
- involvement of patient/service users and carers in strategy and programme development
- training and development for staff in audit skills
- availability of resources to support clinical audit
- implementation of strategy, plans and policies
- monitoring of the results of audit and closing of the audit cycle loop through the implementation of change and the dissemination of lessons learnt.

Pillar Four – Staffing and Staff Management

6

Chapter Contents:

- workforce planning
- leadership
- learning from complaints
- managing poor performance
- mentorship
- an open and participative culture.

Key elements of this include:

- leadership skills are developed at clinical team level
- lessons for clinical practice are systematically learned from complaints made by patients
- problems of poor clinical performance are recognised at an early stage and dealt with to prevent harm to patients
- the culture is open and participative.

This pillar includes the recruitment, management and development of staff. It also covers the promotion of good working conditions and effective methods of work.

In order to assure patients of a standard of care that is acceptable and meets their needs, it is essential to have the right number of staff with the right skills in the right place at the right time. This requires good resource management on behalf of the managers and the knowledge and skill associated with effective workforce planning. Within the scope of this book it is not possible to give more than an overview of workforce planning but it is a very important part of clinical governance.

Workforce Planning

Workforce planning is the contemporary term which has generally replaced the phrase of manpower planning. There are a number of definitions of workforce planning in the literature, each of which differs slightly in emphasis. However, it may be seen as 'A planning process undertaken to ensure that there are sufficient staff available at the right time, with the right skills, diversity and flexibility, in the right place, to deliver high quality care to meet the needs of individuals and communities' (DoH, 2000).

Workforce planning can be simple or very complex, depending on the needs of the trust or healthcare organisation. In the NHS today it can also be seen as quite a challenge. It is a multifaceted and dynamic process that requires information from a variety of sources and at different levels of the organisation. In its simplest form, workforce planning is about trying to predict the future demand for different types of staff and seeking to match this with supply.

Workforce planning ensures that 'the right people with the right skills are in the right place at the right time'. This definition covers a methodical process that provides managers with a framework for making human resources decisions based on the organisation's mission, strategic plan and budgetary resources, and on a set of desired workforce competencies. The trust or healthcare organisation sets about the task of writing a workforce development plan. The framework that follows is based on the Department of Health's *Primary Care Workforce Planning Framework* (DoH, 2002), which has five elements:

- defining the vision
- identifying future demand
- mapping the existing workforce
- developing the future workforce
- developing a workforce action plan.

The Vision

The vision means agreeing the values and goals for developing the service and the workforce. The values are the criteria by which improvements in the service will be judged. Some will reflect national policy, the national vision, and others will be local priorities and issues, the local vision. The national vision is set out in the NHS Plan (DoH, 2000) and in the consultation document *Standards for Better Health* (DoH, 2004), for example:

- fifth domain – Accessible and responsive care: Healthcare organisations ensure that patients with emergency health needs are able to access care promptly (DoH, 2004)
- reduction in health inequalities in terms of service delivery and health outcomes (DoH, 2002).

The local vision translates the national vision into the local need, for example:

- the fifth domain standard above may require the emergency services within a trust to review staffing levels, skill-mix and roles and responsibilities in their accident and emergency department.

The vision requires multidisciplinary and multi-agency staff as it will rely upon a combination of developing professional skills and their contribution within the multidisciplinary teams or networks. It may also require substantial investment. A clear description of what the service will look like and how it is to develop is required to be matched alongside workforce planning to meet the redesigned service. The vision includes new services or services developed to meet the needs of the local population, the local HIMP and national targets such as reducing health inequalities and improving access, public health and outcomes in categories such as coronary heart disease, smoking cessation and teenage pregnancy.

The starting point for looking at future demand is to identify the drivers which are most likely to bring about changes in service delivery or the workforce: the environmental drivers, demographic trends and new technologies policy drivers. Areas where national or local action can be taken to drive change include service targets and priorities such as those in the NHS.

Identifying Future Demand

Workforce planning cannot be undertaken in isolation from service planning, the redesigning of services and the implementation of care pathways that cross organisational boundaries and link with other trusts. The key demand drivers include:

- demographic changes leading to an older population which increases the demand on community services, allied health professional staff, hospitals, and so on
- the NSF programmes to improve clinical care
- clinical governance which impacts on the workload
- changes in the provision of care by the acute trusts, such as shorter lengths of stay in hospital which impact on community services
- new technology resulting in more complex needs for patients.

To assess the impact of the key drivers on the service provision, an assessment of the political, economic, social and technical factors, otherwise known as a PEST analysis, will inform workforce planning, for example:

- identify drivers such as new treatments, or other medical advances
- identify policy drivers such as the standards in the NSFs, the clinical governance agenda, the results of clinical audit and feedback from the appraisal of staff
- include local policies from the SHA, Health Improvement and Modernisation Plans, Local Authorities and other stakeholders in the local health economies
- analyse the impact of each of the drivers on service provision.

To meet the workforce implications, new and existing skills and a perceived need for additional staff and/or new ways of working in skill mix teams that best meet service needs may be identified. A more sophisticated and flexible approach to education and training may be required.

Mapping the Existing Workforce

A good picture of the existing workforce is a prerequisite for understanding what the development needs of the workforce will be if the vision is to be achieved, and the following information is required about each of the demand scenarios identified in the vision. This is done by identifying numbers, skills and roles that already exist in the trust or healthcare organisation, and matching them against those required to meet the vision and identifying the variance, for example:

- the number of full- and part-time staff and a whole-time equivalent (WTE) by class of staff or profession
- an age and gender profile of the workforce according to the profession or function, with possible inclusion of other factors such as ethnic composition
- the proportion of vacancies to relevant workforce number category, for example the number of vacancies to number of agreed or funded posts
- the typical time it takes to recruit into certain types of post
- the typical length of service, starters, leavers, re-entrants and anticipated retirements to indicate turnover rates
- data on where recruits come from and where leavers go
- data on qualifications held, known training needs, training timescales and available training resources.

A skills audit should be undertaken to identify the available skills in the organisation. The skills required should then be identified and matched to those already in the organisation and any gaps noted. The Government's plan is to have National Occupational Standards for all sectors of the health workforce. However, in the meantime a quick assessment can be carried out using functional mapping through self-assessment, where staff are asked to rate their level of competence.

Who Supports Workforce Planning?

The Workforce Development Confederations (WDCs) have a key role in driving forward work to increase staff numbers. There are 27 confederations aligned to the SHAs and they bring together local NHS and non-NHS employers to plan and develop the whole healthcare workforce. They work closely with SHAs and the postgraduate deaneries to deliver on workforce issues in the context of the NHS Plan and local priorities, and the membership includes:

- councils with social services responsibilities and other social care employers
- further-education institutions
- higher-education institutions
- independent-sector organisations
- the Learning and Skills Councils
- the Ministry of Defence
- the National Blood Authority
- NHS Direct
- voluntary-sector organisations.

They also work with Government Offices for Regions and Regional Development Agencies to ensure that strategies reflect the wider labour market issues.

Workforce development starts with the definition of the services and potential services that the public need and then an identification of the skills and competencies required to deliver these identified services, which must be matched to the number and types of staff required. It is important to remember that the skills and knowledge which the staff bring to patient care is more important than simply their professional background and this should be accounted for in the planning process. All clinical staff are involved not just in patient care but in related work that includes teaching, clinical governance, management, and further training and development – all of which take time and skill and form part of the equation. Education and training must be responsive to skills and competencies required for healthcare delivery, including changing roles to those that meet the patients' needs. Service development will highlight changes in clinical practice which must be fed into the system so that the plan is for the workforce required for the future and planners are not simply fighting yesterday's battles! The needs of patients for care drives the workforce planning agenda.

The National Workforce Development Board (NWDB) provides:

■ a long-term focus on workforce planning and development in the NHS. It advises the Secretary of State on workforce development issues and translates strategic aims into an agenda for action
■ a strategic overview at national level of all health service workforce issues and ensures that this is built into the development of local service plans.

There is also the Workforce Numbers Advisory Board which is a technical group which advises the NWDB on the overall numbers of undergraduates and postgraduate education and training places to be commissioned in each staff group. On the basis of information from local plans, it advises the NWDB on the targets for workforce distribution and the number and location of training places that will best support this aim. The Care Group Workforce Teams were established to take a national overview of the workforce implications in terms of numbers, skills and competencies and of delivering national commitment on services, and currently cover:

■ coronary heart disease
■ mental health
■ cancer
■ emergency care
■ older people
■ children
■ long-term conditions (renal and diabetes).

The NHS Modernisation Agency's Changing Workforce Programme (CWP) was set up in 2001. This is a national programme set up to support staff in the redesign of roles and tasks (see also Chapter 1). The aim is to improve services to patients and improve staff satisfaction, retention and recruitment.

Developing the Future Workforce

Before a final action plan can be developed, it is necessary to identify the options for developing the workforce so that the demand scenarios can be met and the vision achieved. These include the labour market supply, the projected local supply, local options for recruitment and retention, new roles and ways of working, perhaps supported by the CWP.

Education

Education must be patient-centred and focused on clinical teams, across traditional professional boundaries and service boundaries. Programmes must meet local service needs as well as the professional and personal development needs of individuals. It is important to make full use of the stakeholders and the range of approaches and methods that they have on offer. The NHS Plan promised NHS staff without a professional qualification access to either an NHS Learning Account or dedicated training to National Vocational Qualification (NVQ) levels two and three as set out in *Working Together – Learning Together* (DoH, 2001). Interprofessional education and training (pre- and post-registration) and common learning programmes ensure that there are core skills in the key areas of communications, NHS principles and organisation, and professional skills are combined to support patient-centred care. Programmes have been and are being developed by partnerships of higher educational institutions and WDCs which focus on professional learning with and from each other. They are often based around a problem-solving model, which allows professionals to understand what they do best separately and what they do best together and how they can maximise their collective skills.

Finally a workforce action plan must be developed. Workforce planning is a by-product of good management and integral service planning which includes:

- succession planning
- skill-mix reviews
- educational training (both purchaser and provider)
- recruitment and retention
- continuing professional development
- career development.

There are four phases to workforce planning:

- setting the strategic direction
- workforce analysis/strategies
- implementing the workforce plan
- monitoring – evaluating – revising.

Leadership

An effective organisation requires clear organisational and clinical leadership. Management and leadership are often confused and essentially they are different. Managers are the people who ensure the efficiency and effectiveness of an organisation but they are not always effective leaders. As Stewart (1996) suggests, for clinical governance to work the NHS needs leaders who can 'make others feel that what they are doing matters and hence make them feel good about their work'. This is a statement that empowers and values staff, which is an essential ingredient in successful clinical governance. The notion of empowering and valuing staff is discussed later in this chapter. Leaders influence others by what they say, how they say it and what they do. An effective leader should, therefore, be:

- a visionary
- a communicator
- a facilitator
- an advocate
- a doer
- an evaluator
- a critical thinker
- knowledgeable
- tactful
- able to inspire respect.

There are different styles of leadership, some of which are discussed in Chapters 13 and 14. However, when looking at clinical governance some leadership styles may have a positive or negative effect on the implementation and ongoing development of clinical governance. Marquis and Hutson (2000), set out the description of each style of leadership (Table 6.1) and it is clear that some styles are more applicable to clinical governance than others.

Table 6.1 Leadership styles

Theory	Description
Autocratic	Strong control Gives commands Communicates downwards only Does not involve others in decision-making Apportions blame
Democratic	Less control Directs by guidance Two-way process of communication up and down Shared decision-making Uses constructive criticism
Laissez-faire	Little control Limited direction Communicates well Devolves decision-making Group-orientated Does not criticise

Source: Adapted from Marquis and Hutson, 2000.

The authoritarian style of leadership:
- requires strong control
- gives commands
- communicates downwards only
- does not involve others in decision-making
- apportions blame.

In the context of clinical governance this type of leadership is destructive and inappropriate as it is not in keeping with the notion of sharing and openness, which is one of the fundamental principles of clinical governance.

The democratic style of leadership:
- requires less control
- directs by guidance
- involves a two-way process of communication – up and down
- encourages shared decision-making
- uses constructive criticism.

This style is the preferred one as it offers a strong approach to breaking down the barriers of resistance through the development of a collaborative, empowering and trusting culture based on effective communication and partnership.

The laissez-faire style of leadership:
- involves little control
- has limited direction
- communicates well
- devolves decision-making
- is group orientated
- does not criticise.

This style contains some of the elements, which are important for the implementation and ongoing development of a clinical governance culture. However, there is a need to use constructive criticism as an essential part of the principle of learning from mistakes. The other areas where this style falls short of the mark is the lack of control and limited direction.

There are also personality types and traits, as set out in Table 6.2, which clearly demonstrate the different strengths that different personalities will bring to a group, a team or indeed to the process of continued development of clinical governance and continuous quality improvement.

Innovators are the people who offer most support to the implementation and continued development of clinical governance, followed by the moderately enthusiastic early adapters. The early majority accept innovations just before

Table 6.2 Personality types and traits

Personality type	Personality traits
Innovators	Curious, enthusiastic and eager
Early adapters	Moderately enthusiastic, well-established group members, with high self-esteem (do not usually introduce radical/controversial ideas)
Early majority	Accept the innovation just before the majorities do
Late majority	View the innovation with scepticism, do not actively resist
Laggards	Suspicious of change, discourage others by their negative attitude
Rejecters	Openly reject change and encourage others to do so

Source: Adapted from McSherry and Simmons, 2001.

the majorities followed by the late majority who view innovation with scepticism but do not actively resist. Then come the laggards with their negative attitude and suspicions of change, their tendency to discourage others. The group that are least supportive of clinical governance innovations are the rejecters, who openly reject change and encourage others to do so. However, it is important to remember that an organisation or a team requires a combination of personality types with different strengths in order to make the team successful. It would be unimaginable if everyone involved in developing clinical governance was a laggard and equally difficult if everyone was an innovator. There is more about leadership and managing change in Chapter 13, working with and facilitating groups in Chapter 14 and project management in Chapter 15.

Effective leaders may be at any level of an organisation but there are some key elements and these leaders:

- are key to the quality of service or care rendered in the organisation and need to see themselves as valued in that role
- choose their results (are proactive)
- create the vision
- as people understand empowerment, and as leaders require an understanding of power, the choice to take power and the skills to build it
- take risks and encourage risk-taking in others
- use a problem-solving approach that focuses on results
- create an environment for success
- develop rather than control others
- respect others

- understand that elitist attitudes are unethical
- model rather than mould
- trust their experience.

Source: Leading an Empowered Organisation Seminar (Creative Health Care Management).

Learning from Complaints

In 1994 a report *Being Heard* (DoH, 1994) was published as a result of the work of a review committee set up to review the NHS complaints procedures and chaired by Professor Alan Wilson. This was followed in 1995 by the Government's proposals to address the issues raised by Professor Wilson in a report called *Acting on Complaints: The Government's Proposals* (DoH, 1995). This policy set out a new procedure for complaints with some key objectives that included:

- providing ease of access for patients and complainants
- providing a simplified procedure, with common features, for complaints about any of the services provided as part of the NHS
- separating complaints from disciplinary procedures
- making it easier to extract lessons on quality from complaints to improve services for patients
- being fair to staff and complainants alike
- providing a more rapid and open process
- providing an approach that is honest and thorough, with the main aim of resolving the problems and satisfying the concerns of the complainant.

In 1996 a new NHS Complaints Procedure was introduced which was intended as a template from which all trusts, health authorities, family health service authorities and GPs would develop their own local complaints procedures (NHS, 1996). Each NHS trust has a designated complaints manager who has an overview of all complaints and is easily accessible to the public. This is sometimes the chief executive or a senior manager; in primary care it could be the lead GP or practice manager. In primary care, where there is a close relationship between the patient and the GP, if this relationship breaks down and the patient is dissatisfied with their GP then a conciliator may be appointed by the PCT to help the two parties discuss the issues and, if at all possible, settle the complaint. This is known as the local resolution process. If a complainant feels that the issue has not been resolved to his/her satisfaction, then he/she may request an independent review from the convenor of the trust or PCT within 28 days of the completion of the local complaints process. The convenor will check that the local resolution process has been followed correctly and, if appropriate, will then set up a review panel. The convenor must have no prior involvement in the complaint. The panel consists of three members: a lay chairman, the convenor and another independent person. If the complaint is clinical, then the panel will be advised by at least two independent clinical assessors nominated by the Strategic Health Authority (SHA) with advice from the relevant professional bodies such as the General Medical Council and the Royal College of Nursing.

The panel investigate the complaint and present a report to the trust. This report is discussed and action agreed as a result of the report. The chief executive then informs the complainant of the result and also advises him of his/her right to take the complaint to the Health Service Commissioner.

In March 2003, the Government issued a paper called the *NHS Complaints Reform: Making Things Right* (DoH, 2003) in which it set out plans to improve the NHS complaints procedure following an independent two-year evaluation of the complaints procedure and listening exercises to gather feedback in relation to suggestions made by a team of researchers.

The paper sets out a comprehensive programme of reforms which are subject to legislation and some of the planned changes include:

- the need to improve support for people who are making a complaint
- better communication and customer-care training for those involved in dealing with complaints
- NHS organisations to be held accountable for the performance of complaints handling
- reform of the independent review panel process by placing responsibility with the Healthcare Commission, the intention being that those who remain dissatisfied with the result or outcome of the complaint from the local resolution process will have access to an independent, neutral and impartial view of their complaint.

It is essential that all staff understand that they have a personal accountability for complaints made against them and, in a wider context, that they should learn from other complaints both locally and nationally. All staff must have a clear understanding of the complaints procedure to support and facilitate patients and their carers in making a complaint. Complaints should be handled efficiently, effectively, in a timely manner, and at source – at local level whenever possible. The key element is that staff should learn from a complaint, investigate the problem and change their practice to 'close the loop' and ensure that it does not happen again. Finally, they should disseminate across the trust the lessons learned and the changes made to prevent a similar problem occurring elsewhere in the trust or organisation. See also Chapter 1 for information about the Commission for Patients and Public Involvement in Health (CPPIH), Patient Advice and Liaison Services (PALS) and Patient Forums.

Managing Poor Performance

Part of the clinical governance framework is the management of poor performance, which relates to devices and/or personnel. As set out earlier in this chapter, the leadership and management style of an organisation has a direct effect on how people perform. It is essential to have an approach that creates an open and honest culture which encourages staff, patients and the general public to share their concerns about the organisation and to promote good performance and manage poor performance. The delivery of healthcare is a complex process and when things go wrong it is often quicker and easier to blame an individual than to spend time reviewing the systems and processes in order to establish the cause of a complaint.

The Royal College of Nursing (RCN, 2000) suggests that:

> A culture that encourages open discussion and reflection on practice allows staff to learn from their experiences. This includes both celebrating what is done well and learning from what is done well. However, if an organisation is going to encourage clinicians to report incidents and learn from mistakes, it must develop a blame free culture, rather than one that revolves around disciplinary procedures.

As stated above, the whole ethos of performance management must be balanced and about managing both good and poor performance. Performance management is through:

- individual appraisal
- clinical supervision
- mentoring schemes
- systems for dealing with cases of poor performance, including whistle-blowing
- effective workforce planning – minimum staff numbers and the correct skill-mix to deliver safe and effective care; getting the right staff in the right place, in the right numbers, and with the right skills to meet identified patient need
- schemes of delegation and supervision
- protocols for staff working in extended roles
- compliance with working time directives
- health and safety and managing risks to staff, such as violence.

Mentorship

Mentorship is a useful and effective method of supporting and developing staff at all levels of a trust or healthcare organisation. There are a number of possible uses for mentoring in an organisation and some of these include:

- induction – to help people become familiar with the organisation
- support for development – to ensure effective learning
- career progression – to assist in identifying and supporting potential
- support for learning on the job – to enhance job-related knowledge and skills
- support in a new project or job
- within change programmes – to help people understand what is involved in the change, and
- as part of clinical governance and the process of supporting and empowering staff.

Mentoring is an exciting yet complex phenomenon that is natural or artificially contrived to benefit individuals within a sharing partnership (Palmer, 1987). It is a dynamic relationship and based on shared values and mutual attraction. It is about shared encouragement and support of personal, career and/or professional development. Mentorship is a relationship that enables, cultivates and empowers an individual in the working environment and is concerned with making the most of human potential.

In healthcare the individuals being mentored are usually described as mentees or students. Levinson's (1978) study of adult development suggests that the mentor is normally older than the mentee, of greater experience and his professional senior. The mentor is seen as a transitional, exemplary figure in the mentee's development (Levinson, 1978).

As suggested by Hagerty (1986), there are numerous definitions of mentorship but Levinson et al. (1978) suggest and interpret the nature of the classical mentor, which supports an exploration of the relationships and the various mentoring approaches.

Common Elements of Mentoring

Morton-Cooper and Palmer (2000) outline some common elements that can be applied to mentoring:

- the character of the relationship is that of enabling and empowerment
- the mentor offers a repertoire of assisting or helper functions to facilitate guidance and provide support
- the mentor role comprises an interplay of personal, functional and relational aspects
- individual purposes and helper functions are mutually set by the individuals involved

- helper functions are mutually determined by individuals
- individuals choose each other and there are identifiable stages in the relationship.

Types of Relationships

It is usual that the two individuals are naturally drawn together because they hold similar values, they have similar characteristics and they enjoy spending time together in order to learn from each other and share experiences. However, this is not always the case as the organisation may have a formal mentoring scheme or system for facilitating mentoring, in which case the match will be arranged.

Mentoring relationships vary depending upon the people and the organisation, so they may be:

- open – able to discuss any topic
- closed – restricted to discussion topics
- public – everyone knows that the relationship exists
- private – few know that the relationship exists
- formal – agreed appointment dates, venues and timings
- informal – a casual arrangement where they can see each other as and when required.

Qualities of a Mentor

The mentee may be a peer, a team member, someone you know well or someone you have never met before. The process of mentoring promotes change in the mentee and helps him/her towards a new view of what is possible. There are some personal qualities that a good mentor will have. These include being:

- enthusiastic – genuinely interested in the mentee's aspirations, concerns and needs
- a motivator and encourager – able to channel the mentee's energy into constructive change, new challenges and overcoming difficulties
- open – honest and open about oneself and about the mentee. Being prepared to share personal experiences of similar issues
- empathetic – able to appreciate how the mentee behaves, thinks and feels
- supportive – a source of emotional support
- positive in outlook – able to appreciate the mentee's point of view
- a good listener – able to focus on what the mentee is saying without one's own thoughts crowding out the mentee's words – a good sounding board
- critical – able to criticise in a positive and supportive way.

There are some key mentoring roles that a mentor can fulfil and these include:

- *adviser*: the mentor offers advice and support in terms of career and social issues. The personal qualities of being open and honest are essential when offering advice and support. It is important for the mentor to use his/her own past experience of similar situations and be able to use this to support the mentee. I have been a mentor to people at all levels in a variety of NHS trusts and health care organisations outside the NHS and one of my mentees was being bullied by a senior colleague. Having lived through a similar experience, I was able to support my mentee in working towards resolving the problem. However, mentoring is not just about advising; the key to effective mentoring is to listen and not jump in with advice that is not asked for. The mentor should resist the temptation to tell the mentee what to do but help him/her to find his/her own solutions. But there will be times when the mentee asks for advice and direction, in which case the mentor should respond and support the mentee
- *coach*: in mentoring the coaching role concerns the mutual setting of guidelines, with the mentor offering advice and constructive feedback. The mentee then tries out the feedback in practical situations in his/her daily working life. Sometimes there is a requirement to move from mentor to coach in order to support the mentee in realising his/her goals: for example coaching or helping someone to prepare for an interview to progress their career or preparing for a presentation to the board. Here the boundaries between mentor and coach begin to blur
- *counsellor*: in the role of a counsellor the mentor acts as a listener and sounding board to facilitate self-awareness and encourage independence. In my experience this aspect of the role of mentor is, certainly at the start of the relationship, the most important as far as the mentee is concerned, particularly if the mentee is in a senior position in the organisation. He/she needs someone to listen, someone who is on his/her side and is not going to run off and tell the world what has been said. One of the ground rules of mentoring is that the discussions and the information exchanged remain confidential and what is said is not reported by the mentor to anyone. This is particularly important if the mentor/mentee relationship is not public knowledge
- *guide/networker*: the mentor introduces the mentee to helpful contacts and groups within the organisation. Networking is an extension of this and the mentor is able to support the mentee through access to a much wider network outside the organisation. If the mentee believes that this sort of support is what he/she requires, then careful research is needed before a mentor is chosen. Often when a mentor is chosen for a mentee who is in a senior management position, such as a director, then this will be one of

the main drivers for choosing a mentor from outside the organisation who can offer this sort of experience and breadth of knowledge

■ *role model*: the mentor provides an observable image and demonstrates skills and qualities for the mentee to copy. This can be at any level of an organisation. This role of the mentor is used extensively for students of medicine and nursing, junior managers, and so on. Also, at a senior level for example, the aspiring manager chooses the chief executive as his/her role model

■ *sponsor*: the mentor as a sponsor will influence career development by introducing the mentee to a potential employer who could enhance his/her career. The mentor may make recommendations within the organisation, which could put forward the mentee for promotion or development

■ *teacher*: the mentor has a role as a teacher in the sharing of knowledge and experience with the mentee in order to promote his/her personal development. Once the mentor has got to know the mentee and his/her individual needs, there will be opportunities to discuss learning opportunities such as reflecting on how well a particular event went, whether it could have been done better or differently, and learning from the experience. I ask my mentees to keep a diary of events and to make a note of what went well and what did not go quite so well. When we meet we reflect on and discuss an event of the mentee's choice, reviewing and reflecting on things that went well and, when things did not go so well, identifying ways of doing things differently that might result in a more positive outcome for the mentee

■ *resource facilitator*: the mentor acts as a resource, as an experienced colleague or practitioner sharing experiences and information to support the mentee. For example, one of my mentees had been asked to write a clinical governance strategy and wanted to see some examples. I was able to offer some contacts and also some examples of well-written strategies, which set my mentee on the right track.

There are different models for mentoring but I use a three-stage approach: getting to know each other, understanding each other, and final action planning. It is important to go through these stages and not to force the action planning until the mentee is ready.

The Three Stages of Mentoring

1. Getting to know each other

Arrange the first meeting at which the mentor takes the lead in building a relationship with the mentee, listening to what the mentee is saying, giving him/her time to talk and encouraging this through asking open questions. Also at this first meeting:

■ establish and write down the aims and objectives of mentoring
■ discuss confidentiality and come to an agreement about the boundaries within which you are going to work
■ establish ground rules such as:
  □ the frequency of meetings
  □ the length of meetings
  □ the location
  □ the system of recording meetings – could be in note or diary format.

During this stage the mentor will negotiate the agenda and begin to support the mentee in thinking about an action plan. This stage could be completed in one meeting or may take several meetings.

2. Understanding each other
At this stage the mentor supports and counsels the mentee, listens to what is being said, challenges as appropriate and gives constructive feedback. As the mentor gets to know the mentee, his/her strengths and weaknesses become apparent and it is possible to identify the needs of the mentee and to offer information and advice. This is a time for sharing experiences, getting to know each other, exploring ways forward, agreeing ideas for an action plan, reflecting back and clarifying the mentee's developmental needs, goals and aspirations.

The next stage begins when the mentor and mentee have reached a point where they understand each other and the issues.

3. Action planning
The mentor examines the options for actions and the consequences. He/she encourages new and creative thinking, and supports the mentee in making decisions, resolving issues and solving problems. The action plan is agreed and implemented, with ongoing monitoring of progress towards meeting the aims and objectives of the mentee. Sometimes the action plan is straightforward and is discussed, documented and agreed at the end of the first session, but sometimes it takes days, weeks or even months to get to this stage because of the complexity of the issues.

An Open and Participative Culture

Much of what has been said already in this chapter is about creating an organisation that is open, honest and participative through effective leadership and management, involving patients and their carers and good communication. However, there is another element, which is empowerment.

Empowerment

Empowerment may be defined as the process by which individuals have control over the resources, decisions, structures and other factors that can affect the quality of life. This results in an individual having a strong voice and being actively involved in decision-making processes. The process of empowerment implies interdependence, engagement, information, goals, collaboration, confidence and change, which result in the wellbeing and development of the individual.

An individual who is empowered can be said to have:

- decision-making power
- access to information and resources
- a range of options with which to make informed choices
- assertiveness
- hope – a feeling that he/she can make a difference
- critical-thinking ability – able to see things differently, for example learning to redefine who he/she is, what he/she can do and his/her relationships with hierarchical power
- an understanding about anger and how to express it
- a feeling of being part of a group, not isolated and alone
- an understanding that everyone has rights
- the ability to effect change both in his/her life and in the life of the organisation
- the ability to learn new skills that he/she sees as important
- the ability to change the perception of others about competency and the capacity to act
- self-initiated growth and change that is ongoing
- a positive self-image.

Some of the lessons learned through the development of successful Practice Development Units (PDUs) give useful insight into empowering both staff and patients. A PDU is a multidisciplinary approach to evidence-based clinical care for patients, and the drivers of a PDU are:

- clinical leadership
- shared multidisciplinary vision and philosophy
- the empowerment of patients
- the empowerment of staff

- the identification of a need to change, with a planned approach to change
- a strong commitment to quality
- the development of research-based practice
- the dissemination of good practice
- the evaluation of practice
- the evaluation of change.

Empowering Staff

Staff are empowered when an environment has been created which encourages and facilitates all staff of all grades and disciplines to be actively involved in debates and decision-making processes. To enable staff to be involved in these processes there must be a programme of education and development to meet their identified needs and to support their participation in these activities.

A PDU provides a culture and environment where all grades of staff and disciplines are involved in debates and decision-making processes. Great importance is placed on the development of all staff to enable them to participate effectively in the development of the PDU. The ethos is one of a work-based approach to learning through reflection on practice, and project-based learning supported by learning contracts and mentorship. Also management and leadership functions are designed to be facilitated across professional boundaries and to reduce the superiority of one profession over another.

As Casley et al. (1998) show, in the past one of the features of the NHS culture was the rigid distribution of power through the hierarchy of the hospital organisation. At the top of the 'pecking order' were those in the medical profession, with everyone else placed beneath them. Nursing, therapies, pharmacy, management, and so on were all organised into separate departments which facilitated accountability but isolated these groups and created divisions. The Seacroft PDU (Casley et al., 1998) broke down these barriers and created a team approach which valued the contributions of all staff, devolved the decision-making closer to the patient and enabled critical review and the development of processes of care across departmental boundaries. One of the main principles of a PDU is that the 'power' is delegated downwards, ensuring that the decision-making is as close to the clinical situation as possible.

The empowerment of staff is through the development of new skills and knowledge, and the facilitation of the multidisciplinary team, building on the strengths and overcoming weaknesses. This is achieved through reflection on practice and the creation of new opportunities for participation in debate and decisions about future services, approaches to the delivery of care, and so on.

The PDU offers an environment where these barriers can be broken down and the team work together to improve or develop practice through open discussion and each team member being valued equally for his/her contribution.

The culture of a PDU is to support the development of skills and knowledge of all staff by any means at its disposal, from personal development through multidisciplinary project work, personal development programmes and shadowing to formal study days and courses. There is more about practice development and quality improvement in Chapter 7.

Empowering Patients

Patients are empowered when they have enough information with which to make informed decisions, particularly in the area of consent for an intervention. Decisions are made by the patient and not by professionals on behalf of the patient. It is about making informed choices such as whether or not to consent to a treatment, to able to choose between options and come to a conclusion based on sound information. Today patients are encouraged to ask questions, read supporting literature, be involved in health education, access their health records and express their views.

Patients are empowered when they are involved in the decision-making of the organisation such as when participating in focus groups, completing patient-satisfaction surveys, and working as part of a steering group of a PDU; indeed, in any situation where they are part of the debate, and ultimately their views influence the decisions taken.

Conclusion

This pillar of clinical governance contains some of the most crucial elements essential to the structure of a trust or healthcare organisation. For example, without effective workforce planning there may be a lack of staff skills and knowledge, which would threaten the core business of the organisation, which is the provision of good-quality clinical care. The issue of leadership at all levels of the organisation and not just at the top is key to the delivery of well-planned, well-managed care.

In any healthcare organisation there will inevitably be complaints, and the more patients are empowered the more likely they are to feel confident in expressing disatisfaction and any concerns about the delivery of care. The process of managing complaints must be efficient, timely and effective but it is perhaps even more important to have learned from the events that led up to the complaint and to make sure that it is not repeated anywhere in the organisation.

Identifying and managing poor performance is a difficult and sensitive area, but must be tackled to ensure patient safety. To support this, the culture must be open and participative by listening to staff and patients and having systems in place to improve practice and prevent patients being put at risk.

Making It Happen

Staffing and Staff Management

The trust needs to ensure that:

- strategy and workforce planning for staffing is in place (working together and improving working lives)
- human resources employment processes are in place
- employee support services, such as occupational health services, independent confidential advice services and support for staff against bullying and harassment, are available
- systems of induction, appraisal, clinical supervision and mentoring, and managing poor performance are in place
- workforce planning is in action
- training and development of all staff in all processes above are available.

Pillar Five – Education, Training and Continuing Personal and Professional Development

7

Chapter Contents:

- professional development
- practice development and quality improvement (Brendan McCormack, Helen Chambers)
- continuing professional development
- reviewing practice.

Key elements of this include:

- all professional development programmes reflect the principles of clinical governance
- there is monitoring of all clinical staff to ensure that they meet professional requirements for updating or reregistration, for example Continuing Medical Education (CME) and Post-Registration Educational Practice (PREP)
- there is a forum for discussing all clinical practice and for agreeing/reviewing new practices.

This covers the support of available education and training to enable staff to be competent at their jobs, whilst developing their skills and the degree to which staff are up to date with developments in their field.

Professional Development

Clinical governance and continuous quality improvement in the delivery of healthcare can only be achieved in an organisation where the culture values their staff, as demonstrated through the provision of and support for ongoing learning and development. The trust or organisation must have a structure in place for education and training for all staff, both clinical and non-clinical, but the responsibility also lies with individual members of staff who must keep themselves up to date and well-informed of best practice.

There are three levels of education and training for clinical governance:

- *trust or organisational level*: at this level there is a responsibility for the provision of induction programmes for all new staff and this provides an opportunity to give an overview of clinical governance, what it means, how the trust is meeting the clinical governance agenda, and the role that each member of staff is expected to undertake in ensuring that the trust has a culture which embraces the ethos of clinical governance. There is also a need for the organisation to respond to educational and training needs identified through appraisal, professional development plans (PDPs) and all mandatory training such as fire, manual handling, resuscitation, infection control, and so on
- *directorate or team level*: education and training for clinical governance should be:
  - ☐ in response to learning needs identified from a complaint and the introduction of new practice to improve on the practice that was the basis of the complaint
  - ☐ identified by means of appraisal, PDPs, and so on
  - ☐ an opportunity for learning through reflective practice
  - ☐ identified through the process of clinical audit
  - ☐ through sharing good practice and innovations by means of networks such as the Practice Development Unit network
  - ☐ through case studies, and so on.
- *individual level*: learning needs should be identified after performance review, through appraisal and as part of the process of personal development plans and provided through attendance on a workshop, course or seminar.

In order to reflect the principles of clinical governance, all educational programmes should be multidisciplinary or multiprofessional, evidence-based, competency-based and regularly evaluated.

At the University of Leeds Susan Hamer has led a very successful approach to improving practice, ensuring that practice is evidence-based through a network of accredited PDUs. The ethos of a PDU is to empower staff to explore innovative and creative ideas; to develop, research, implement and then disseminate and share their findings to improve patient care. Practice development is an essential part of clinical governance, and Brendan McCormack and Helen Chambers from the Royal Hospitals NHS Trust, Belfast have contributed the following thoughts on Practice Development and Quality Improvement.

Practice Development and Quality Improvement

In a healthcare context that is continuously changing, finding the best approaches to achieving sustained change in practice is a key challenge for organisations. In healthcare developing practice and services has adopted a variety of approaches. The most common of these are practice development and quality improvement. Ultimately, both these approaches are about developing quality patient care, but there is considerable misunderstanding about the meaning of practice development.

A Definition of Practice Development

Practice development is a continuous process of improvement towards increased effectiveness in patient-centred care. This is brought about by helping healthcare teams to develop their knowledge and skills and to transform the culture and context of care. It is enabled and supported by facilitators committed to systematic, rigorous, continuous processes of emancipatory change that reflect the perspectives of service users (Garbett and McCormack, 2002a).

This definition has been developed from ongoing research work with practising nurses and nurses in practice development roles (Garbett and McCormack, 2001; 2002a). The definition reflects the central purpose of practice development, that of the development of patient-centred care. It further highlights the need for development work to be undertaken rigorously and systematically, set within a continuous culture of improvement. Practice development, according to this approach, differs from traditional notions of bringing about change in that the emphasis is not just on changing a particular practice, but also on transforming the culture(s) and context of care settings.

Practice Development and Quality Improvement in Context

The current impetus to improve practice can be attributed to a wide range of influences. Government policy provides the context for directions in the development of practice. For example, *Health of the Nation* (DoH, 1992) and *A Vision for the Future* (DoH, 1993) underpinned NDU work in Graham's (1996) work. Professional conduct (Draper, 1996; McMahon, 1998) and the development of accountability frameworks add further impetus to this work. For example, Kitson (1997) argues that nurses need to determine the structure and function of nursing care in order to demonstrate its value and to be able to influence and shape the broader issues in changes to the delivery of healthcare, especially in the light of the increasing emphasis on practitioners of all healthcare disciplines providing evidence of their quality of care contained within policy documents such as *A First Class Service* (DoH, 1998b). These policy drivers set the scene for an approach to the development of practice that incorporates the development of individuals. In addition, there is increasing emphasis on reprofiling services in response to needs identified by service users. Approaches to addressing the skills and knowledge requirements of practitioners are concerned with addressing the issue of competence, the nature of knowledge, and skills development. It is argued that for professional development to be effective, it needs to be explicitly concerned with the needs of the client group catered for. Nonetheless, professional development is a strategy for demonstrating commitment to teams who are being asked to change their practice (Binnie & Titchen 1999) and one that is firmly embedded in clinical governance strategies (DoH, 1998b).

Transforming Contexts and Cultures of Care

The emphasis on the development of patient care means that the nature of the transformation and the ways in which it takes place must be considered. Two main trends can be described: the first addresses the direction that changes in care should take and concerns the drive towards patient-centred models of care provision; the second reflects beliefs about the ways in which lasting change can best be brought about.

The increasing importance of the individual patient within healthcare is founded both on an emergent professional ideology within nursing (and other healthcare professions) and on a 'customer care' model of consumerism that has developed within the NHS as a whole. Both trends challenge a dominant mode of organisation within the NHS characterised by bureaucratic and industrial models of organisation, which resulted in task orientation and a lack of responsiveness to the needs of individuals. A major focus of practice development, therefore, is on the transformation of healthcare environments to ensure that they cater for the needs of individual patients (for example, Vaughan and Edwards, 1995; Graham, 1996; Kitson et al., 1996; Ward et al., 1998; Binnie and Titchen, 1999; Jackson et al., 1999; McCormack et al., 1999). This entails an environment in which practitioners can make and act on decisions about the care given to individuals without being stifled by hierarchical models of reporting and approval. This in turn entails the development of knowledge, skills and decision-making in individuals and cultures that allow such attributes to be applied with regard to the safety and dignity of individual clients (McCormack et al., 1999).

Given the radical nature of the transformation being tackled, the methods employed to effect such a change need to be chosen carefully. The dominant theme in the literature is for a model of change that inculcates the attitudes and skills necessary for a more person-centred form of care through the process of change itself.

Research by Garbett and McCormack (2002a) recognised that practice development involved the development of an environment in which changes to practice could be accepted. The research also emphasised the need to encourage people to think differently about their work, for example talking about supporting risk-taking, valuing practitioners' ideas and 'realising capabilities that have been crushed' by bureaucratic models of organisation.

Practice development is associated with questioning the way in which practice takes place in order to attempt some change or improvement – something that is consistent with clinical audit. Similarly, the policy agenda within the NHS clearly has an impact on perceptions of practice development issues, such as the importance attached to clinical governance and evidence-based practice.

Practice developers increasingly talk of the necessity to adopt a multi-disciplinary focus in their work. The necessity to think beyond the practice of one group and consider the developmental needs of all those whose work has an impact on patient care has been evident in the shift from nursing development units to practice development units (see, for example, Williams et al., 1993). More recently, the Promoting Action for Clinical Effectiveness project (PACE) at the King's Fund supported multidisciplinary teams in addressing clinical issues in ways that sought to promote broad involvement across organisations (Dunning, 1998). Practice development that is concerned with the development of one group alone may be limited in its potential for success. Making a difference to the experience of people receiving healthcare is likely to require work at a range of organisational levels, involving people working within a number of disciplines (McCormack and Wright, 1999). The conceptualisation of practice development occurring at different levels (individual, team and organisational) (McCormack et al., 1999) reflects the need to work at a number of levels to transform the context of care. It could be argued that development work in nursing has, historically, been hampered by its focus on nursing practice alone. Defining practice development as being concerned with the development of the care delivered to patients implies that the practice of all those involved with providing such care should be scrutinised. The notion of 'transforming the culture and context of care' (McCormack and Wright, 1999; McCormack et al., 2002) should be seen as inclusive of all practice that affects patient outcomes.

Systematic Approaches to Practice Development

The dominant trend in the literature is towards the presentation of practice development as systematic in nature. However, it is most usually presented as a systematic process that engages with the 'messy' and context-specific nature of the environment in which practice development takes place (for example, McCormack et al., 2002; Kitson et al., 1996; Cutcliffe et al., 1998; McCormack, 1998).

The importance of systematic approaches to practice development has been identified at a policy level; for example, *A Vision for the Future* (DoH, 1993) sets out the need for clearly specified goals, end points or outcomes and mechanisms for dissemination. Kitson and Currie (1996) surveyed practice development activity in one regional health authority. While acknowledging that informal approaches to developing practice were not without value, Kitson and Currie observed that without a systematic approach being taken there was little prospect of deriving a satisfactory account of how practice development might best be approached.

There are two broad areas of reasoning behind the idea that practice development should be systematic. The first concerns the argument that a systematic approach is more likely to result in a successful outcome (for example, Marsh and MacAlpine, 1995; Vaughan, 1996). The second concerns the credibility of a systematic approach to external observers (for example, Luker, 1997; McMahon, 1998) and the establishment of cost-effectiveness (McCormack et al., 1999). The need to demonstrate the quality and cost-effectiveness of care is central to more recent government policy. It is not surprising, therefore, that clinical governance, as outlined in *A First Class Service* (DoH, 1998b), is recognised as an important consideration within practice development work.

However, practitioners do not readily accept adopting a systematic approach to practice development. For some, change in practice that occurs within a systematic framework differentiates practice development from the kind of attention to improving care that should be part and parcel of clinical practice. However, there is also acceptance of the logic of using systematic approaches. Practice developers accept the adoption of systematic approaches as a strategy for meeting particular aims (funding or other forms of support) as a kind of necessary evil. Being able to account for progress and improvement is one of the principal reasons given for using systematic approaches to practice development. For this reason it can be extremely valuable to find out what systems have been developed to help automate the quality assessment process.

There are two main areas of discomfort, one concerning the extent to which there is a mismatch between the demands of systematic approaches and the 'real world' of practice and another to do with the practical difficulties inherent in systematic approaches. Formal structures are sometimes seen as stifling creativity and innovation rather than encouraging it. In research by Garbett and McCormack (2002a) there was an expressed concern that systematic approaches to practice development risked missing out on work that everyday practitioners valued. Some participants described their work as reactive to issues that were arising in practice, resulting in the perception that formal approaches could hamper their ability to be responsive to the needs of practitioners. It was accepted that an approach to practice development which used no systematic frameworks to gather information could not account for progress. However, systematic approaches were also seen as inadequate for capturing all progress within practice development; for example, 'traditional systematic approaches do not capture all that happens, do not capture shifts in people's horizons when they are part of practice change'. Moreover, for some practitioners the lack of organisational strategic commitment to planning for practice development, as well as limited or non-existent structures to support such work, set up difficulties for systematic work.

The Importance of Facilitation

Kitson et al (1998), considering the conditions that need to be in place in order for evidence-based practice to take place, suggest that the context of implementation and its facilitation are of equal importance to the nature of the evidence itself. They argue that features such as a lack of investment in individuals, poor leadership and lack of performance feedback indicate a context which is unlikely to foster successful change. By contrast, an environment in which people are valued, have a clear sense of what they are doing and have feedback about their performance is a more fertile environment for progress. Such an environment is more likely to be developed where individuals experience respect for their opinions and ideas, feel involved in changes to their work and where development reflects their individual needs rather than in a setting where such qualities are absent (Kitson et al. 1996).

Practice developers adopt a range of facilitative approaches, including getting practitioners to think creatively and more broadly and helping them put their ideas into action. But they also see their facilitative roles as being required at a variety of organisational levels (Garbett and McCormack, 2002b). Participants frequently refer to their roles as being situated 'in the middle', working with practitioners but also with managers at middle and senior levels and increasingly with representatives from other members of the healthcare team and user groups.

Facilitation is associated with more than the successful completion of a single project. It is an activity concerned with the development of individuals in groups in such a way as to help foster greater initiative, self-reliance and motivation (Harvey et al., 2002; Titchen, 1998). The investment is, therefore, not only about achieving the goals of a particular project but also about equipping people with experience, skills and knowledge (Thomas and Ingham, 1995). Facilitation requires a range of qualities, skills and abilities; for example Titchen (1998) identifies openness, supportiveness, approachability, reliability, self-confidence and the ability to think laterally and non-judgementally in a model derived from work in an acute medical unit called critical companionship. A fuller discussion of facilitation can be found in Harvey et al. (2002). See Chapter 14 for more information about facilitation.

The Consequences of Practice Development

The consequences of practice development can be seen as concerned as much with process outcomes as they are with more traditional forms of clinical outcome.

The primary purpose of practice development is increased effectiveness in patient-centred care. Logically it can therefore be argued that a consequence of practice development should be to reflect that purpose. It is, however, difficult always clearly to demonstrate that impact. The complexity of organisations within which practice development takes place means that unambiguous cause-and-effect relationships cannot always be inferred with confidence. As has been discussed above, the pace and scope of change within the health service implies the need to help practitioners become more flexible and responsive in order to be able to adapt to and assimilate change. These are the intended outcomes of the approaches talked about in the practice development literature by practice developers themselves and attested to by practitioners. Adopting a facilitative approach also implies helping practitioners to identify organisational factors that impede progress and helping them find ways around such barriers. Another consequence of practice development can therefore be construed as being concerned with promoting awareness of the impact of organisations on practice.

The consequences associated with practice development are clearly congruent with the clinical governance agenda within the NHS at the present time. Clinical governance has been established to address the need to identify the activities involved in delivering high-quality care to patients (DoH, 1998a). Within clinical governance the need to recognise the contextual and situated nature of such a project is acknowledged. Practice development approaches explicitly address these concerns.

The Government's NHS Plan (DoH, 2000) has placed firmly the experience of the patient at the top of professionals' agendas. Being responsive to people's experiences of health services lies at the heart of recommendations for both day-to-day activity and strategic planning. This message is reinforced by the recommendations of the public inquiry into children's heart surgery at the Bristol Royal Infirmary (DoH, 2001).

Practice development is an activity concerned with achieving increased effectiveness in providing care that is centred on patients' needs. This is echoed by Unsworth (2000), who carried out a concept analysis of practice development, and Gerrish (2001), in an evaluation of nursing/practice development units. Both authors also refer to the need to sustain effective clinical practice as well as bring about innovations, reflecting a concern of practice developers in Garbett and McCormack's (2002b) research.

The integration of learning, practice and knowledge development (or research) in practice development strategies can be seen in Manley's work on a London intensive care unit (see, for example, Manley, 2000). Manley employed practice development strategies within an action research framework to develop a consultant nurse role over a period of some twelve years. Her analysis of the outcomes of this work demonstrates the impact of her work on the culture of the unit and organisation in which she was working. Evaluative data drawn from a range of stakeholders in the project supported the claim that values and beliefs developed by the team were demonstrated in practice, for example patient-centredness and openness to change. Manley (2000) argues that two processes were central to bringing about and sustaining cultural shifts: first, clarifying the values and beliefs of team members about their own roles and that of the unit; secondly, highlighting the contradictions between espoused values and practice. In addition Manley argues, drawing on literature about successful cultures in commerce and health services, that organisational values such as participation, devolution, promoting accountability and leadership at all levels of the organisation, and supporting learning and adaptability are vital in sustaining effective workplace cultures.

There are clear areas of congruity between work being undertaken by practice developers and the kinds of practice being promoted in national healthcare policy. England's Chief Nursing Officer launched a publication in the wake of the NHS Plan (Mullally, 2001) that emphasises the importance of learning from practice, being responsive to patients and developing adaptability to change. Staff working in the many and varied practice development roles across the UK are clearly central to the wholesale cultural shift that is being demanded of the NHS.

Practice Development, Quality and Audit

Quality within the health service was, until the late 1970s, never openly addressed. Nursing practice focused on tasks until models of nursing were introduced but, even so, the task-based approach to nursing was never far removed. Quality conjures up a plethora of terms such as excellence, standards, best in class, and superior (to other services). However, it is important to consider the value of a service to the customer. Often healthcare professionals have looked at the outcome and forgotten about the process; for patients the outcome is less of an issue but the process is very important, something that is at the heart of practice development. Their experience of care will formulate their opinion of the type of service provided. This concept has been a difficult one for some in the health service to grasp, just as the idea of a patient being a customer has seemed ludicrous to others. However, the gradual cultural changes throughout the last 25 years have tried to make quality an explicit issue. Changes such as commissioning, the formal introduction of audit and accreditation processes are all very real examples of the drive to make quality a more important aspect of patient care and experiences.

This has required healthcare professionals such as nurses to develop an enquiring mind into the standards and processes of the service they deliver. In many organisations audit was initially medically focused, few were trained in the process and a full understanding of this as a cyclic process was, therefore, not always reflected. The very essence of practice development is, as already stated, about transforming contexts and cultures of care. This cannot be achieved without an enquiring mind, a patient-centred approach and a belief in the fundamentals of care. The most recent of government initiatives – clinical and social care governance and the Essence of Care benchmark standards, bring quality improvement into sharp focus. It brings control and it reawakens fundamentals of care but there is a danger that once again fragmentation will occur unless through informing practice we develop and move forward the culture of patient-centredness. (Donaldson and Gray, 1998)

Over the years a number of quality assessment tools have been developed to assist with the audit process. These range from the Royal College of Nursing's Dynamic Standard Setting System to Len Goldstone's Monitor Series, amongst others. However, as previously discussed, practice development is an activity aimed at increasing effectiveness in providing care that is centred on patients' needs (Garbett and McCormack, 2002a). It is, therefore, more than audit but needs to encompass the benefits that can be delivered by the objective view that a comprehensive audit programme offers. Nursing audit can be seen as part of a cycle of quality assurance involving the systematic and critical analysis of the planning, delivery and evaluation of nursing and midwifery services. Issues such as the use of resources, quality of care delivered, service outcomes and patient outcomes have been the major foci of audit analysis. The dominant focus was on efficiency and effectiveness. Nursing care audit is a system which allows nurses to measure their performance, recognise good care practice and, if necessary, make changes.

Engaging Front-Line Staff

Engaging front-line staff, from all disciplines, not just nursing, is absolutely crucial to delivering the change in practice that can come about from a thorough, comprehensive and consistently implemented audit programme.

Quality development work, when executed via such an audit programme, is much more rewarding and positive than is often realised. In particular, it can empower teams to make great strides toward quality, and it can energise colleagues' work as it removes inefficiencies, improves processes, decreases frustration and boosts satisfaction (American Academy of Family Physicians, 1999). It can bring about substantial, lasting, positive change in practice. It all begins with front-line staff identifying the opportunities and routes to success and recognising that without local ownership change will not be sustainable.

Currently, clinical and social care governance clearly lays down organisations' statutory duties of quality. So how do we transform the culture of care that ensures the delivery of patient-centredness, that is not just about nursing but about multiprofessional practice development? Cultural change can only come about when the patient is the central focus. Healthcare professionals must embrace the role that patients play in shaping their care, something that is key to the approach proposed by Garbett and McCormack (2002a).

Mahatma Gandhi wrote, 'Customers (patients) are the most important visitors on our premises ... They are not an interruption of our work – they are the purpose of it ... They are not an outsider of our business – they are part of it.' His words are more valuable today than ever before. Once health professionals recognise and acknowledge this fundamental principle, the first movement towards culture change is achievable.

A systematic approach, therefore, to the monitoring of the statutory duty for quality is necessary to deliver consistent patient care. The great benefit of taking such a systematic approach, and one that is often overlooked, is that problems are unearthed before they impinge on patient wellbeing, something that the complaints department will certainly appreciate, and something that the modern health service should make the highest of priorities. Such a systematic approach will also make sense of the wealth of quality initiatives, accreditations and reporting mechanisms that flow these days from the Department of Health and other related bodies at such an astounding rate.

There are various options for tackling how best to implement such an approach and it is most important that new technologies and IT systems are given due consideration and that time is taken for a thorough assessment. The reader should recognise the need to create the systematic approach that is being discussed and consider all the options available.

Informing practice development comes from a soundly based, systematic approach to nursing and midwifery audit, professional development and enquiring research. This can best be achieved through an organisation-wide initiative for developing practice and its facilitation. The consequence of practice development and quality being driven in this way is the increased sharing of good practice. A 'getting it right first time' culture can only influence the practice of other health professionals and the future outcomes expected.

Contributed by Brendan McCormack, Director of Nursing Research and Helen Chambers, Quality Manager of a PDU, at the Royal Hospitals Trust in Belfast.

Continuing Professional Development

To ensure that a trust or a healthcare organisation and their staff deliver good-quality care, they must have well-developed knowledge, skills and competencies. To keep staff up to date and maintain their skills at an acceptable level, there must be systems that support lifelong learning and ongoing continuing professional development (CPD). The Department of Health (DoH, 1998a) defines CPD as: 'A process of lifelong learning for all individuals and teams which meets the needs of patients and delivers the health outcomes and healthcare priorities of the NHS and which enables professionals to expand and fulfil their potential.'

Doctors, nurses, therapists and all other clinicians are responsible and accountable for their clinical practice and must ensure that their practice is current, evidenced-based best practice. The responsibility for CPD is theirs but the trust or organisation has a responsibility for ensuring that there is a system of annual appraisal for all clinical staff.

The CPD cycle has four stages:

- an assessment of the individual's and the organisation's needs
- the compiling of personal development plans (PDPs)
- implementation and dissemination
- an evaluation of the CPD process and its benefit to the individual and to patient care.

An annual appraisal is a review undertaken by the manager with the employee who reviews the year's progress against agreed objectives. In an NHS trust all staff are part of an appraisal system which includes the chairman and the non-executive directors.

Personal development plans (PDPs) are linked to the individual's annual appraisal and a SWOT analysis identifies his/her strengths, weaknesses, opportunities and threats to his/her performance or achievement of objectives. These are discussed, a personal development plan is worked out for the following twelve months and review dates are agreed. In primary care the practice professional development plan (PPDP) addresses the learning needs of the whole practice and all the staff within the practice based on an identified service development plan, local and national objectives, and identified educational needs, all of which feed into the practice strategy. All health service staff were expected to have a PDP by April 2000. The PDP must be a comprehensive document that records the outcome of appraisal, a summary of educational needs and discussion with the appraiser about how these needs will be met, and the dates agreed and set for the completion of the PDP.

To ensure that patients only receive care from appropriately qualified staff, the trust or organisation has a responsibility to check the registration details of all staff employed, including locums and bank staff. It is the responsibility of the professional to keep a portfolio of evidence with which to maintain their registration.

Reviewing Practice

There are a variety of ways of discussing and reviewing practice, for example:

- reflective diaries, journals and profiles
- small-group case discussions
- critical-incident analysis
- random case analysis
- clinical supervision
- research and development.

Reflective Practice and Critical-Incident Analysis

Reflective practice encourages self-awareness and addresses both case-specific errors and generic error weaknesses. It is a valuable approach to reviewing care given to patients and an essential part of a system of clinical governance.

Significant events can be medical, clinical, managerial, administrative or any combination of these and are those:

- in which intervention really made a difference to patient outcome, either directly or indirectly
- which did not go as planned or anticipated
- that are really very ordinary, typical or routine
- that are particularly demanding or satisfying
- that were unusual, interesting or unexpected.

Critical incidents are those:

- deemed as serious incidents
- which are formally reported, for example reporting systems for adverse incidents
- which will often have action plans associated with them.

An ongoing review of significant events and critical incidents is part of the process of learning from mistakes and making changes to improve practice.

Clinical Supervision

Clinical supervision is an exchange between practising professionals to enable the development of professional skills. A system of clinical supervision offers a framework for staff to discuss the quality of care delivered to patients and to identify education and training needs to support staff in improving their clinical skills and competence as part of continuous quality improvement.

Poor Performance

When discussing poor performance it is important to recognise that the majority of NHS staff deliver a more than satisfactory standard of care and that it is a small minority who can be said to be poor performers. The Chief Medical Officer (1995) set out a requirement for health organisations to put in place procedures to identify and deal with performance issues early rather than later in order to prevent harm to patients. This document was the basis of a procedure set out by the British Association for Medical Managers and was sent to all medical directors. One of the roles of the clinical governance committee is to follow up early signs of poor performance gathered through reports on complaints, accidents, incidents, near misses, morbidity, and so on to avoid repeated untoward incidents and protect patients from harm. See also Chapter 4.

Research and Development

Research and development is an integral part of clinical governance and the research and development agenda is closely linked to clinical audit, clinical risk and the development of service standards, education and training. Evidence-based practice is research in action and is discussed in Chapter 8. To promote evidence-based practice there must be a system that supports staff in accessing, implementing, monitoring, supporting, supervising and disseminating research findings.

Conclusion

Although clinical staff have always kept themselves up to date through courses, journals, conferences and so on, under clinical governance there must be a systematic approach to ensure that all staff are offered professional development programmes which reflect the principles of clinical governance. Trusts and organisations must ensure that all staff are appraised and set objectives for the year to come which will be reviewed and evaluated.

Clinical staff need to reflect on their practice, and identify what went well and not so well, in order constantly to improve their practice. The organisation has a responsibility to provide the resources to support education, training and continuing personal and professional development.

Making It Happen

Education, Training and Continuing Personal and Professional Development

The trust will need to:

- put organisational structures in place to support education, training and CPD issues
- establish links between training, CPD programmes, quality improvement programmes and individual PDPs
- establish partnerships with educational establishments, and joint training programmes with partners including other health organisations, social services, and so on
- ensure there are budgets to support professional development, education and training
- ensure that mandatory training is in place
- ensure that work-based training schemes are in place and that there are schemes for obtaining relevant professional or further qualifications
- ensure time, financial and other support for staff undergoing formal education and for individual CPD activities.

Pillar Six – Clinical Effectiveness

8

Chapter Contents:

- clinical effectiveness
- critical appraisal
- clinical guidelines
- evidence-based practice
- integrated care pathways
- good practice ideas and innovations.

Key elements of this include:

- evidence-based practice is in day-to-day use with the infrastructure to support it
- good practice, ideas and innovations, which have been evaluated, are systematically disseminated within and outside the organisation.

Clinical effectiveness is the degree to which the organisation is ensuring that 'best practice', based on evidence of effectiveness where such evidence exists, is used. The Department of Health (DoH, 1996b) defined clinical effectiveness as 'the extent to which specific interventions, when deployed in the field for a particular patient or population, do what they are intended to do, for example, maintain and improve health and secure the greatest possible health gain from available sources'. Professor Alison Kitson at a conference in London in 1995 on 'Clinical Effectiveness from Guidelines to Cost Effective Practice' described clinical effectiveness more poignantly as 'doing the right thing' and 'doing the thing right'. She went on to say, 'The former requirement relates to the effective utilisation of research through mechanisms such as clinical guidelines, which are rigorously developed. The latter requirement relates to how such information is implemented.'

The concept of clinical effectiveness is that healthcare treatments should be clinically effective and cost-effective, supported by a well-researched evidence base. The Royal College of Nursing (RCN, 1995) outlined the main elements of clinical effectiveness as the:

- production of evidence through research and scientific review
- production and dissemination of evidence-based clinical guidelines

■ implementation of evidence-based, cost-effective practice through education and change management
■ evaluation of compliance to agreed practice guidance and evaluation of patient outcomes, including clinical audit.

Cost-Effectiveness

Cost-effectiveness is only one of a number of criteria that should be applied to purchasing decisions, which should include equity, needs and priorities. A cost-effectiveness analysis will compare the costs and health effects of an intervention or treatment to establish whether or not it is worth using in terms of an economic perspective.

Critical Appraisal

Critical appraisal is an essential part of the delivery of clinically effective care. It is the skills needed to establish which research will result in effective clinical care for patients in the care of professionals within their own hospital or trust. Today trusts and healthcare organisations support staff with in-house education and development to help staff critically appraise research. Hill and Spittlehouse (2001) define critical appraisal as:

■ the process of systematically examining research evidence to assess its validity, results and relevance before using it to inform a decision
■ an essential part of evidence-based clinical practice that includes the process of systematically finding, appraising and acting on evidence of effectiveness
■ that which allows clinicians to make sense of research evidence and begin to close the gap between research and practice.

The work of Crombie (1997), Sackett et al. (1997) and Swage (1998) suggests that it is possible to break down the process of critical appraisal into some simple points that summarise what critical appraisal is all about:

■ considering the relevance of a research question
■ evaluating the evidence to answer the question
■ assessing the relevance of the conclusion and the recommendations for practice
■ reviewing the research through the stages that make up the process of research which include the title, abstract, introduction, literature review, methods, results, discussions and recommendations.

Then consider the following questions (Crombie, 1997):

- is the research of interest?
- why was it done?
- how was it performed?
- what did it show?
- what are the possible implications for practice?
- is the research for information only or can it be used to support practice?

Clinical Guidelines

The work on guidelines has been developed since the publication of the Department of Health document, *Clinical Guidelines: Using Clinical Guidelines to Improve Patient Care within the NHS* (DoH, 1996). Clinical guidelines are systematically developed statements to assist practitioner and patient decisions about appropriate health care for specific clinical circumstances. The key words here are 'assist decision making', as guidelines do not replace the decision-making processes concerning individual clinicians and patients. The definition of local clinical guidelines or protocols is that they are locally adapted versions of the broad statement of good practice contained in national guidelines. They include more operational detail (RCN, 1995).

Clinical guidelines have been identified as the approach to promoting good clinical practice since 1993 (DoH, 1993). It is important that patients receive care that is clinically proven to be both sound and cost-effective. To ensure that this is the case, the Government has introduced the National Institute for Clinical Effectiveness (NICE) and National Service Frameworks (NSFs), to establish national standards. See Chapter 1 for more information. Trusts and healthcare organisations are expected to ensure that the clinical teams have access to available evidence on which to base their practice and have a good understanding of research and development (R&D). The R&D activity is linked to clinical risk management, clinical audit and the development of standards and education and training to ensure good quality outcomes for patients.

Since 1999 for major areas of care and disease groups, NICE has produced and disseminated clinical guidelines based on relevant evidence of clinical and cost-effectiveness. See Chapter 1 for more information.

As well as NICE, other organisations also develop clinical guidelines. Some examples include:

- the Medical Royal Colleges
- the NHS Management Executive
- academic institutions
- the Royal College of Nursing

- the Royal College of Midwives
- the National Institute for Nursing, Oxford
- the professional organisations representing professions allied to medicine
- patient representatives' organisations.

Developing local clinical guidelines is very time-consuming and requires a lot of skilled research to ensure that they are accurate and evidence-based. There are very probably national guidelines that have been developed which could be adapted to meet local requirements. However, if there are no national guidelines for the particular area of care then the following ten steps to implementation, adapted from those developed by the Royal College of Nursing (RCN, 1995) demonstrate a well-structured approach which include guideline development, spreading the information, implementation, evaluation and review (see Figure 8.1):

Step one:
- decide on the subject to address
- set up a group to develop a strategy

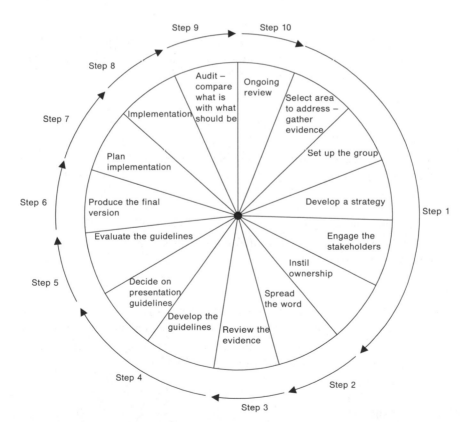

Figure 8.1 Clinical guidelines – implementation

- involve other members of the multidisciplinary team as well as management and patient/client representatives
- ensure the backing of the key players
- instil a sense of ownership of the guidelines among those who will be using them. Otherwise, no matter how good your guidelines are, they will not be successfully implemented.

Step two:
- spread the word among all those who will be affected
- explain how the change will benefit patient care
- use meetings, conferences, publications and any other means of raising awareness.

Step three:
- review the evidence
- when developing guidelines or adapting national guidelines to suit local conditions it is important to take account of any other quality improvement initiatives – don't work in isolation.

Step four:
- decide in what form to present the guidelines, for example a booklet, a computer program, a poster or a quick reference pocket-card. Be clear who the target audience is and how best to reach them
- develop the guidelines.

Step five:
- evaluate the guidelines
- check the guidelines using a reliable evaluation tool and make any necessary adjustments.

Step six:
- produce the final version
- brief staff on the final version of the guidelines and set a date when the changes come into effect.

Step seven:
- devise a plan for implementing the changes assigning responsibility for various actions. Support staff carrying out the changes in every way possible – offer incentives, use 'opinion leaders' among the staff to get the message across and get feedback on how things are going.

Step eight:
- carry out the plan
- reinforce the message. Remind people what it is all about.

Step nine:
■ carry out an audit comparing the outcome with what was happening before.

Step ten:
■ take action to ensure improvements are maintained by periodic review of the guidelines.

There is potential for developing local guidelines in areas:

■ where guidelines have been developed nationally and are available for adaptation, for example asthma, diabetes, head injury, management of leg ulcers, cancer, hospital infection
■ of high volume, high risk, high cost
■ where there are variations in practice with potential to improve.

Benefits of Clinical Guidelines

■ they support the provision of a high level of standardised health care
■ they reduce unacceptable or undesirable variations in clinical practice
■ they provide a basis for clinical audit
■ they offer a way of implementing research findings
■ they provide a means of ensuring research-based practice
■ they facilitate agreement between professionals about treatment
■ they offer an interface between purchasers and providers that will establish cost-effective practice
■ they help the purchasers of care to make informed choices
■ they give managers useful data for establishing treatment costs.

Clinical Guidelines – Issues

■ the adoption of clinical guidelines, which reflect evidence-based practice, will improve safety and quality but does not limit good professional judgement which is always required when there are multiple disease processes which occur simultaneously
■ they make clinical staff justify their reasons for not keeping to the guidelines
■ they provide a framework for clinical staff to structure their decisions and should support rather than direct care
■ the development of evidence-based guidelines should be at a national level to ensure the most effective use of resources and prevent duplication of effort

■ it is essential to have local consensus for the implementation of guidelines by translating them into operational clinical protocols or pathways for use in a trust or healthcare organisation.

Problems with Clinical Guidelines

■ they are expensive to develop
■ there is not always clear evidence of best practice
■ there are medico-legal problems – guidelines may well be disclosed in legal proceedings where there is an alleged medical negligence. The plaintiff may attempt to demonstrate that guidelines were available but not followed by the clinical staff, in which case the hospital would be in the position of having to justify not following the guidelines in the best interests of a particular patient. The completion of comprehensive documentation of a variance from the guidelines is, therefore, vital, not only for medico-legal purposes but also for clinical audit
■ the guidelines need to be well implemented. The plans for implementation need to start at a very early stage to ensure that the key players are on board, that clinical staff are clear about the benefits for the patient and they are involved in the process, resulting in ownership of the guidelines. If this is not the case, then the guidelines will not be used, which will jeopardise the continuity and quality of care
■ there needs to be multidisciplinary collaboration. The collaborative and multidisciplinary content of the group that develops and/or adapts local guidelines is vital to the success of the development and implementation of the guidelines. Poor multidisciplinary teamworking will need to be addressed through the process of developing or adapting guidelines. If well facilitated, it can strengthen multidisciplinary teamworking through discussion about the care that is given by the professionals involved and the expected outcomes for the patient.

Summary of Clinical Guidelines

If clinical guidelines are to work, then in some instances it will be essential to change the culture to one of 'lifelong learners' with a willingness to learn. To support this, trusts must invest in equipping professionals with the skills to access and critically appraise information and evidence, and provide an environment that encourages and responds to learning. Grimshaw and Russell (1993), in their discussion of guideline development, argue that clinical guidelines must be scientifically valid, based on the best available scientific evidence and worthwhile.

Clinical guidelines provide an important route to promoting evidence-based practice and the basis for systematic audit. They are multidisciplinary, evidence-based, focused on service priorities and reflect patient interests. In summary clinical guidelines must be:

- valid
- reliable
- reproducible
- clinically applicable
- clinically flexible
- clear
- multidisciplinary
- regularly reviewed
- well-documented.

Ultimately guidelines should be shared with the patients and their families so that they are able to make informed choices about care options. Later in this chapter the development of integrated care pathways demonstrates how guidelines support the delivery of evidence-based practice as part of a pathway for specific areas of care.

Evidence-based Practice as the Basis for Patient Care

Since the early 1990s there has been a growing interest in using the results of research to improve patient care. Over the last decade this work has been advanced under a variety of titles including clinical audit, clinical effectiveness, implementation of research and evidence-based practice.

Evidence-based practice is defined by Long and Harrison (1996) as 'the process of systematically finding and using contemporaneous research findings as the basis for clinical decision-making'. Evidence-based practice is an essential part of clinical governance which requires the trust or healthcare organisation and staff to use the principles of evidence-based practice to support good-quality outcomes for patients and service users. As Belsey and Snell (2001) suggest, evidence-based medicine forms part of the multifaceted process of assuring clinical effectiveness the main elements are:

- the production of evidence through research and scientific review
- the production and dissemination of evidence-based clinical guidelines
- the implementation of evidence-based, cost-effective practice through education and management changes
- the evaluation of compliance with agreed practice and patient outcomes this process includes clinical audit.

Implementing Evidence-based Practice

Sackett et al. (1997) advise that there are four stages to implementing evidence-based practice, as set out in Figure 8.2, which are as follows:

■ identifying the problem
■ finding the answers through literature search and critical appraisal
■ implementing the changes
■ evaluating the changes.

In order that evidence-based practice becomes part of the culture of the multidisciplinary team, it is important that the environment of the organisation be one that supports and nurtures evidence-based practice. As stated earlier in this chapter, in the section about clinical guidelines, it is about the provision of access to information and research; the provision of training and development to acquire or develop skills such as critical appraisal, searching the literature and evaluating the research.

Searching through the library, the journals or one of the organisations listed at the end of this chapter may be fairly straightforward. Once the research has been done, then evaluating it can be the first major stumbling block. Evidence-based practice requires the practitioner critically to appraise and review the

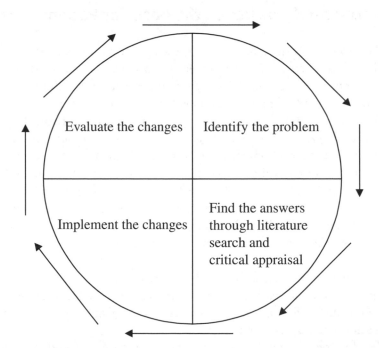

Figure 8.2 The four stages to implementing evidence-based practice

research to establish if the findings were valid in the setting in which they were conducted and, more importantly, if they could be applied in the chosen clinical setting. If the answer to this fundamental question is 'no', then move on to the next piece of research. If the answer is 'yes', then the next step is to establish if the approach used was comprehensive, if there were sufficient data, and so on. From the work developed by Milne and Chambers (1993) some key questions emerge:

- are the literature search strategies explicitly designed and stated?
- is the search strategy comprehensive?
- is the issue of publication bias addressed?
- are the methodologies of the individual studies appropriately reviewed?
- is sufficient data given on the individual studies, (patients, diagnoses, therapies and outcomes)?
- if a quantitative overview is provided, is such an overview justifiable, given possible sources of heterogeneity (not of the same type)?
- are appropriate conclusions drawn for treatment recommendations (beneficial, equivocal, harmful) and for future research?

Having successfully completed this process then research findings may be incorporated into practice through clinical guidelines and integrated care pathways and evaluated though clinical audit to establish if expected outcomes were achieved.

Benefits of Evidence-Based Practice

- there is a greater understanding of the area of care/practice
- practice is evidence-based
- it is cost-effective
- it leads to improved quality of care
- it leads to standardised care
- it allows ongoing monitoring of the quality of care
- it reduces unacceptable or undesirable variations in clinical practice
- it facilitates agreement between professionals about treatment
- it offers an interface between purchasers and providers that will establish cost-effective practice
- it helps the purchasers of care to make informed choices
- it leads to a desire to learn more about research and a commitment to evidence-based practice.

Bassett (1993), McSherry (1997) and May et al. (1998) state that there is a vast amount of information in the academic journals which suggests that the theory–practice gap continues to widen. If this is the case, then professionals need to address the issues if they are to meet the standards set by the Government and the Healthcare Commission (previously known as the CHAI).

Problems Implementing Evidence-Based Practice

- lack of commitment. The implementation of the Culyer Report (DoH, 1996b) recommendations challenges trust managers to nurture a climate that supports research and development initiatives. There must be organisational commitment and leadership if research and development is to become part of the normal day-to-day business of the trusts
- lack of evidence. The amount of evidence available to some professions, including nursing, is often small and not always reliable or valid. Work undertaken by Appleby, Walshe and Ham (1995) established that more than 70 per cent of available information related to acute care treatments and these were dominated by pharmaceutical interventions. They also established that 79 per cent of the activities related to the medical profession and only 15 per cent concerned nursing
- lack of dissemination of the findings of research
- lack of knowledge about the NHS Research and Development strategy
- lack of training in research skills for both managers and clinicians
- lack of support in gaining these skills
- time constraints
- activity additional to an already heavy workload
- lack of multidisciplinary team working
- lack of knowledge and experience
- problems in making changes in the light of research.

Once evidence-based care has been implemented, it is important that the outcomes be evaluated through systems of clinical audit, benchmarking, and so on.

Integrated Care Pathways

Integrated care pathways (ICPs) are a vehicle for turning the concept of clinical governance into reality and incorporate many of the elements of clinical governance. A care pathway is the route to delivering evidence-based practice as part of everyday patient care. They are not packages of care that are taken 'off the shelf' but are developed by a multidisciplinary team focused on the delivery of a particular aspect of care such as an ICP for stroke patients which could cover the patient's care while in an acute hospital and also on transfer to the community for continuing rehabilitation. This process of development of an ICP leads to involvement in the process and ownership of the pathway.

ICPs — Their Origins

Berwick (1989) wrote about an approach to quality improvement that is not just about dealing with the problems and deficiencies in health care but is rather about finding systems that work better, which allow readjustments and continuous improvement to take place. ICPs have been in use in the USA since the late 1980s where they were also known as anticipated recovery paths and critical pathways. The pathway is part of the US system of managed care. Kongstevedt (1995) defines managed care as 'a system of care delivery that manages the costs, the quality and the access to welfare services'.

Managed care in the USA was developed in response to high hospital costs, an ever-increasing number of new hospitals and a system of reimbursing hospitals for the care provided for patients on a 'dollar-for-dollar ' basis. The care was paid for whether or not it was necessary and there were more and more patients without insurance or the means to pay for their care. The US government then changed the system to one that reimbursed the hospitals according to diagnostic related groups (DRGs). This meant that a single fee was paid for the patient based on a diagnosis and not on how long the care continued, what care the patient received or how many tests were required. The hospitals responded by making sure that the care was managed, resources were managed, in-patient stays were as short as possible and patients received the care and tests that they needed to provide and support a good standard of care. The ICP is part of this process of managing care. The pathway informs the hospital about the resources, tests and treatments that are necessary for a specific episode of care. The written criteria in the pathway are all evidence-based and ensure that the care is organised, co-ordinated and can be tracked, monitored and costed. It is interesting to note that a computerised nursing system called Excelcare was implemented in a group of wards in an acute trust in West Dorset in the late 1980s. The system was designed on these principles and allowed the nurses to print out the care pathway for a patient and evaluate the care against pre-set outcomes on an ongoing basis. This pathway also identified the staff skills required to deliver the care to the required standard and had the capability to be developed into a system for managing care using multidisciplinary integrated care pathways. On a daily basis, or more fre-quently as required, Excelcare produced an ICP for a specific diagnosis or problem, which was evidenced-based, and each element of care had been timed, assigned an appropriate skill level and validated against pre-set outcomes.

At the end of each 24-hour period Excelcare generated reports that included:

- the number and skill-mix of staff required for the patients
- the variance against the actual number and skill-mix on duty that shift/day
- the outcomes against which to monitor the patients' care
- the variance of actual to desired outcome
- the cost of care.

The main problems associated with Excelcare were:

- the large amount of paper generated through the printing of updated care plans on a shift-by-shift basis
- the time spent at the computer, which was at the nurses' station, to the detriment of time spent with patients
- the belief that patient care could not be individualised if every patient with the same diagnosis used the same care pathway
- the storage of data and the time required to track and analyse data generated by the system as part of continuous quality improvement.

Today many of these problems would be easily rectified with advances in technology, hand-held terminals, scanners, increased computer literacy and changes in attitude to the concept of managed care and multidisciplinary record-keeping. In fact, a system a few years ahead of its time would have been an ideal clinical governance tool.

What is an ICP?

Essentially a pathway is intended as collaborative guidelines which time and sequence the major interventions of doctors, nurses and other key professionals and services for a particular case type or condition. An ICP represents specific practice patterns, patient populations and limits on length of stay. Included in a co-ordinated sequence of events, in the form of guidelines, are the assessments, investigations and interventions that should occur to achieve the desired outcome.

According to the National Pathways Association newsletter of 1988: 'An integrated care pathway determines locally agreed multidisciplinary practice, based on guidelines and evidence where available, for a specific patient/client group. It forms all or part of the clinical record, documents the care given and facilitates the evaluation of outcomes for continuous quality improvement.'

A care pathway sets out the care that should be given to the patient by all professionals and services involved in his/her episode of care (Zander and McGill, 1994). The care is described, tracked and monitored to ensure that outcomes set along the pathway and the final outcomes are achieved. Tracking the care follows the patient-care journey from wherever it may start, for example home, GP, acute hospital, community hospital and then back home. If at any point the pathway is not followed then the person delivering that particular aspect of care records the reason for the deviation from the pathway as a variance. Analysis of the variance provides a system for ongoing monitoring of the quality of care and the pathway. Part of the ongoing review of the pathway is the analysis of the variances which may lead to changes being made in the pathway.

Care pathways are developed from evidence-based guidelines and are therefore a vehicle for implementing evidence-based practice into everyday patient care. The pathway is developed into a multidisciplinary record of care, which is used by every professional to record and evaluate care given. Pathways are not only multidisciplinary but may also include multi-agency collaboration.

In summary an ICP:

- is a daily plan of care
- identifies anticipated progress based on guidelines, protocols and evidence
- incorporates risk management
- facilitates the evaluation of goals and outcomes by the professionals who deliver the care
- requires deviations from the pathway to be recorded as variances. The analysis of the variances results in ongoing monitoring of the quality of care
- is a multidisciplinary plan of care
- is a legal record
- presents a format that helps patients have a better understanding of their care and encourages greater patient involvement and informed decision making
- reduces paperwork and improves the accuracy of record-keeping by all the multidisciplinary team.

An ICP Cycle

The approach to implementing an ICP is a cycle, which is set out in Figure 8.3.

Five Steps to Implementing an Integrated Care Pathway

Step one – Select an area in which to develop a care pathway:
Get the multidisciplinary team together, review current practice and decide on a suitable area for a pathway. The following points may contribute to the selection process:

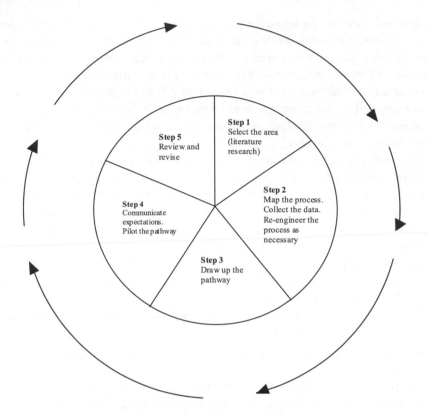

Figure 8.3 Implementing an integrated care pathway

- a high-volume area, for example if the area of speciality is orthopaedics then a high-volume area might be first-time hip replacements
- a high-risk area such as the urgent referral of a patient with a breast lump and the need for early referral, diagnosis and treatment
- an area of high cost as a result of an extended length of stay
- an area of care where an enthusiastic leader will help to progress the process of developing care pathways
- an enthusiastic consultant/opinion leader
- a problem identified through a complaint or an area where professionals believe that a pathway would improve the quality of care by reducing duplication of care between professionals.

Step two – Map the process of care:
- agree the area to be mapped, set the boundaries around the episode of care
- gain the support of 'Directors' and Senior Clinicians for the process
- gather the scientific literature through the clinical journals, the Internet, the National Pathway Association, the Regional Care Pathway groups and so

on. Gather together any pathways that have already been developed for your chosen topic. Review the evidence

- meet with a selection of representative staff to talk through the process and define and agree objectives and goals. Trust staff with a quality assurance background or staff from the education or training department often help by facilitating these meetings
- choose the team to drive the process – include all disciplines
- decide who in the team will see the process through, who will drive the process, agree and meet deadlines, and so on
- identify and map current practice either by talking through the process using group discussion or brainstorming (see Chapter 16 for information on brainstorming) or by direct observation and mapping the process
- process mapping is about following the patient's care journey from its start to the end. This can either be achieved by group discussion or by direct observations, either way every aspect of the care journey must be mapped a bit like a road map, noting names, places and road numbers on the way to the final destination. In my experience the simplest way to do this is to observe the process of the care journey and note each step of the way on a separate 'post-it'. Then stick the 'post-its' on a wall or a board in the order that the care actually happened. The observers note only what they see and hear and do not make decisions about what should or should not have happened.

Once the process of the patient's care journey has been mapped, then it should be compared with what should be, based on sound, proven evidence (see Figure 8.4). The processes can then be discussed and changes made to improve the patient's care journey, for example by reducing the length of stay or rehabilitating home quicker, and so on.

Process mapping is an effective way of establishing what really happens and not what people think is happening. Experience shows that groups that used process mapping were able to:

- improve the patient's care journey
- reduce the length of stay
- identify activities that did not contribute to care
- identify those that were repetitious
- identify those that were of no real benefit
- identify those that were duplicated by others, often from different professions.

The role of the team who undertake the process mapping is to give feedback to the area where mapping has occurred and to challenge practice so that it can be discussed and compared with the reviewed evidence. This will start the process

DAY SURGERY ENDOSCOPY – ADMISSION

Process map of current practice	Issues for consideration based on research findings and good practice
Patients arrive in unit - some have the same admission time, some are staggered	• To have better control and planning of lists to enable all patients to have a staggered admission time • Health Questionnaires to be sent with admission letter and detailed information regarding sedation or cord spraying *Pre Endoscopy Questionnaire - Form 1, Mobile Gastroscopy Service, Exeter & District Community Health Service NHS-Trust (considered good practice)*
↓	
Patients are met by Ward Clerk or Recovery Nurse – who arranges a collection time with relative or friend	• Use of Videos to inform patient about the procedure to be undertaken • To produce a pathway for Endoscopy patients to ensure that each patient receives the same standard of care
↓	
Some patients are asked to wait in Day Room whilst others are shown to trolley area	• Consider a named nurse for each patient to build relationships during short stay *Panting A. (1998). Preparing Patients for Endoscopy. Nursing Times; 94:27,60.*
↓	
Ward Clerk checks details for PAS	
↓	• Send a consent form with patient to enable informed consent to be obtained after explanation by a 'Knowledgeable Practitioner' *Alexander, J. (1997). Types of consent and the means of obtaining consent. Clinical Risk **Management** in Day Surgery. IBC UK Conferences Ltd.*
Patient's admission details taken by Nurse	• Obtain consent if not carried out in OPD • Ensure that patient is fully informed to reduce stress and that the information given is current, researched and looks good *Murphy, D. (1993). Managing Patient Stress in Endoscopy. Society of Gastoenterology Nurse and Associates.*
↓	
Procedure explained to patient by theatre nurse Patient asked to decide whether they wish to have sedation or cord spray Patients for sigmoidoscopy have an enema in the trolley room* Patient informed of approximate time into theatre	• Consider greater privacy especially for those having an enema • Surgeon to consent patients in a quiet area • Walk patients to theatre
↓	
Patient prepared for theatre and taken to theatre on trolley	

* Trolley room is a small room with eight trolley spaces

Figure 8.4 Process-mapping
Source: Sale, 1998

of change management and lead to a consensus on the agreed way forward. Once the process has been mapped, then the next stage is to re-engineer the process in the light of the evidence base and the resulting discussions with the group.

Step three – Draw up the pathway:
- follow the process systematically, ensuring that all the professionals who deliver care are included
- make sure that the timings of interventions are correct
- ensure that the interventions are evidence-based and the outcomes are recorded within the pathway
- incorporate standards, clinical guidelines and outcome measures
- develop the pathway into a single multidisciplinary document to support the recording of interventions completed and include space for recording variances and outcome measurement. Time-based documentation is the easiest, for example day by day.

Step four – Communicate expectations:
- decide on a minimum period over which to pilot the pathway, for example three months or a specified number of patients
- decide where the pathway document will be located, offering easy access for all the team, and include this in your written guidelines for staff.

The project group should take responsibility for:

- developing and circulating the guidelines on using the pathway to all staff involved in the pathway
- discussing the pathway with all the staff in all the departments involved in its use
- devising ways of ensuring that locum doctors and bank and agency nursing staff are alerted to the use of the pathway
- deciding on ways of providing training for staff to gain their commitment and ensure it is used correctly
- piloting the pathway.

Step five – Review and revise:
- discuss the pathway with all members of the group and identify any problems
- analyse the variances, the completeness of the documentation, alterations that were made, comments from the users, and so on
- review at least thirty sets of records to validate the pathway. To do this you will need to identify thirty patients who have been discharged and who used the pathway. Then audit each set of records to establish if the

documentation was completed by all members of the team and, if not, why not. Also make a note of all the variances and establish:

- [ ] if in several patient pathways the same variances occurred. This may indicate that the pathway needs to be reviewed; for example, 90 per cent of patients scheduled for discharge on day six were actually discharged on day five, so the pathway length of stay should be reduced
- [ ] the reasons for the variances, which may be patient-centred or related to staff not following the pathway owing to lack of understanding of the system
- [ ] if the variances are patient-centred, a clinical audit or a review of the process would resolve the problem
- [ ] the patient's views on the care received
- develop and implement the final pathway
- plan the ongoing review of the pathway.

Problems with Pathways

There are a few problems associated with pathways, one of which is that some staff lack the skills critically to appraise the evidence or research, and this may need to be supported by additional training. See Chapter 7 for more information on critical appraisal. Another very common problem is that the documentation is not completed. There are several reasons for this but the most common is that out of habit some professionals continue to document care within their own system of record-keeping. Locum doctors write in the medical record because they were not involved in the process and may be unaware of the existence of the pathway and the same applies to bank and agency nursing staff. A further reason for non-completion of the pathway documentation may be the location of the pathway. If it is not in the right place at the right time it may not be completed. For instance, if the patient receives physiotherapy in the department and the pathway documentation stays on the ward, the physio-therapist may write in the record in the department.

There could be medico-legal problems if the care prescribed in the pathway is out of date or results in poor practice. This issue needs to be thought through as the ICP is developed. Some medical staff are concerned about individual professional autonomy and describe this as 'cookbook medicine'. Nursing staff may also express concerns that the care is not individualised. These concerns need to be addressed early in the process.

A further problem is perceived as the lack of time to devote to the development of a pathway but this is time well spent, as can be seen in the list of benefits further on in this chapter. Finally, the project group may resent any criticism of the pathway but need to be encouraged to be open to suggestions and change.

Successful Pathways

Success will depend upon:

- a demonstration of commitment at senior management and clinical levels
- the composition of the team that develops the pathway: for example, a group of people that like each other, an opinion leader, a completer and finisher, a good communicator, a scribe, a strong chairperson and a senior clinician. See Chapters 14 and 16 and the appendix for more information on working with groups
- the choice of topic area. Choose an area of care that is simple, straightforward and fairly predictable in the first instance. However, complex processes and procedures often show most benefit from the development of a pathway and so in the long term are more beneficial to the trust. For many patients, such as those admitted for elective surgery, the stages of care are predictable. Medical conditions are less predictable but often follow a common pattern, for example a patient admitted with a myocardial infarction
- the choice of high-volume areas of care, because if you want to make changes to the delivery of care there must be a substantial number of patients using the pathway to make valid changes.

Benefits of Pathways

A well-planned care pathway will:

- ensure that every patient receives care, from all the healthcare team, that is planned, consistent and evidence-based
- rationalise the process of care
- promote efficiency, for example less time wasted on unplanned activities and less duplication of care
- prove useful for training and developing staff
- empower staff
- encourage critical-process analysis
- reduce the impact of staff rotation
- through shared structured documentation, reduce the paperwork and improve record-keeping and communication
- provide a basis for operational research
- improve the continuity of care, for example the removal of variations in care patterns and outcomes that do not benefit patient care
- link the process of care to clinical outcome and the monitoring and evaluation of outcome

■ support team building as the various members of the team become aware of each other's role within the care pathway

■ support the analysis of variations from the pathway to facilitate clinical audit, which is more dynamic than previous approaches to implementing changes as a result of clinical audit

■ improve multidisciplinary teamworking through professionals working to shared goals

■ increase patient understanding – patients can follow the pathway giving them greater insight into their care and leading to greater co-operation and more informed decision making

■ facilitate the patient's informed participation in the care journey.

There are a number of organisations that support this type of work including the National Pathways Association (address at the end of this chapter) and the Modernisation Agency.

Integrated care pathways are a systemic approach to incorporating many of the elements of clinical governance through:

■ full participation in audit by all clinical staff – ICPs can act as a framework for clinical audit providing both concurrent and retrospective data for audit purposes. The ICP acts as a standard against which actual practice may be monitored. The identification of trends, which deviate from the standard allows for changes and revisions to be made to the pathway ensuring that clinical practice is changed as required, thus completing the audit cycle

■ evidence-based practice supported and applied routinely in every day practice – the baseline review of practice prior to the development of the ICP requires the professional staff to revise practice against the evidence supporting best practice, for example whether or not investigations, treatments and therapies are appropriate and evidence-based. The ICP is developed using investigations, treatments and therapies that are evidence-based and appropriate to the delivery of care. Routine monitoring of patient outcomes and variations allows the multidisciplinary team to make decisions about the effectiveness of the evidence for their local patients. Where no evidence exists, the ICP encourages the team to discuss the care and reach a consensus as to whether or not it constitutes best practice with positive outcomes

■ ensuring the clinical standards of NSFs and NICE recommendations are implemented – the development of an ICP and in particular the outcome standards will be informed by the NSFs and NICE

■ workforce planning and development, for example the recruitment and retention of an appropriately trained workforce, fully integrated within the NHS organisation's service planning. The ICP defines the roles and responsibilities of the different members of the team involved in the delivery of care

- effective monitoring of clinical care with high-quality systems for clinical record-keeping and the collection of relevant information – the ICP is a single multidisciplinary document which supports the notion of a comprehensive outcome-based record of care that reflects all the care that the patient has received. It identifies care that has deviated from the ICP and the actions that were taken
- processes for assuring the quality of clinical care are in place and integrated with the quality programme for the organisation as a whole – ICPs can be used to integrate a system of quality assurance. Their use can demonstrate the quality and appropriateness of care, and the routine review of variances and assessment of outcomes demonstrates a dynamic approach to quality assurance
- clear policies for managing risk – ICPs can be used to identify risk during the process of their development and then any identified risk management through the competed pathway
- clear lines of responsibility and accountability for the overall quality of clinical care – an ICP sets out individual roles and responsibilities with clearly defined outcomes.

Good Practice, Ideas and Innovations

The trust or healthcare organisation must encourage and support good practice, new ideas and innovations through working groups, regular team meetings, appraisal, clinical supervision, and so on. Ideas and innovations need to be rigorously evaluated and then, if the results are positive, disseminated across the organisation. Empowerment is an essential ingredient if staff and patients are to feel confident enough to put forward ideas and suggestions. Empowerment is discussed in detail in Chapter 6.

Principles for Achieving Best Practice

Best practice is the best achievable practice in a given setting. It is influenced by social, economic, political and environmental factors. It is dynamic, as the boundary of 'achievable' is constantly redefined as a result of developments in practice. Achievable incorporates the principles of efficiency and effectiveness. Best practice can only be achieved by empowering the patient. This empowerment is dependent on a strategy that is focused on the patient's participation in individualised plans of care. It incorporates developing staff, facilitating risk-taking, and encouraging innovation and evaluation of the impact of new or changed practice on the patient's wellbeing and self-direction.

There are several principles involved in achieving best practice:

- the process of achieving best practice should be strategically planned.
- the strategy should centre on empowering the patient
- it requires a multitude of approaches
- all approaches should incorporate the dissemination of practices which have been tried, tested and evaluated as successful
- developments in practice must be seen to be led and owned by clinical staff
- all approaches should have links with research and higher education, and have organisational support
- the strategic focus on empowering patients through developing practice should enable the development of education, research and management
- developments in practice should incorporate interagency and multi-disciplinary collaboration
- the achievement of best practice is not a competitive process but is dependent on networking
- the strategy should incorporate the process by which best practice influences and is integrated into policy-making.

Achieving best practice is fundamental to a trust or healthcare organisation that is committed to continuous quality improvement and often requires the culture to change. There is also a culture change required to support an open, 'no blame' organisation, as has been discussed throughout this book, but there are some key issues that, if addressed, have a very positive effect and go a long way to supporting individuals whether they are staff or service users. These include:

- treating people in a friendly and approachable way
- listening and hearing
- giving time
- recognising people as unique individuals
- giving the right information at the right time
- seeing each individual as valuable and worthy of respect
- involving people being open to their opinions and suggestions
- seeing each person as a whole.

Conclusion

This pillar of clinical governance is about ensuring that the care delivered to patients is evidence-based and will result in positive outcomes. It is also about ensuring that the healthcare team deliver care that is based on sound evidence which leads to patients receiving the same care for specific problems, resulting in consistency of approach and predicted outcomes.

Making It Happen

Clinical Effectiveness

The trust will need to ensure that:

- the strategy and programmes are in place for clinical effectiveness to work, including research to identify effective practice
- the clinical effectiveness strategy and programmes are integrated into the wider clinical governance and quality improvement programmes
- patients, service users, carers and partners are involved in the development of the clinical effectiveness strategy
- research projects are in action to identify effective clinical practice
- there is implementation of effective clinical practice through integrated care pathways and evidence-based guidelines for disease management
- there are systems for the collection and distribution of evidence-based practice to the relevant teams and staff, including the results of the trust or organisation's own research and the published evidence of effective practice including NSFs and guidance issued by NICE
- there are systems for monitoring the effectiveness and application of evidence-based practice, including a cycle of data collection and the use of performance indicators, clinical audit, team discussions and guideline amendments
- the research results and evidence of effective practice are made available to staff through libraries, the internet, journals, intranet, and so on
- budgets are in place to support research, development and the implementation of effective clinical practice
- there is training for staff in critical and appraisal skills, literature, and database and internet search skills.

Useful Websites

http://www.nice.org.uk
National Institute for Clinical Excellence

http://www.sign.ac.uk
The Scottish Intercollegiate Guidelines Network (SIGN) develops and publishes evidence-based clinical practice guidelines for use by the health service in Scotland. This website also includes SIGN's criteria for the appraisal of guidelines.

http://www.healthcentre.org.uk/hc/library/guidelines.htm

UK and worldwide guidelines available on the internet (not necessarily formally appraised or reviewed).

http://www.sghms.ac.uk/phs/hceu/nhsguide.htm
The Health Care Evaluation Unit's critical appraisal instrument is available on the internet. Its aim is to encourage the systematic development of clinical guidelines in the UK and to provide a structured and transparent approach to their appraisal. It can be used by independent appraisers to assess existing guidelines or by guideline developers as an aide-mémoire.

http://www.medlib.com
A collection of databases including the full text of the Cochrane Database of Systematic Reviews, critical commentaries on selected systematic reviews that have been assessed for quality by the NHS Centre for Reviews and Dissemination, and brief details of more than 170,000 randomised controlled trials. These are also available from Update Software, Summertown Pavilion, Middle Way, Summertown, Oxford, OX2 7LG.

http://text.nlm.nih.gov or http://www.ahcpr.gov:80/news/press/ngc.html
A series of clinical guidelines based on thorough reviews of research evidence. The agency is now focusing on producing evidence reports, (reviews and analyses of scientific literature designed to provide the basis for guidelines, measures of performance, and other tools for quality improvement), as well as working with the American Medical Association and the American Association of Health Plans to develop an on-line clearing house for practice guidelines. The on-line service will have electronic mailing lists to keep users informed about the implementation of guidelines.

http://www.york.ac.uk/inst/crd
Reports of systematic reviews presented in a readable and accessible format, produced by the NHS Centre for Reviews and Dissemination.

http://www.jr2.ox.ac.uk/Bandolier
UK newsletter alerting readers to key evidence about effectiveness in healthcare.

http://www.york.ac.uk/ins/crd
Summaries of published research on a single topic, which emphasise presenting clear messages on effectiveness. These are also available from the NHS Centre for Reviews and Dissemination, University of York, York, YO1 5DD.

http://nhscrd.york.ac.uk/Welcome.html or http://www.hcn.net.au/
Critical assessments of published economic evaluations, produced by the NHS Centre for Reviews and Dissemination. These are also available from the NHS Centre for Reviews and Dissemination, University of York, York, YO1 5DD.

Pillar Seven – Clinical Information 9

Chapter Contents:

- the quality of data
- information for health strategy.

A key element of this chapter is to establish that the quality of data collected to monitor clinical care is itself of a high standard.

This chapter covers the systems in place to collect, collate and interpret clinical information which is used to monitor, plan and improve the quality of patient care.

The Quality of Data

Clinical governance requires a trust or organisation to establish a framework which ensures all clinicians and staff are engaged in addressing and implementing a wide range of key targets. See Chapter 11 for more information. Essential to this process is good information and effective reporting systems which make the process open. In order to deliver the care agenda, trusts must have good-quality, timely and accurate information with which to monitor their performance against standards and benchmarks.

Historically the collection of information has been around management and financial data rather than clinical data such as that which might be held on an electronic patient record. At national level in England and Wales there are information management and technology (IM&T) information strategies, which set out the information needs for healthcare professionals, managers, planners, the public and patients within a timescale of 1998–2005.

Information for Health Strategy

In 1998 the Government launched a national infrastructure development programme for information, management and technology (IM&T strategy) called *Information for Health* (Secretary of State for Health, 1998) which set out as strategy for the NHS until 2005. The aims of the strategy are:

- to ensure that information is used to help patients receive the best possible care
- for health professionals to have the information they need to provide that care
- to provide accurate information for managers to support the local Health Improvement and Modernisation Programme and the NHS Performance Assessment Framework.

The IM&T strategy objectives for 1998–2005 include:

- lifelong electronic health records for every person in the country
- round-the-clock on-line access to patient records and information about best clinical practice for all NHS clinicians
- genuinely seamless care for patients from GPs, and hospital and community services sharing information across the NHS information highway
- fast and convenient public access to information and care via on-line services and telemedicine
- effective use of NHS resources by providing managers with the information they need.

There have been some updates on the IM&T strategy but the targets have mainly stayed the same. The key developments include the following (DoH, 2001; 2002):

- the NHS Information Authority is a special health authority set up to head the implementation of the *Information for Health* strategy
- an electronic patient record is the record of an episode of care which has been provided by one healthcare organisation, for example a period in an acute hospital for cardiac surgery or an episode of care in a mental health NHS trust
- an electronic health record is the record of all healthcare, wherever it is delivered, over the whole life of an individual. These electronic records will eventually replace the paper-based system that has been the method of recording care in the NHS since its inception in 1948. The result will be the integration of care across the various NHS health organisations. It will improve accuracy, and the record will be legible, provide information for clinical audit, research and the monitoring of the quality of care, and support clinical governance
- the NHS number is a unique number that identifies a patient using the NHS. The number is given to an individual and then kept for life and used whenever he/she visits his/her GP or uses any NHS hospital service

- the NHS strategic tracing service is a service for the NHS which enables staff to obtain an individual's NHS number
- the NHS-wide clearing service
- the NHS net is a communications network which supports electronic communication between NHS users. It is only accessible by the NHS and is quick and secure
- NHS Direct is a telephone service for the public which covers the UK and provides advice on health matters
- telemedicine, which is usually found in a hospital or practice setting, or telecare, which is transmitted to the patient's home, is a service that links a patient with a healthcare professional when they are geographically separated. Alternatively, it can be used to bring together health professionals to support discussion or for advice on diagnosis and treatment
- the national clinical information programme is a programme that includes confidentiality issues, Read codes, clinical record management, data quality, education and professional development.

The Welsh Office (1999) defines a clinical information system as:

> one which will contain all the administrative, demographic and person based information relating to an individual's health care which the clinician needs, when and where needed, to provide relevant, evidence based care to the patient. The agreed information that is derived from this enables the clinician to manage and review the quality of the clinical service provided ... Management information can then be extracted and derived from these systems without introducing burdensome data collection procedures on clinical staff, as has happened in the past. Implementing systems, which truly support clinical activity, should be the main focus for IM&T activities in provider organisation.

The success of these initiatives will depend on training for staff to develop their keyboard skills and IT knowledge and support to overcome some of the negative attitudes to some of these changes.

Information required for clinical governance will include clinical indicators and the National Performance Framework to support clinical audit and comparison with other organisations to support clinical practice. See Chapter 11 for more information on measurement and benchmarking.

Conclusion

The quality of information is very important if it is to be used effectively to measure performance. Essentially there are two types of data:

■ those associated with quantitative analysis, for example statistical and numerical information
■ qualitative – patient and staff experience.

This information may be found separately or in combination, for example:

■ activity:
  ☐ casemix data – healthcare resource groups (HRGs) which give information on patient type, diagnosis and treatment
  ☐ finished consultant episodes (FCEs)
  ☐ average length of stay (LOS)
■ contract minimum data set – patient demographic details which is basic information about the patient's stay, including admission and discharge dates, mode of admission and discharge, diagnosis and procedural codes
■ readmission rates – patients returning to the hospital after discharge or back to intensive care or coronary care after transfer to the wards
■ outcome measures – data relating to the patient's improved quality of life, for example pain control using a valid pain measurement tool, Barthel Index, and so on
■ infection control rates
■ incidents of pressure ulcers
■ clinical incidents – any untoward or serious incidents that affect the outcome for the patient
■ health and safety incidents such as accidents, falls, and so on
■ benchmarking – comparing information with another similar organisation or ward or unit, for example the stroke sentinel audit.

Making It Happen

Clinical Information

The trust must ensure that:

■ IM&T strategy and plans are in place
■ clinical and other information needed is supplied to the board, executive team, management teams and clinical teams to support clinical governance and the delivery of heatlhcare
■ the staff and budgets are in place to support the implementation of IM&T
■ information is used to monitor performance, and support performance review and improvement. Information is used to review and improve clinical practice
■ information is used to inform clinical governance activities

- information is used to support the implementation of policies and guidelines
- systems link with other organisations and support sharing of information
  - □ there are healthcare record systems, including electronic healthcare records, in place
  - □ there are processes to ensure confidentiality of information such as Caldicott guardianship, compliance with the data protection act, and so on
  - □ there are processes and systems for assuring data quality
  - □ training and support for staff in the interpretation and use of clinical information, is available
  - □ there is analytic support to users of information.

Useful Address

National Pathways Association, Priory Hospitals Group, Broadwater Park, Denham, Uxbridge, UB9 5HB. Telephone 01895 836339.

A Strategy for Clinical Governance

10

Chapter Contents:

- developing a strategy for clinical governance
- an example of a clinical governance strategy for a primary care trust.

Developing a Strategy for Clinical Governance

A strategic planning approach is essential in order effectively to manage clinical governance across an organisation. A strategic plan provides a set of actions and is aimed at giving the trust a clear direction and focus both now and in the future. Successful strategies are those that are dynamic and keep

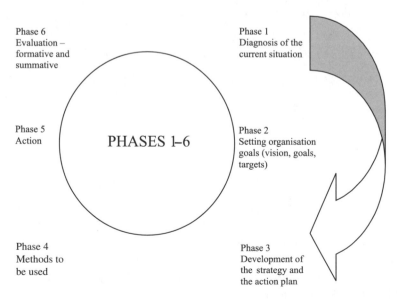

Phase 6
Evaluation –
formative and
summative

Phase 1
Diagnosis of the
current situation

Phase 5
Action

PHASES 1–6

Phase 2
Setting organisation
goals (vision, goals,
targets)

Phase 4
Methods to
be used

Phase 3
Development of
the strategy and
the action plan

Figure 10.1 The phases of a strategic plan

abreast of the continuous changes in healthcare today. The model for developing any strategy, but in particular a clinical governance strategy, requires strong leadership and commitment from all levels of the organisation. The strategic plan is a cyclical process and this model is based on the quality assurance cycle (see Figure 10.1) which consists of six phases:

- Phase 1: diagnosis of the current situation
- Phase 2: setting organisation goals (vision, goals and targets)
- Phase 3: development of the strategy and the action plan
- Phase 4: methods to be used
- Phase 5: action
- Phase 6: evaluation – formative and summative.

Phase One: Diagnosis of the current situation

This is the beginning of the cycle and starts with the identification and review of the current situation in the organisation. This phase answers the question, where are we now? It sets the baseline for the trust or healthcare organisation and includes clinical governance activities that are already in existence, such as policies and procedures for corporate governance, risk management, clinical audit, clinical governance committee structure, their agenda and plans, and so on. Information from the organisation's business plan will help establish the baseline, together with any external reports, from, for example, the Healthcare Commission, the Care Standards Commission and external consultants, local and national policies and guidelines, National Service Frameworks, internal clinical audit reports, and so on.

The business plan

The business plan will give the writer of the strategy information concerning the mission statement, the philosophy of the organisation, which will outline the purpose and direction of the organisation. The business plan will also provide detailed information about the organisation's values and beliefs, the current service provision and its plans for the future.

The customers

It is also important to identify who are the customers of the trust or healthcare organisation, the patients, their carers and families, the different directorates, departments and services, external providers of services and the staff. Having identified who the customers are, then the next step is to look at their requirements, what the trust is required to provide for them and to establish what the customers think of the service.

The workforce

It is necessary to establish and develop a profile of the numbers and skill-mix of the workforce and seek their views and understanding of clinical governance. Gaining their views on clinical governance and in particular their involvement is essential if the trust is to be in the position to say that clinical governance is at the heart of its organisation. Some of the areas on which the trust requires information from the staff are:

- their understanding of clinical governance and their role in ensuring that clinical governance is in place
- their current knowledge and skills and any education and training requirements to support clinical governance
- clinical governance activities, in their clinical area or department, both current and completed
- their ideas concerning clinical governance projects, approaches and activities that they would like to see in the future.

Management style, ethos and culture

Clinical governance requires a management style that is approachable, consultative and empowers staff to take responsibility for their actions and to work in partnership with management. If the current management style is authoritarian and controlling then there will be a need for training and development, so a baseline assessment of the current management style is also required.

Resources

There needs to be a baseline assessment of the financial and human resources available to use in developing, implementing and evaluating the clinical governance strategy.

The final part of this first phase incorporates all this baseline information in a SWOT analysis, looking at the strengths, weaknesses, opportunities and threats as compared to those in similar trusts.

Phase Two: Setting organisation goals (vision, goals and targets)

This phase looks at the vision, goals and targets, the 'where do we want to be?' factor. The trust must establish a clear vision of where the organisation wants to be and identify some goals for clinical governance. The goals should be linked to the business plan and based on the factors outlined with the objective of helping members of staff to understand what is expected of them. The goals then become the benchmarks for the trust against which to measure its success in achieving the clinical governance strategy. The goals must be:

- consistent with the overall objectives and the clinical governance agenda
- measurable
- achievable
- relevant to clinical governance
- clear, precise and understandable.

Phase Three: Development of the strategy and action plan

The lead for clinical governance, the clinical governance committee and senior staff within the trust should be involved in the development of the strategy, which should include the mission statement or philosophy of the trust's approach to clinical governance, the goals, and the long-term plans with timescales. The role of the clinical governance lead and the committee should be determined, so that there are clear lines of responsibility and accountability throughout the trust.

This phase describes the actions required to achieve the goals. It involves identifying the key tasks and actions that need to be undertaken, who will do them, in what order and by when. The order should follow a logical sequence as one activity or project builds on another. For example, if one of the goals is to have an integrated care pathway for the management of patients with suspected breast cancer, this should be preceded by an action that supports education and training for all staff who are part of the development of the care pathway.

When developing an action plan there are some key questions to ask and address, for example:

- how will we know when we have clinical governance in place?
- what framework will we use for clinical governance?
- how will activities be co-ordinated?
- how will we measure and monitor our progress and effectiveness in implementing clinical governance across the trust?
- what tools or systems will we use to measure clinical governance?
- how will we get support from people in the trust?
- how will we motivate people to meet the clinical governance agenda?

Key people and groups will have specific areas of responsibility and these should be clearly defined: for example, clinical governance co-ordinators will be responsible for working with directorates' and departments' management teams to ensure that the staff support the strategy and develop local clinical governance plans to ensure that their part of the trust's strategy is met. They should identify training and education needs, collate consumer feedback and ensure that results are fed back to the clinical governance committee along with progress reports against the action plans. Other roles and responsibilities within teams and groups are discussed in depth in Chapter 14.

Phase Four: Methods to be used

There are some key issues that need to be addressed to ensure that the strategy, when operational, meets the present goals within the timescales. These include education of staff in the objectives, tools and techniques of clinical governance, communication, documentation and co-ordination of all other initiatives such as peer review, clinical supervision, quality circles, risk management, and so on.

Phase Five: Action

This phase describes the actions required to implement the strategy and the action plans to achieve the goals. The first issue is often one of resistance to the implementation of something new. When clinical governance was introduced there were groups who felt it was unnecessary, added to their workload, would not benefit patients, and was just a paper exercise and another management tool inflicted upon them. This sort of resistance needs to be overcome through good communication, information and support, and involving people in the formulation and implementation of the particular activity (Towell and Harries, 1979). Helping people to understand and accept the need for change and the management of change is discussed in more detail in Chapter 13. There is also further information about working with groups and facilitator training in Chapter 14, project management in Chapter 15 and empowerment in Chapter 6, all of which help the written strategy become a reality.

Phase Six: Evaluation – formative and summative

The evaluation stage uses:

1. formative evaluation – how will we know we are getting there?
2. summative evaluation – how will we know when we get there?

The first step is to plan the evaluation and in order to do this to consider the following (Morton-Cooper and Bamford, 1997):

- for whom the evaluation is being done
  who wants the information
  who will benefit from it
- the purpose of the evaluation
  why the evaluation is being conducted
- the scope of the evaluation
- whether everything in the plan needs to be evaluated
- what the key success criteria are
- what resources there are to do the evaluation.

The formative evaluation involves monitoring the goals set and the action plan, checking at regular intervals that the trust is on track, that actions are being completed by the time specified and that the outcomes on target for being achieved.

The summative evaluation comes at the end of the cycle when actions have been completed, targets have been met and a judgement is made as to the success or failure of meeting the goals set in the strategy by their target date.

The goals in the strategy will produce a wide range of quantitative and qualitative data that can be used for evaluation and may include the output from questionnaires, patient-satisfaction surveys, results of audit, monitoring of care pathways, and so on. The annual report should incorporate progress to date against the action plan and goals with an evaluation of how well the goals were met.

A strategy, whether it has been written for clinical governance, quality assurance or risk management, should be seen as part of the existing quality improvement agenda, business planning and organisational development, and not as just another initiative demanding time and resources.

A clinical governance strategy is the blueprint with which to meet the clinical governance agenda and the example that follows was written by Barbara Merricks who is the Director of Primary and Community Services and Lead Director of Clinical Governance for North Dorset PCT. The strategy is included in this chapter with the kind permission of North Dorset PCT.

North Dorset Primary Care Trust – Clinical Governance Strategy

1. Background

1.1 The former Dorset Community NHS Trust largely fulfilled its obligations for Clinical Governance via its investment in Practice Development Units.

1.2 The erstwhile North Dorset Primary Care Group unpicked Clinical Governance to expose its constituent elements. Such elucidation revealed the basic familiarity of those elements and so thereby reduced anxiety and threat and facilitated engagement with them.

1.3 One organisation retained a sense of embodiment of Clinical Governance at the expense of scope, detail and application whilst the other, although it embraced a good deal of detail, never satisfactorily drew everything together into a composite whole.

1.4 Building on what has been learned nationally and locally it is now necessary for the North Dorset Primary Care Trust (NDPCT) to both define the scope of Clinical Governance detail and to draw all the disparate elements back together into a unified whole set in the context of overall Trust performance.

1.5 There is a need to support this contextualisation with a clinical governance culture; an environment:

- in which every member of staff continuously identifies and acts out their contribution to Trust-wide quality improvement;
- in which imposed, top-down, quality measurement activity and leadership is matched by a voluntary, bottom-up, relentless pursuit of excellence in healthcare activity.

2. Definition

2.1 Clinical Governance is:

A framework through which NHS organisations are accountable for continuously improving the quality of their services and safeguarding high standards of care by creating an environment in which excellence in clinical care will flourish. The New NHS: Modern, Dependable December 1997.

The keywords for this strategy are:

- framework;
- continuously improving;
- environment.

3. Purpose

3.1 The purpose of this strategy is:

- to describe the NDPCT 'framework' for Clinical Governance;
- to specify the process whereby the NDPCT will demonstrate year on year, continuous improvement in quality of services;

▣ to mobilize and enable leadership and management at all levels to build a culture throughout the NDPCT in which excellence is relentlessly pursued by all.

3.2 The overall aim is to describe the comprehensive structured management of Clinical Governance in its entirety throughout the NDPCT.

3.3 Two separate and subordinate strategies detail the Trust's management of clinical audit and clinical effectiveness – two of the seven pillars of clinical governance.

4. Framework

4.1 The NDPCT framework for Clinical Governance consists of 4 separate structures:

▣ the Clinical Governance organisational structure;
▣ the Clinical Governance activity structure;
▣ the Clinical Governance planning, reporting and co-ordinating structure;
▣ local Clinical Governance structures.

Clinical Governance Organisational Structure

4.2 The organisational structure for clinical governance within the NDPCT is not included in this chapter but it is largely, but not entirely, based on the operational management line of accountability and displays:

▣ all appropriate teams, groups and sub-committees;
▣ a continuous line of accountability for clinical governance matters from individuals to the Trust Board. The plan of the organisational structure has not been include in this chapter.

4.3 There is responsibility and accountability at every level. Of significant note:

▣ the NDPCT Trust Board has responsibility for:
  ☐ ensuring that clinical governance principles, processes and systems are embedded within itself and throughout the organisation;
  ☐ ensuring compliance with their statutory duty for the quality, principles of clinical governance and patient safety of services commissioned from other providers;

- [ ] ensuring the implementation of national quality imperatives, e.g. National Patient Safety Agency reporting, National Institute for Clinical Excellence (NICE) guidance, National Service Frameworks (NSF) standards;
- [ ] ensuring participation in National Confidential Enquiries;
- [ ] ensuring that all clinicians are involved in regular review and clinical audit of clinical services;
- [ ] developing an open culture within the organisation where incidents, mistakes and omissions are reported and lessons learned;
- [ ] ensuring effective risk management processes and accounting for clinical governance responsibilities when signing their statement of internal control;
- [ ] monitoring trends in key clinical quality and clinical outcome measures;
- [ ] maintaining a focus on continuous, demonstrable improvement in the quality of the patient experience and improvement in healthcare outcomes;
- [ ] involving partners in service provision in clinical governance activities;
- [ ] assuming and making clear, the joint accountability for services, which are provided on a multi-agency, multi-sector basis;
- [ ] reporting as necessary to the Strategic Health Authority on clinical governance activity and progress;
- [ ] publishing on the Internet and within the local community the Annual Clinical Governance Report in abbreviated and lay terms;
- the Chief Executive is accountable to the Trust Board for ensuring that both the structure and processes for implementing clinical governance are appropriate and adequate for the Board to meet its obligations;
- the Clinical Governance Subcommittee will meet monthly and has responsibility for:
  - [ ] acting as the co-ordinating body for all aspects of Clinical Governance throughout the NDPCT;
  - [ ] leading on, authorising and monitoring all aspects of day to day Clinical Governance;
  - [ ] ensuring the necessary information and advice is continuously and regularly set before the Trust Board in a clear, concise manner, such that the Board is enabled to properly discharge its responsibilities;
  - [ ] overseeing the establishment, maintenance and co-ordination of robust and effective clinical governance arrangements throughout the Trust and which embrace all elements and activities;

- ☐ setting, monitoring, reviewing the necessary targets, indicators, trends and standards as appropriate for all clinical governance activity;
- ☐ drawing up the contents of the annual Clinical Governance Development Plan, ensuring it shows demonstrable continuity and improvement and that it includes action on any feedback from the Trust Board as well as including action in response to specialist advice both from within and without the Trust;
- ☐ maintaining a three year clinical governance plan;
- ☐ overseeing the work of the Clinical Effectiveness Group and approving the annual Clinical Audit Plan;
- ☐ delegating appropriately to the Clinical Effectiveness Group those responsibilities set out in the strategies for Clinical Effectiveness and Clinical Audit;
- ☐ agreeing annual work programmes;
- ☐ agreeing the Annual Clinical Governance Report and interim reports to Trust Board;
- ☐ ensuring the necessary feedback and encouragement to all clinicians;
- ☐ agreeing the Annual Clinical Governance Report expressed in abbreviated and lay terms for the Trust Board to publish within the local community and on the Internet;
- ☐ reviewing local clinical governance arrangements, activity and evidence on a team by team basis;
- ■ the Director of Primary and Community Services is responsible for:
- ☐ acting as Lead Director for Clinical Governance;
- ☐ advising the Clinical Governance Subcommittee on all aspects of clinical governance, both strategic and operational;
- ☐ providing specialist advice to the Clinical Governance Subcommittee concerning clinical governance arrangements and activity in Primary and Community Care;
- ☐ leading, and facilitating clinical governance throughout Primary and Community Care including all nurses and therapists;
- ☐ acting as lead support to the Clinical Governance Subcommittee.
- ■ the Director of Mental Health Services is responsible for:
- ☐ leading and facilitating clinical governance throughout Mental Health Services;
- ■ the Clinical Director Mental Health Services is responsible for:
- ☐ providing specialist advice to the Clinical Governance Subcommittee concerning clinical governance throughout Mental Health Services;
- ☐ chairing the Mental Health Forum.

- the Director of Public Health is responsible for:
  - ☐ providing specialist advice to the Clinical Governance Sub-committee concerning clinical governance from a Public Health perspective;
  - ☐ ensuring Public Health activity contains appropriate clinical governance arrangements;
  - ☐ leading the work of the Clinical Effectiveness Group and for the responsibilities set out in the North Dorset Primary Care Trust Strategies for Clinical Audit and Clinical Effectiveness;
  - ☐ leading the Trust quest to capture, evaluate and implement appropriate evidence-based practice in accordance with the North Dorset Primary Care Trust Clinical Effectiveness Strategy;
- the GP Lead on Clinical Governance/Prescribing is responsible for:
  - ☐ providing specialist advice to the Clinical Governance Subcommittee concerning clinical governance arrangements and activity in Primary Care;
  - ☐ providing specialist advice to the Clinical Effectiveness Group;
  - ☐ providing specialist advice on prescribing;
  - ☐ leading, encouraging, facilitating appropriate and cost-effective prescribing throughout the Trust (supported by Clinical Director Mental Health Services and Pharmacist).
- the Chair of the Professional Executive Committee, through the Primary Care Management Group, and the Chair of the Mental Health Forum are responsible for supporting the implementation of clinical governance throughout Primary Care and Mental Health Services respectively
- all Leaders, Managers and Supervisors throughout the Trust are responsible for:
  - ☐ mobilising and enabling their teams to create the necessary structures and dynamics to implement clinical governance generally and the Annual Clinical Governance Development Plan/Work Programme in particular;
  - ☐ building a culture in which excellence is relentlessly pursued by all;
  - ☐ reacting constructively to all feedback from whatever source;
  - ☐ reviewing, measuring, evaluating clinical activity within their teams in accordance with the principles of Clinical Governance. (*Note*: this is in addition to work set out in the Annual Clinical Governance Development Plan/Work Programme)
  - ☐ maintaining a permanent record of all local clinical governance activity for inspection by Directors, Clinical Governance Sub-committee and external review teams;

- ☐ supporting individual team members and turning every incident, mistake, error, omission, example of poor performance into an opportunity for positive improvement.
- individuals are expected:
  - ☐ to engage with all clinical governance activity, including some by their own volition, as appropriate;
  - ☐ to support every activity with a personal focus on quality and safety;
  - ☐ to be open and honest in relation to incidents, mistakes, errors, omissions and poor performance.
- the Director of Planning and Modernisation is responsible for effecting Clinical Governance:
  - ☐ amongst Dentists;
  - ☐ amongst Pharmacists (supported by Pharmacy Advisor);
  - ☐ amongst Optometrists;
  - ☐ within the Intermediate Care Team.
- the Director of Human Resources, in consultation with the Chief Executive, Clinical Governance Subcommittee, and appropriate managers and individuals is to ensure that all job descriptions reflect the principles of clinical governance and specific responsibilities where necessary.
- the Director of Finance supported by the Risk Manager is responsible for:
  - ☐ the implementation and regular review of a robust risk management policy;
  - ☐ the management of indirect patient risk;
  - ☐ the management of health and safety issues;
  - ☐ directing Controls Assurance activity;
  - ☐ the management, evaluation and analysis of adverse incidents.

Clinical Governance Activity Structure

4.4 There is as yet no definitive list of exactly what constitutes Clinical Governance. The concept does not easily define itself by disciplines and elements, but rather by principles and objectives. From October 2003 the Clinical Governance Subcommittee has incorporated the Risk Committee and is known as the Clinical Governance and Risk Committee.

4.5 The Commission for Health Improvement's Review Structure is based overall on Clinical Governance and consists of '7 Pillars'. This framework of 7 pillars is used for the regular formal reporting of plans and achievements associated with Clinical Governance. The 7 Pillars are:

- Patient and Public Involvement;
- Risk Management;
- Clinical Audit;
- Clinical Effectiveness;
- Staffing and Staff Management;
- Education and Training;
- Use of Information.

4.6 Wherever possible clinical governance activity within the NDPCT should be contextualised by reference to this framework. Clinical Audit and Clinical Effectiveness are the subjects of two supporting strategies.

4.7 In order to provide practitioners, managers and Trust leadership with some sense of boundary and with tangible, familiar activity Clinical Governance is unpicked into constituent elements, disciplines and activity. The list is not exhaustive; it possibly never can be. The arrangement is to a large degree arbitrary and done on the basis of perceived general appropriateness. There is no reason why the arrangement should not be altered or added to in light of experience and consensus.

North Dorset Primary Care Trust – clinical governance unpicked

The Patient Experience

Including the environment, planning and organisation of care:

- develop a range of external single performance indicators for the overall Trust and units, hospitals and practices;
- complaints – regularly review robust procedures to respond to complaints in a timely, structured way; overall Trust and Practices;
- patient literature and notices – regularly review range, authenticity and display;
- the Patients Charter – consider display; ensure all staff know it;
- patient's rights and responsibilities – ensure all staff know them;
- patient confidentiality – ensure all staff know and understand the rules; review regularly;
- Caldicott Guardian arrangements;
- patient's access to their medical records – ensure all staff know and understand the rules; review regularly;
- Random Case Analysis;
- patients' 'suggestion' mechanisms – develop a Trust wide and local range of mechanisms including a procedure to process them properly;

- stakeholders' 'suggestion' mechanisms – develop a Trust wide and local range of mechanisms including a procedure to process them properly. Having to put them in writing will ensure that suggestions are better thought through;
- regularly define and review the full complement of strategies, policies, protocols, directives etc., to be held locally throughout the Trust;
- every Practice, hospital, team, unit, etc., to share all manner of healthcare information. Good and effective innovations are not to be kept hidden from others;
- identify and offer to share special expertise and experience throughout the Trust;
- identify and develop a range of care pathways throughout the Trust and with other healthcare partners. Records to be retained including audit activity;
- Practice Professional Development Plans – design a proforma for use. Retain records to demonstrate progressive continuity of Plans for service development;
- Clean Hospital Indicators – continue to develop the scheme internally;
- infection control policies – reviews and evaluation;
- vaccine storage arrangements and monitoring;
- maintenance of 'cold chain';
- Controlled Drugs stored and recorded in accordance with Home Office instructions;
- records management policy; local records managers;
- regular audits of the quality of records;
- records storage and security;
- electronic data security;
- the principles of informed patient consent – implied, verbal, written – understood by all staff – common application throughout Trust;
- p;atient consent for videoing consultations for training purposes; the presence of a student, etc.;
- all controls Assurance Standards applied and progress monitored;
- seek security advice from local Crime Prevention Officers/Security Firm as appropriate;
- Risk Management Strategy;
- Risk Management Policies;
- a framework for safe practice – the relentless pursuit of designing out the possibility of mistakes being made;
- reviews of matching qualifications, skills, experience and assessments against the work being undertaken;
- system whereby all staff can report concerns or 'near-misses', without fear or favour for deliberation by trusted panel;
- use of message books;

- telephone enquiries to be recorded in patient's notes;
- regular review of patient call and recall systems; the system for advising patients of adverse test results must be totally reliable;
- Immunisations/Drug administration – always check the data sheet for side-effects, contraindications, recommended injection site. Record: date; batch number; type of injection; injection site; dose given; information to patient – signature!
- GPs and nurses become suppliers when they dispense a product, e.g. local anaesthetic, ointments, suture material. Record names of products, suppliers, batch numbers and dates. Records should be retained for 10 years and 4 months;
- being aware of medico-legal issues such as those surrounding the 'prescribing', 'referring' and recommending of exercise.

Use of Information

Including information about resources, processes, the patient experience and outcomes of care:

- clinical audits of structure – develop and record a progressive programme. Include suitability and sufficiency of instruments, equipment, spares. Also maintenance, re-calibration, re-charging routines;
- develop a range of internally derived indicators of general performance;
- utilize indicators of good and cost effective prescribing;
- formulary – use and regularly review;
- regular patient surveys – analyse, interpret, evaluate results. Feedback and invest in lessons learned;
- patient group directions, protocols, procedures – define the range to be held locally. Regularly review. Maintain records;
- ensure advice from Strategic Health Authority and others is disseminated and implemented as necessary;
- ensure all equipment routinely maintained;
- storage and recording of all medicines and controlled drugs;
- stock control;
- regular, effective Health Needs Analysis of all types.

Processes for Quality Improvement

- clinical audits of process – develop and record a progressive programme;
- clinical audits of outcome – develop and record a progressive programme;
- develop a range of disease centred process indicators;

- National Service Frameworks – demonstrable implementation;
- the Essence of Care – demonstrable implementation;
- National Institute for Clinical Excellence – demonstrable implementation of directives, advice, etc.;
- draw up definitive list of local policies, guidelines, standards, codes, etc. Monitor implementation and authenticity;
- evidence-based practice – develop a reliable structured process for capturing all appropriate information followed by evaluation, dissemination, implementation and further evaluation;
- research appraisal skills – education programme for all practitioners;
- reflection-in-action – encourage the development of intuition in senior practitioners;
- Critical Incident Analysis – develop a reliable, robust, structured procedure for analysing, evaluating incident and re-investing lessons learned throughout the Trust;
- Significant Event Analysis – require all teams to undertake this practice frequently. Maintain records;
- complaints – a reliable, robust and structured procedure to analyse, evaluate and learn from complaints, mistakes and incidents be they local or national;
- Research and Development Strategy;
- Research Governance Policy;
- Risk Management;
- PCT Risk Register, reviewing and updating.

Staff focus

- develop a range of summative and formative assessments for appropriate purposes;
- staff surveys – analyse, evaluate and learn from results;
- communication strategies – Trust wide and local;
- encourage honesty and authenticity in all communication;
- develop a range of ways to disseminate innovation and best practice;
- team meetings – regular and recorded, focused and controlled;
- clinical meetings – regular and recorded, focused and controlled;
- capturing and acting on advice from professional bodies;
- professional portfolios and profiles – arrangements to ensure all practitioners are maintaining one;
- maintenance of Professional Registration and authority to practice – personal responsibility. Trust to carry out checks;
- reflective self-assessment – expectation perhaps prior to annual appraisal;
- local measures for the recruitment and retention of nursing staff;

- Personal Development Plans – everyone required to have one;
- annual, structured Learning Needs Analysis;
- formal academic courses;
- workshops, study days, seminars, conferences – insist on learning outcomes, evaluations, overviews, etc;
- formal evaluations of formal education and training;
- Pre and Post education/training interviews;
- formal evaluations of effect on performance and service following education and training;
- critically review the effective use of budgets with respect to education, training and continuing professional development;
- develop range of cost benefit indicators;
- reliable system for GP appraisals;
- introduce peer and work based assessments;
- annual job reviews;
- Job Description reviews;
- nurses to familiarize themselves with GMC Guidelines good practice with respect to financial awards/gifts/inducements from pharmaceutical companies, etc;
- effecting Primary Health Care Team (PCHT) working – develop indicators?
- effective integrated nursing team working – develop performance management indicators;
- multi-disciplinary, multi-professional team working;
- networking;
- reflection-on-action – recorded and retained in reflective diaries, journals, profiles, etc., by local teams or individuals;
- small group case discussions/Ballint Seminars;
- professional conversation and tutorials – reflective practice pieces written up;
- Clinical Supervision – guided reflection. Supervisor's annual report of trends etc;
- identification of poorly performing practitioners;
- whistle blowing policy;
- identified procedures for protecting patients, protecting practitioners from making (further) mistakes, supporting them and using action plans to address identified weaknesses;
- policy to manage non engagement/compliance with Clinical Governance;
- local plans to identify and support/protect colleagues deemed to be stressed;
- address all matters of concern in a deliberate and responsible manner – endeavouring to effect correction before critical or crisis situation arrived at;
- induction processes;

- mentorship schemes;
- preceptorship schemes;
- occasional job swaps, shadowing, etc;
- Compulsory Training (Manual Handling, CPR, Breakaway, etc.);
- Personal/Practice Accreditation: Royal College of General Practitioners (membership by Assessment of Performance; Fellowship by Assessment; Quality Practice Award); Practice Development Units; Designated Training Practices; Awards and Scholarships;
- Practice Receptionist's training programmes;
- training for newly appointed Practice Nurses;
- initial training and regular updates for Cervical Cytology, Defibrillation, etc.;
- 'Improving Working Lives' accreditation;
- family friendly policies, etc.;
- Workforce Planning – critical, realistic, linked to identified service need;
- Practice Professional Development Plans – design a proforma for use. Retain records to demonstrate progressive continuity of plans for training and education component.

Leadership, Strategy and Planning

- regular review of organisational performance;
- organisational development – planned and progressive;
- positive promotion of NHS and NDPCT;
- develop public disclosure of all appropriate information;
- public meetings;
- partnership with patient support groups;
- set up client care focus groups;
- set up a Patient Forum;
- liaison with Community Health Council;
- partnership with Patient Advice and Liaison Service;
- partnerships with neighbouring and other health communities, social services, local government, patients and public – one example of this is the multi agency approach necessary to deliver the National Service Frameworks;
- management development programme;
- leadership courses;
- central register and portfolio of all clinical governance activity throughout the Trust;
- effective communication strategies throughout the Trust;
- a 'No Blame' culture of openness;
- use of Intranet, electronic bulletin boards; grapevines';

- newsletters;
- written communications in 'house style';
- limiting distribution of communications and e-mail to appropriate staff; beware information overload;
- accurate identification of health inequalities and variations in service – take into account vulnerable or marginalized groups;
- contribution to and use of Local Delivery Plan;
- remaining aware of the wider NHS picture.

4.8 Clinical Governance is a performance management tool but a complex one. Increasing engagement with it and increasingly skilful use of it will be led by experiential learning and measured experiment. Ultimately a large amount of information will be generated and the organisation must learn how to manage that information and indeed how to use it.

4.9 Even gentle perusal of 'The Patient Experience' reveals the existence of three alternative perspectives;

- one sets clinical governance activity in context, usually the context of actual healthcare, the patient or identified need;
- another uses clinical governance activity more directly for its own sake to build professional wisdom, capability, confidence and assurance throughout the Trust's body of practitioners;
- the third is straightforward implementation of directives from higher authority.

4.10 Therefore although part of the clinical governance agenda is set for the Trust there remains significant scope for the Clinical Governance Subcommittee when drawing up the remainder.

4.11 As the principal lead, co-ordinating and evaluating body for the Trust the Clinical Governance Subcommittee is to set the agenda and draw up and agree the annual clinical governance development plans and associated work programmes. In doing so:

- it should refer to the three-year clinical governance plan;
- it should remember that clinical governance development plans are a key (perhaps the key) performance monitoring tool. Plans should be based on a self-assessment of the organisation's strengths and weaknesses and must be designed to improve the quality of local clinical care;
- it should use 'The Patient Experience' as an aide-mémoire to further develop local processes across the full range of clinical governance activities and provide service-related quality objectives for the coming year;

- it should ensure that for each action point, development plans clearly identify lead responsibility and target date for completion;
- it should ensure development plans incorporate any actions resulting from a Commission for Health Improvement clinical governance review or investigation, assessment, inspection by any other external authority;
- it should ensure development plans address any clinical, patient or staff issues identified by the performance measurement processes of current clinical governance activity;
- it should ensure development plans incorporate local learning from national enquiries and National Patient Safety Agency alerts;
- it should bear in mind the capacity and capability of the Trust to manage and productively use increasing volumes of information. In this context organisational development is a significant element of overall clinical governance;
- it should ensure that as far as is practicable each activity is designed, structured and kept as simple as possible. The simple structure should not end at data collection but continue with collation, analysis, evaluation and ultimately interpretation into meaningful form;
- wherever possible it should assign the target, indicator, trend or standard expected. There is much to learn here. The Trust needs to learn how to measure things that cannot presently be measured. The Trust needs to design new indicators. The ability to demonstrate continuous improvement will thereby become easier;
- it should include scope for activity to be generated at local practice or team level. Leaders, managers and supervisors need to assume a measure of local ownerships of Clinical Governance. They need to be encouraged to develop the insight and skills to manage micro-clinical governance at local level; to seek out, identify and address local weaknesses;
- it should insist that portfolios of clinical governance activity, evidence, results and information are built up both at local level and centrally within the Trust;
- it should always endeavour to balance and optimise the challenge, support and supervision elements of implementing Clinical Governance;
- it should ensure that appropriate education and facilitation is made available to match the increasing sophistication of Clinical Governance within the Trust, over time;
- it should ensure that any and all information that constitutes feedback is indeed passed back to local teams with plaudits, encouragement and support as appropriate;

■ it should remember that its starting canvas is essentially blank. In some areas development can build on what has been already achieved. In other areas a start-up standard may need to be stipulated or a baseline assessment made;

■ it should as far as is practicable always set clinical governance in context, making it applicable and meaningful. Those activities, such as Clinical Supervision, which can be considered as isolated and pure, usually have their own separate and applied identity. Always match activity with a reason;

■ It should ensure that partners in service provision, e.g. dentists, community pharmacists, optometrists and other partner organisations are taken into account.

4.12 As far as is practicable the various contents of the annual clinical governance development plan are to be merged with any action plans from other sources into single overall Annual Work Programmes appropriate to each individual healthcare site or team.

Planning, Reporting and Co-ordinating Structure

4.13 the basis of the Planning and Reporting Structure is the continuous, progressive cycle of annual clinical governance plans and reports required by the Trust Board and the Strategic Health Authority. (Annual Clinical Governance Development Plans incorporate annual clinical audit plans)

4.14 the annual clinical governance development plan and report have specific annual schedules set out by the Department of Health. All internal processes and reporting must be geared to these schedules

4.15 below is an outline annual programme embracing all known clinical governance activity. As the Trust learns and its engagement with and use of Clinical Governance grows, so more input will no doubt be added to the yearly cycle.

North Dorset Clinical Governance Outline Annual Programme

Main Activities

■ Annual Clinical Governance Development Plan
■ Annual Work Programmes for all Health Care Sites
■ Quarterly Progress Reports – Work programmes, Risk Management activity, NSF Milestones.

■ Annual Clinical Governance Report
■ Annual Clinical Governance Public Report
■ Maintenance of central Clinical Governance register and portfolio
■ Annual Audit Plan

Supporting Activities

The Patient's Experience

■ complaints analysis with identification of trends
■ patient/ Stakeholder suggestion analysis
■ review of Care Pathway Register
■ clean Hospitals Indicators Reports
■ patient Survey analysis
■ equipment maintenance schedules
■ patient/ public involvement – review and analysis
■ PALS activity report

Use of Information

■ external appraisals and reports, e.g. Audit Commission, Mental Health Act Committee
■ Caldicott Report
■ adverse Incident Reports – analysis and evaluation
■ NICE guidance directives
■ National Patient Safety Agency guidance
■ Significant Event Analysis – evaluations
■ Critical Incident Reviews – outcomes
■ Public Health alerts
■ National Conference attendance feedback
■ external funding resources
■ medical and Surgical Supplies and Equipment Committee recommendations

Processes for Quality Improvement

■ review of clinical audit programme – analysis and evaluation
■ Essence of Care benchmarking
■ Controls Assurance Standards – application and monitor progress, RPST/ CNST moving up levels
■ prescribing activity reports
■ Patient Group Directions – register, review and reissue

■ evaluation of evidence based practice
■ research activity reports
■ review local clinical governance activity on a unit by unit basis

Staff Focus

■ Leadership and Management – regular assessment
■ Professional Bodies guidance
■ Staff Survey analyses
■ Annual Learning Needs Analysis – overview
■ overview of in-house programme relating to workshops, study days, seminars and conferences
■ evaluation of purchased education and training including effect on service and performance
■ Clinical Supervisors' annual report – overview of uptake and any identified trends
■ compulsory training – overview report
■ Practice Teachers'/Practice Educators' – overview report
■ staff leavers' interviews – overview
■ Academic Centre in Practice annual report
■ policy to identify and support health professionals whose performance gives cause for concern.

Leadership, Strategy, Planning

■ programme to ensure continuous review of all Strategies and Policies, etc.
■ identification and review of health needs analyses, health inequalities, variations in service and health improvement/local delivery plans
■ overview of Practice Development Plans
■ Practice Health Plans/Annual Reviews
■ North Dorset PCT 3 Year Business Plan – 3 Year Clinical Governance Plan
■ Workforce Development Plan
■ Clinical Governance Strategy

4.16 The Trust is also expected to simplify and express its annual clinical governance report in layman's terms for release to the public and stakeholders.

4.17 Nevertheless, this report is expected to provide concise details of systems and processes, illustrated by examples, and how they have resulted in change and quality improvement during the year.

4.18 All areas of the Commission for Health Improvement Review Framework are to be addressed in the annual report. Where other sources of information are available to the public the Trust must ensure consistency across all reports and may wish to consider including the development plan for that year and any action plans arising from a Commission for Health Improvement review as part of that report.

4.19 The clinical governance annual report should also be available on the Trust's website;

4.20 The Trust will also maintain a three-year Clinical Governance Plan to support strategic direction and seamless continuity.

Local Clinical Governance Structure

4.21 General practices, wards, teams and units are expected to have identified lead doctors and nurses for Clinical Governance. These may or may not be the team leaders;

4.22 General Practitioners, matrons, ward sisters, leaders, managers and supervisors are expected to ensure that each local team has a structure to support Clinical Governance and every member's participation. Normally this can be the existing primary healthcare team, ward, nursing or therapy team together with its normal dynamics and processes.

4.23 Local team leaders are expected to ensure:

- every team/clinical meeting includes an agenda item to review and evaluate the team's current clinical governance activity;
- clinical governance activity, especially clinical audits, is the product of team wide contributions and not the sterling work of one individual stalwart!
- records, held electronically where practicable, of all their clinical governance activity are retained within a growing portfolio available for inspection by line managers, Clinical Governance Subcommittee, Directors and external assessors;
- teams frequently apply themselves to reflective self-assessment and identify perceived local weaknesses in performance or service;
- teams address those weaknesses by taking appropriate measures and by seeking support when necessary perhaps via the annual Learning Needs Analysis;
- they draw up a local clinical governance development plan using 'The Patient Experience' as necessary to compile it. This is in addition to the Trust Development Plans/Work Programmes but will complement them.
- this plan includes straightforward and routine items such as clinical supervision, core skills, CPR resuscitation, job reviews, annual appraisals, etc., and also reflective practice, significant event analysis and clinical audit, etc.

■ instructions, procedures, duties and the like are reviewed and rewritten to better reflect the principles of Clinical Governance.

5. Demonstrable continuous improvement

5.1 At first reading this appears to be a simple aim. In reality it could be one of the most challenging aspects of clinical governance. Measurement is implicit in the phrase.

5.2 Audit (healthcare performance measurement) is:

> The systematic, critical analysis of the quality of (health) care, including the procedures for diagnosis and treatment, the use of resources, and the resulting outcome and quality of life for the patient.

Secretary of State for Health (1989); Cmd 555; Working for Patients London, HMSO.

5.3 Measurement, especially in the form of 'audit', with its undertones of financial control and being called to account, can produce negative feelings. The reality can all too readily become censorious and dispiriting; a focus for sanction and discontent; a means of only searching for errors and a tool for monitoring deviations from contractual norms.

5.4 Instead the Trust should deploy the 'kaizen' approach of Japanese industry at its most successful. Instead of sanction there should be a sense of discovery, pride and achievement brought about by creative leadership. It should provide encouragement and education to improve performance.

5.5 Together with others, if the NDPCT is to be scientific in its orientation and honesty, it must become creative in its search for good standards and apt measurement and remain its own sternest critic in searching for error without undue blame and sanction.

5.6 Donabedian, perhaps the most influential theorist in the field of healthcare quality assurance, believes every healthcare-related activity can be divided into: Structure; Process; Outcome (Donabedian, 1990):

■ structure refers to the physical and personal resources of an organisation and is probably the easiest to measure. The presence of structural attributes increases the chances of good quality care but does not assure it;

■ process describes the actions taken by all those involved in the aspect of care. It is what is done for the patient and reflects the knowledge, skills and attitudes that lie behind that action;

■ outcomes are the definitive indicators of the effectiveness of healthcare and are difficult to measure especially in primary care and mental health services.

5.7 Each of the NDPCT healthcare sites and teams is unique and brings to the PCT a rich diversity of experience, talent and expertise – and problems! Measurements of quality and performance should be flexible enough to accommodate this. Different sites and teams will develop at different rates at different times. The patient has a right to expect reasonable timely, seamless care to a common high standard but the Clinical Governance Subcommittee may need to remember the requirement for the Trust to be a cost-effective, flexible, responsive, sensitive and caring organisation.

5.8 Measurement in the context of assessment can be looked at as opposite ends of continuum, as set out below.

Formative		Summative
Informal		Formal
Continuous		Terminal
Process		Outcome
Divergent		Convergent
Quantitative		Qualitative
Case-Specific		Generic
Objective		Subjective
Direct		Indirect
Definitive		Abstract
Criterion-Referenced	Norm-Referenced	Self-Referenced
Internally derived		Externally derived

5.9 When drawing up the Clinical Governance agenda and development plans the Clinical Governance Subcommittee should bear in mind the following guiding principles (Rowntree, 1987):

- assessment should motivate teams and sites to achieve and should judge the efficacy of any facilitation being applied;
- goals etc., should be realistic and achievable with the resources to hand;
- measurement and assessment should execute a diagnostic function not one of sanction;
- assessment criteria should be varied and appropriate;
- affirm:
  - □ why assess
  - □ what to assess
  - □ how to assess
  - □ how to interpret
  - □ how to respond
- with all its faults the divergent assessment that reflects the real decision-making processes of the professional, individual or team,

that are competent and reliable, and that are executed in context and culture, are usually more preferable and meaningful within an organisation than the convergent assessment based on objective criteria and standards preferred by external authority.

Measures

5.10 The Clinical Governance Subcommittee should develop:

- a growing central portfolio of clinical governance activity;
- registers of clinical audit and clinical effectiveness activity;
- seamless continuity of clinical governance development over successive years; (The Three Year Clinical Governance Plan will support this);
- a model or profile of Trust clinical governance performance;
- an ever evolving picture of that model or profile;
- a continuous assessment of the strengths and weaknesses of the healthcare sites and teams that constitute the Trust;
- the ability to take a snapshot of the model or profile at any time;
- systems whereby measurement and assessment information is accrued and evaluated throughout the year and so avoids peaks at busy times;
- a range of targets, indicators, trends, standards and criteria as appropriate for use in the model or profile. Creativity will be required.

6. Mobilisation

6.1 Like so much else, the keys to a successful regime of clinical governance will be vision, inspiring leadership and sound management. Leaders and their teams to be galvanised into uniting behind an outward corporate aspiration to serve the local population with unrelenting vigour and application.

6.2 Prior to the current reforms, many managers and leaders retired to the comforts of the administrative element of their roles, which largely served the internal bureaucracy of the NHS. Many now need encouragement to resume their outward leadership function and in particular to develop a pioneering spirit in relation to clinical governance.

6.3 The organisation needs to build a body of clinical governance knowledge that is embodied first in the actions of practitioners and then in the knowledge that informs those actions. Currently clinical governance remains as an end in itself in the eyes of many; an onerous additional chore. In reality, it is a means to an end; a performance management tool.

6.4 Certainly as far as its principles and subjective perspectives are concerned both doctors and nurses are largely familiar with the activities and elements that make up Clinical Governance (see 'The Patient Experience'). They have been part of education and professional health service literature for some time. However, until very recently, there has been reluctance to acknowledge the objectives and objective perspectives of Clinical Governance. There has been a reluctance to put theory into practice and where implementation has occurred there has been a tendency to protect practitioners from reality. Implementation has not always been rigorously consolidated nor linked to services and outcomes for patients.

6.5 Traditionally, doctors have been able to be reasonably collectivist in their approach to healthcare whilst nurses have remained steadfastly individualist. Both have distanced and protected themselves from open empirical measurement, assessment and comparison.

6.6 Thus there are significant cultural barriers to creating the 'environment' of Clinical Governance (para. 2.1).

6.7 This 'environment' will have to be worked for and leaders emboldened with the ability and confidence to really lead and engage with Clinical Governance.

6.8 Measures:

- in the shorter term, the provision of as much technical facilitation and day-to-day management of clinical governance as the Trust thinks it can afford;
- the creation of an on-going training and facilitation programme for appropriate leaders and managers that complements the Trust's Management Development Programme. The new programme to focus on renewing familiarity and building ability in relation to implementing clinical governance by means of successive, specific action plans that gradually and progressively move the teams towards real achievements;
- annual job reviews to specifically review and evaluate the individual's engagement with Clinical Governance and their commitment to its objectives and principles;
- a review of job descriptions and duties throughout the Trust to better reflect the principles and objectives of Clinical Governance;
- more regular and effective critical feedback to teams specifically and the organisation in general;
- provision of regular and attractive newsletters for Clinical Governance in general and Prescribing in particular;
- all new service, practice and activity to have objective clinical governance built in at the outset;

▪ an insistence that managers and leaders always set clinical governance in context; that 'structure' and 'process' are always supported by a demonstrable focus on 'outcome'.

7. Conclusions

7.1 Once its definition is left behind, Clinical Governance remains a difficult concept for individual health practitioners to grasp and most certainly a challenging management process for any NHS organisation.

7.2 Nevertheless, the organisation that successfully meets that challenge is almost certainly going to be a successful and happy organisation all round. No wonder the Commission for Health Improvement bases its reviews on a clinical governance framework. The ability and capacity of the organisation, to lead and manage all aspects of clinical governance satisfactorily, almost certainly guarantees mastery in other areas.

7.3 Managed well, Clinical Governance can be a significant bonding agent in the development of an esprit de corps. Managed badly it could be divisive and corrosive.

7.4 Clinical Governance all but embodies the whole purpose of the Trust. With its ultimate aims of achieving patient satisfaction and assuring the quality of service outcomes, it supports the outward orientation of the Trust and works against any tendency to focus inward to structures, process and general bureaucracy. Patient satisfaction should be the function of every role and the purpose of every job.

8. Review

8.1 This strategy is to be reviewed by the Clinical Governance Subcommittee annually.

Barbara Merricks Director of Primary and Community Services. January 2003

Monitoring Performance and Organisational Quality Assurance

11

Chapter Contents:

- performance indicators
- the NHS Performance Assessment Framework
- NHS performance ratings
- star ratings
- standards for Better Health
- benchmarking
- Essence of Care
- Essence of Care – A Project Manager's Experience
- Organisation-wide Measurement of Quality
- Total Quality Management (TQM)/Continuous Quality Improvement (CQI)
- accreditation.

Performance Indicators

Performance indicators were introduced into the health service in September 1983 and developed to measure and indicate the efficiency and effectiveness of an organisation. These indicators were grouped under the headings of clinical activity, finance, manpower, support services and estate management. They consist of numerical values which assess certain aspects of a system. When they were first introduced it would be fair to say that neither health authorities nor professionals were very interested in them. However, the planning and financial departments used them with more enthusiasm. In 1985, 1986 and 1988 new performance indicators were introduced and used more widely as new initiatives such as resource management and medical audit were implemented by the Government.

Performance indicators are used by managers to assist them to review systems and examine results both within their own organisation and externally against the results of other organisations. They are often seen as a centralist tool where poor performance can be identified and managers held accountable for their performance. Performance indicators may be held in the following areas:

- service provision such as activity levels, actual versus targeted performance, targets such as numbers of hip operations, waiting times, list sizes, pressure ulcer prevalence indicators and infection rates
- manpower and financial controls
- human resource management.

Vetter (1986) successfully applied performance indicators in the care of the elderly and Caddow (1986) used performance indicators in the area of infection control. However, Reid (1986) felt that performance indicators posed more questions than answers but stressed that computerised performance indicators, such as the DHSS package relevant to clinical activity, can be useful analytical tools but should not be used in isolation from other information.

The purpose of measuring performance is:

- to improve the health of the population
- to provide better care and outcomes for people who use the NHS.

It also supports the link between service agreements with the clinical work carried out by clinicians, and provides a structure for meetings between local healthcare providers by focusing on specific areas. The framework uses indicators of measurement. The Joint Commission on Accreditation of Healthcare Organisations (JCAHO, 1990) defines an indicator as

> a quantitative measure that can be used to monitor and evaluate the quality of important governance, management, clinical and support functions that effect patient outcomes ... an indicator is not a direct measure of quality. Rather a tool that can be used to assess performance and that can direct attention to issues that may require more intense review.

The NHS Performance Assessment Framework

The NHS Plan (DoH, 2000) put forward the idea of a system to measure NHS organisations to help the public make a judgement about the performance of NHS trusts in England. The NHS Performance Assessment Framework identifies six main areas in which to measure performance, which includes the following indicators:

■ health improvement
■ fair access
■ effective delivery of appropriate care
■ user/carer experience
■ health outcome of NHS care.

The Framework assesses NHS services across:

■ a population group and as an ethnic group or geographical area
■ a condition or client group such as coronary heart disease, diabetes, older people, children
■ a service organisation such as an NHS trust or PCT.

The Framework is continuously developed in line with government policy indicators. At the time of writing there are 49 indicators which are linked to the National Service Frameworks, those based on the outcomes of the national survey of NHS patients and primary care indicators (NHS Executive, 2000). See also Tables 11.1, 11.2 and 11.3.

All these indicators are based on statistics which are collected through the Common Information Core, Cancer Registries, Waiting Times Returns, the

---

Table 11.1 NHS Performance Indicators – health authority levels (2000)

1 *Health improvement*
  ■ Deaths from all causes (for people aged 15–64)
  ■ Deaths from all causes (for people aged 65–74)
  ■ Deaths from cancer
  ■ Deaths from all circulatory diseases
  ■ Suicide rates
  ■ Deaths from accidents
  ■ Deaths from injury from accidents

2 *Fair access*
  ■ In-patient waiting list
  ■ Adult dental registrations
  ■ Early detection of cancer
  ■ Number of GPs
  ■ Practice availability
  ■ Elective surgery rates
  ■ Surgery rates – coronary heart disease

3 *Effective delivery of appropriate health care*
  ■ Childhood immunisations
  ■ Inappropriately used surgery
  ■ Acute care management
  ■ Chronic care management
  ■ Mental health in primary care

Table 11.2 NHS Performance Indicators – trust levels (2000)

1 *Effective delivery of appropriate health care*
 ■ Returning home following treatment for a stroke
 ■ Returning home following treatment for a fractured hip

2 *Health outcomes of NHS health care*
 ■ 28 day emergency readmission
 ■ In-hospital premature deaths (30-day perioperative mortality – emergency admission)
 ■ In-hospital premature deaths (30-day perioperative mortality – non-emergency admission)
 ■ In-hospital premature deaths (30-day mortality following acute myocardial infarction)
 ■ Deaths following fractured neck of femur

Table 11.3 NHS Performance Indicators – primary care trusts

Area	Example indicator
Key targets	Percentage of patients offered an appointment to see a GP within two working days. Number of patients waiting more than 26 weeks for an outpatient appointment.
Access to quality services	Emergency readmissions to hospital following a stroke Percentage of patients with HIV appropriately receiving highly active anti-retroviral therapy.
Improving health	Death rates from circulatory disease Percentage of patients aged 25–64 yrs screened for cervical cancer
Service provision	Emergency admission rates for asthma and diabetes Percentage of resolution of patient complaints within four weeks.

Prescription Pricing Authority, the Office for National Statistics, and so on. Data collected around these indicators gives trusts the opportunity to benchmark their performance against other trusts.

NHS Performance Ratings

NHS performance ratings were proposed in the NHS Plan as a system of measurement to help the public assess the performance of the NHS trusts.

(DoH, 2000). The Government sets the priorities and targets and the Healthcare Commission develops the methodology and publishes the ratings. See Chapter 1 for more information on the Healthcare Commission. The targets cover the key areas of the NHS Plan including:

- waiting times
- cancelled operations
- hospital cleanliness.

Star Ratings

At present the star ratings are given based on the trust performance against targets and the reports from the CHI (now known as the Healthcare Commission) reviews. Some of the performance ratings are based on the performance indicators. Trusts are rated in four categories:

- three stars – trusts with the highest levels of performance
- two stars – trusts that are performing well overall, but have not quite reached consistently high standards
- one star – trusts which generate cause for concern
- zero stars – trusts which have shown the poorest levels of performance (DoH, 2001).

The Healthcare Commission performance ratings continued for 2003/04 and 2005/06 based on the criteria published at the end of November 2003. However, the Healthcare Commission plan to consult during Autumn 2004 with a view to changing the system.

Standards for Better Health

Standards for Better Health (DoH, 2004) is a consultation document which was published in February 2004 and the consultation period ended in May 2004. The basis of this document is set out in Chapter 1. There are two sets of standards and, as John Reid, Secretary of State for Health, explains in the document:

- the standards are easier to understand and apply. There are 24 core standards which are intended to establish a level of quality of care which can be expected by all NHS patients, regardless of where they are treated. The effect will be that, in meeting each core standard, NHS services will find themselves in compliance with what should be happening in the NHS

■ the second group of standards are developmental standards. They are designed to enable the overall quality of healthcare to rise as the additional resources being invested in the NHS take effect. They are broad, they recognise new trends in healthcare, and new public attitudes to, and expectations of, the service we offer. They express our aim for the long-term quality of healthcare in England, and our ambition for a service that pursues quality improvement on a continuous basis

■ the consultation document offers people an opportunity to make their views known through a consultation process which ended in May 2004.

The suggested timescales are for formal publication of standards and for the English NHS bodies and cross-border SHAs to take the standards into account in 2004/05. The Healthcare Commission inspection programme will be based on the new criteria to be rolled out in 2005/06 and for the Healthcare Commission to assign and publish ratings based on criteria developed for the Secretary of State's standards in 2006/07. See also Chapter 1.

Benchmarking

Benchmarking can be traced back to the early Egyptians when they used rigorous quality control measures in the building of their pyramids (Zairi, 1999). Modern-day benchmarking has its roots in industry; one of the first experts in quality control or Total Quality Management was W. Edwards Deming.

During the 1990s a number of Benchmarking Clubs were set up and a number of NHS healthcare organisations of similar size, population and activity collected data. Aspects of the service where data were being collected routinely included length of stay, infection rates, staff sick levels, turnover rates, numbers and skill-mix, etc. These data were then compared and a hospital or healthcare organisation could see where they were placed against the others in the group. At the time this was a very useful tool to establish whether your hospital was in line with others and, if not, whether there was an acceptable reason for this or whether the hospital should work towards the club benchmark. This was a useful exercise to an extent but as there was no measurement of outcomes, the benchmark was based on what was common practice rather than best practice.

In 1999 *Making a Difference* (DoH, 1999) acknowledged that the majority of patient care in the UK was excellent but some was below an acceptable standard. Reports from the Health Advisory Service and Health Service Commissioner identified that areas which were often neglected were fundamental and essential aspects of patient care, including the main elements of care essential to a patient's wellbeing, recovery to health or dignified death. These fundamentals are still key issues within healthcare and continue to attract media coverage, the latest being the right to food and nutrition, with suggestions that the law may be changed to make it illegal for patients to be denied these essentials, whether it be hydrating though the subcutaneous or intravenous routes as appropriate or ensuring that when, for example, patients are asleep during a mealtime their nutritional needs are not neglected and food is given when they are awake. This often means a change in the approach to care where mealtimes are set times and there are no supplementary foods available for those who do not or are unable to conform to the set timeframes. *Making a Difference* (DoH, 1999) identified benchmarking as one way in which standards could be raised.

Benchmarking was defined by the National Benchmarking Club as 'using structured comparisons to define and implement good practice'. It is the practice of a formal comparison of processes and systems with those of other organisations as the basis for improvement. It can be used internally by comparing similar processes and outcomes or externally between organisations looking at the same areas of clinical care, for example lengths of stay for specific groups of patient such as those undergoing a hip replacement, or to benchmark staffing numbers and skill-mix, staff sickness and absence rates, cost per case, and so on. The technique for benchmarking is:

- to identify key characteristics to be benchmarked; for example in an accident and emergency department, an area for benchmarking might be door-to-needle time for thrombolysis treatment for a patient diagnosed with a myocardial infarction
- identify partners (similar size accident and emergency department, number of patients per year, number of staff, and location such as urban)
- to design data collection methodology (if the department has a computerised accident and emergency system then the key times, such as the time the patient arrived in the department, the time seen by a doctor, the time thrombolysis commenced, and so on, are likely to be recorded)
- to select tools such as process mapping
- to implement changes.

Benchmarking concentrates on understanding processes and putting right any points of failure in the care or system being benchmarked. It uses performance indicators and comparative databases to identify best practice and performance gaps. Overall, benchmarking requires senior management commitment, particularly in supporting actions arising from the results, and subsequent exploration. It requires staff to be trained and guided through the process to ensure that maximum benefit be obtained. It requires time resource to enable the process to be completed.

Essence of Care – A Project Manager's Experience

Carole Annetts is a project manager for North Dorset PCT and South and West Dorset PCT and has been responsible for the implementation of Essence of Care (DoH, 2001) in the Community Hospitals within these two PCTs. In the information that follows Carole describes the essential elements of Essence of Care and the process of implementing it across the PCT.

Background

Essence of Care was originally designed and promoted as a tool to improve nursing care. The standards set within it have implications for all healthcare

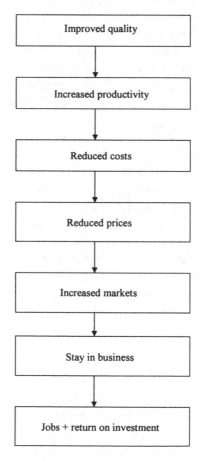

Figure 11.1 Increasing efficiency and competitiveness
Source: Deming, 1986

and support staff in all care settings and should be viewed as a multi-professional/multi-agency tool.

When the NHS was created in 1948, national standards of care were not thought to be necessary. It was generally believed that standards of care for patients would rise automatically all over the country and so it was left to individual health authorities to set the required standard to be achieved (DoH, 2000). However, in reality many professional groups carried out their own evaluations of treatment and care, which over time has lead to a healthcare system often described as a 'postcode lottery', Different values of care and access to treatment have multiplied, often dependent on the preferences of key individuals rather than a need for the most efficacious care and treatments. The Government through the NHS Plan (DoH, 2000) identified this approach to care as being unacceptable in the twenty-first century and planned to 'reduce the unjustified variations and achieve a truly National health service'. As stated earlier in this chapter, benchmarking has its roots in industry, and one of the experts, Deming, developed a model of continuous quality improvement which became known as the Deming (1986) cycle or the PDCA (Plan, Do, Check (study), Act) Cycle. The four phases of this process underpin Essence of Care (see Figure 1.6).

Table 11.4 Healthcare processes

Improve quality	All patient care delivered is evidence-based – ritualistic practice disappears. Care is patient-centred and organisational systems support this approach.
Increased productivity	Delivering evidence-based care enables staff to work efficiently and effectively: 'the Right Person is carrying out the Right Care to the Right Patient at the Right Time' (DoH?)
Reduced costs	Staff time and resources are being used effectively.
Reduced prices	All services have been reviewed and streamlined to work at effective levels not unsafe levels.
Markets increased	Greater opportunity to provide services responsive to patient need and attract more funding to develop new services.
Jobs and return on investment	Job satisfaction, motivation and morale is increased, healthcare staff are working collaboratively for the benefit of the patient. Patient satisfaction increases as they receive high-quality and timely care.

Source: Zairi, 2000

At that time, in industry, Deming saw the need for and the importance of relevant research linked to regular customer-satisfaction surveys and close observations of changes within the marketplace. He saw these as 'pillars' of change which, when supported by effective planning and the implementation of the plan, enabled an increase in efficiency and competitiveness. Deming saw the process as set out in Figure 11.1. In healthcare this process could be translated (Zairi, 1999) as set out in Table 11.4.

Benchmarking in the public sector is relatively new and there are two main approaches to benchmarking:

- *metric (performance) benchmarking*: a quantitative process which helps Organisations to compare performance data such as staffing and sickness levels
- *process benchmarking*: a qualitative approach where there is 'systematic analysis and comparison of the processes used to deliver services' (Audit Commission, 2000).

Using the Essence of Care Benchmarking Tool

There are eight standards within the toolkit:

- principles of self-care
- personal and oral hygiene
- food and nutrition
- continence and bladder and bowel care
- pressure ulcers
- safety of clients/patients with mental health needs in acute mental health and general hospital settings
- record-keeping
- privacy and dignity.

The Essence of Care manual sets out the benchmarking process along the lines of Deming's PDCA model. It is divided into seven phases, as seen in Figure 11.2.

The first step is to identify an area of practice to benchmark and then form a comparison group. This group is made up of healthcare staff and non-healthcare staff, as appropriate, who come together to compare and share best practice and to agree practice which constitutes an 'A' (excellent) score. The members of this group can be diverse but all have a common interest or expertise in the standard being benchmarked or are the stakeholders. The information included in the manual shows that comparison groups can be

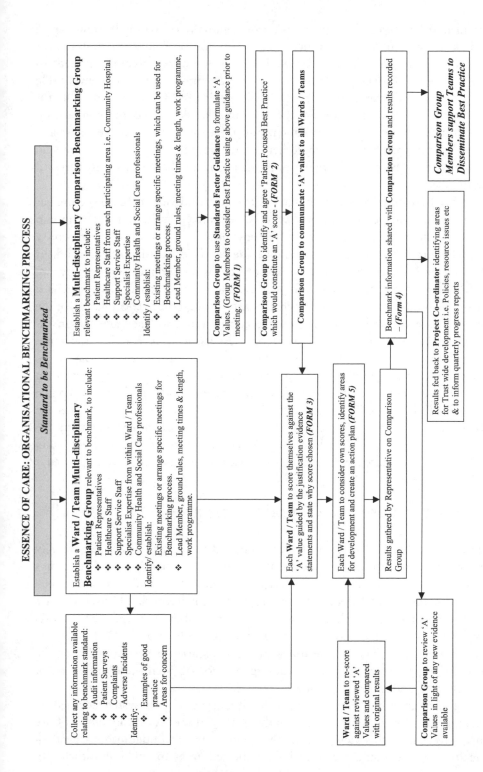

ESSENCE OF CARE: ORGANISATIONAL BENCHMARKING PROCESS

Standard to be Benchmarked

Collect any information available relating to benchmark standard:
❖ Audit information
❖ Patient Surveys
❖ Complaints
❖ Adverse Incidents
Identify:
❖ Examples of good practice
❖ Areas for concern

Establish a **Ward / Team Multi-disciplinary Benchmarking Group** relevant to benchmark, to include:
❖ Patient Representatives
❖ Healthcare Staff
❖ Support Service Staff
❖ Specialist Expertise from within Ward / Team
❖ Community Health and Social Care professionals
Identify/ establish:
❖ Existing meetings or arrange specific meetings for Benchmarking process.
❖ Lead Member, ground rules, meeting times & length, work programme.

Establish a **Multi-disciplinary Comparison Benchmarking Group** relevant to benchmark to include:
❖ Patient Representatives
❖ Healthcare Staff from each participating area i.e. Community Hospital
❖ Support Service Staff
❖ Specialist Expertise
❖ Community Health and Social Care professionals
Identify / establish:
❖ Existing meetings or arrange specific meetings, which can be used for Benchmarking process.
❖ Lead Member, ground rules, meeting times & length, work programme,

Comparison Group to use **Standards Factor Guidance** to formulate 'A' Values. (Group Members to consider Best Practice using above guidance prior to meeting. *(FORM 1)*

Comparison Group to identify and agree 'Patient Focused Best Practice' which would constitute an 'A' score - *(FORM 2)*

Comparison Group to communicate 'A' values to all Wards / Teams

Each **Ward / Team** to score themselves against the 'A' value guided by the justification evidence statements and state why score chosen *(FORM 3)*

Each Ward / Team to consider own scores, identify areas for development and create an action plan *(FORM 5)*

Results gathered by Representative on Comparison Group

Benchmark information shared with **Comparison Group** and results recorded – *(Form 4)*

Results fed back to **Project Co-ordinator** identifying areas for Trust wide development i.e. Policies, resource issues etc & to inform quarterly progress reports

Comparison Group Members support Teams to Disseminate Best Practice

Ward / Team to re-score against reviewed 'A' Values and compared with original results

Comparison Group to review 'A' Values in light of any new evidence available

Figure 11.2 The seven phases of the benchmarking process

formed at any level of an organisation or regionally or nationally, comparing and sharing at all levels. Consumer representation is of utmost importance at every level and stage of the process. The inclusion of representatives needs to be handled sensitively, as many staff and patients find it an uncomfortable experience to discuss and review the delivery of care. One way would be for patient focus groups to review the benchmarks as well as the comparison group initially in a safe environment and then share the outcomes, agreeing best practice together. This would help to integrate the two points of view and establish trust between the two groups achieving a collaborative way forward for subsequent benchmarking.

After best practice has been agreed, teams or individuals score themselves against the evidence statements, which constitute 'A' values. The continuum or scale ranges from 'E' (poor) to 'A' (best practice). The team must identify which score it has attained, providing evidence which justifies why it thinks it has achieved the chosen score. Essence of Care is not a punitive process where all 'E' scores are disciplined for providing a poor standard of care; it is a growth and development model where staff, through the cyclical nature of the process, see themselves moving up the continuum until they achieve an 'A' score. Following scoring, each team considers its own score and carries out a gap analysis, focusing on the areas which need most attention and sharing its experiences and practices where it has achieved high scores. Each team then develops an action plan and with an implementation timeframe to enable practice to develop. The loop of the benchmarking cycle is closed when the benchmarking cycle is repeated at an agreed time, commencing with the review of current best evidence and proceeding through the process again when it is anticipated that the quality of care provided will have improved.

Essence of Care and Clinical Governance

The importance of Essence of Care within healthcare has slowly but steadily risen up the healthcare agenda; its move into the Modernisation Agency has assured that its prominence has never been greater. John Badham the national co-ordinator for the Essence of Care Programme, believes that Essence of Care is the foundation of clinical governance and often uses the CHI (2002) definition of clinical governance to emphasise the point: 'A framework through which NHS organisations and their staff are accountable for the quality of patient care. It covers the organisations' systems and processes for monitoring and improving patient services.'

Clinical governance may be seen as a quality assurance system focused on management systems rather than on the quality of the service. Essence of Care helps to redress this view, linking the quantitative and qualitative aspects of healthcare. It encompasses four interconnected areas to enable healthcare to

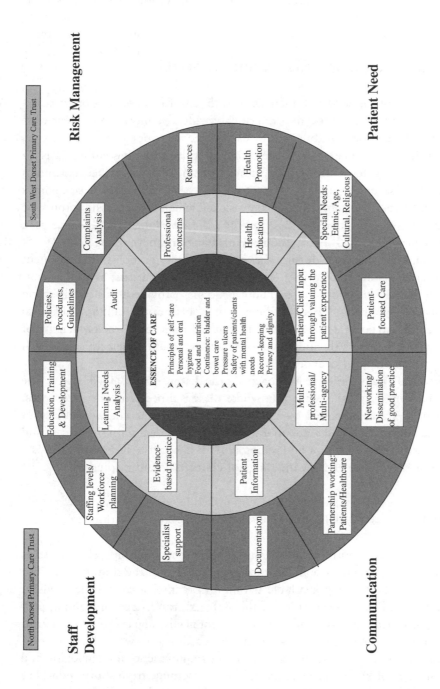

Figure 11.3 Essence of Care: clinical governance in practice

Source: Lang, 1976

develop collaboratively and effectively. These areas can be seen as risk management, staff development, patient need and communication, as set out in Figure 11.3.

Essence of Care and Risk Management

Essence of Care supports risk management though the identification of issues from the complaints procedures, critical-incident analysis and near-miss analysis. These issues can be used for each standard to identify best practice, which helps to eliminate any further complaints of the same nature. It is an opportunity to review existing support mechanisms such as policies, guidelines and protocols, and to update to meet current best evidence. These updates and adjustments then filter though the risk management process and provide evidence to patients and to the trust board that clinical governance is a dynamic process, which is continuously evolving and developing.

Information gathered during the benchmarking and risk management processes assists in the identification of professional concerns, as well as considering the patient point of view. Both processes provide a positive learning experience supporting the development of a blame-free culture and with Essence of Care being a self-assessment or team assessment, the ownership of the outcomes lies with the individual or team, making it a proactive approach to the management of change.

Where an organisational approach to the Essence of Care is taken, the benchmarking process may identify where there is a need for extra resources. This can then be addressed on an organisational basis. The availability of accurate information and a collaborative strength to deal with the issues, and with a variety of both junior and senior staff taking part ensures that there is a wealth of knowledge and a wide range of contacts to aid resolution.

Essence of Care and Staff Development

One of the most important considerations when benchmarking the standards from a staff development point of view is an analysis of the training gap. The gap between the training available within an organisation, and the needs of the patient and the current skills of the staff. All too often the training provided is historical and not responsive to current needs. The information gained during the benchmarking process should be used in two ways. First, to provide the organisation with baseline training requirements for clinicians and non-clinicians alike for each standard. These may range from short updates to postgraduate courses. Healthcare personnel have rarely considered whether the skills they attain are the skills which the patient views as essential.

Nurses may be able to perform minor surgery as an extended role but what the patient may see as most important is excellent communication and customer service skills. Second, if the baseline skills are identified (they should be multi-professional and include the medical profession) and available for all to view, then individuals and teams can carry out a self-assessment to identify the discrepancy and access the relevant training through the appraisal or individual performance review process. Teams are then able to provide their organisation with an accurate training-needs analysis, which has taken minimal time to produce and accurately reflects the true training requirements of the team.

Essence of Care and Communication

It could be argued that communication is a fundamental element of health-care. However, poor communication is the cause of the majority of incidents and complaints within the health service. When Essence of Care was developed it was thought that communication ran through each of the eight benchmarks and that a separate benchmark was not required. However, in 2002 a ninth benchmark has been added and addresses two aspects of communication: that between carers and healthcare personnel and that between patients/clients and healthcare personnel.

Clarity and accuracy of documentation and availability of up-to-date rationalised and well-presented information were all areas of concern raised during the benchmarking process. When teams come together to benchmark, they often find that the organisation is producing different information on the same subject because each unit makes its own or has seen someone else's example. This is an opportunity to decide organisationally which information gives patients confidence in its accuracy and quality. The same issues occur with documentation where several variations of the same form are in use. Rationalisation, where appropriate, ensures familiarity between units when staff interchange or when bank and agency staff are used and guarantees that they are evidence-based.

The importance of sharing information has already been discussed. However, the vehicle for doing this effectively is not so clear. One method is networking, a technique not well used by most healthcare professionals, and yet a concept which has been incorporated into many government documents over the last decade or more (NHSE, 1994). If healthcare professionals are to meet the requirements of the Government's ambitious modernisation programme, then the development of networking skills is essential. Networking is seen as having five main functions:

- building good relationships
- exchanging information

- achieving greater understanding of your organisation
- increasing productivity through clinical effectiveness
- developing skills and careers.

It now needs to be recognised as a formal component of learning, not just a peripheral, social activity; a proactive approach to enable healthcare staff to respond to the evidence-based challenge, which has arisen from the Government's drive for clinical effectiveness.

Essence of Care and Patient Need

How often do staff have the opportunity to stop and really consider whether the care that they provide within their service is the care that their patients currently need or will need in the future? With ever-changing demographics, it is necessary to consider what the health needs of the population within the team's catchment area services will be. The increasing elderly and multi-cultural populations, the 24-hour society and the expert patient all require careful consideration as to how their needs will be met. Essence of Care may be a useful tool to support future team developments. Patient Advice and Liaison Services (PALS) are excellent sources of information on patient need; they are seen as the catalyst for change and improvement within the NHS, they are the patients' and carers' advocate and they are a source valuable information and feedback to organisations to enable them to provide responsive services aligned to patient need. It is this information and feedback which will play an important part in identifying gaps in service provision and helping to evolve a plan for future services. Patient and carer involvement is integral to each stage of the Essence of Care benchmarking process.

Once current and future healthcare needs have been identified, then health education and health promotion programmes can be reassessed to ensure that they meet the identified need. The longer-term view, perhaps through rose-tinted spectacles, is that careful planning and linking of health education and health promotion to the benchmarking process will improve the wellbeing of the population, reduce the pressure on current services and reallocate resources to new services.

Essence of Care – A Personal Account

As Project Manager for Essence of Care, I had listened to a presentation on how to develop a benchmark and the Essence of Care processes. However, there was a lack of clarity about how to take forward the process and about timeframes, and concern as to whether the format in the manual had to be adhered to rigidly, as well as lots of other questions.

The manual was daunting: lots of words and no pictures. My first step was to try to translate the folder into a more meaningful tool. I could already see the value of the information contained within, but found it difficult to explain the process to other people. I was regularly asked to give presentations and found it extremely difficult to present the process with any clarity, which was confirmed as the eyes of the audience glazed over. I could not see how the process affected their patients or themselves. Many staff saw it as a nursing tool, a hospital tool which did not affect large chunks of the organisation. How wrong they were! Essence of Care has something for everyone, clinical or non-clinical.

I then produced two packs, one for comparison groups explaining their role and the process, and developing simple pre-meeting preparation sheets so that when the comparison group had its first meeting it could hit the ground running. A similar pack was developed for benchmarking teams, taking them through the process and providing them with supportive documentation to make the whole process more understandable. See Figures 11.4 and 11.5.

A major step forward for the communication of Essence of Care was when I was asked to provide a poster presentation at the forthcoming Nurses' Day Conference on Celebrating Best Practice. Displaying the content of the folder would attract few visitors to my stand, so in desperation I developed an A4 leaflet relating to each benchmark. These have proved exceedingly popular not only locally but also regionally and nationally.

I decided to focus the first benchmarks on the community hospitals within our organisations and to use the matrons' meetings for each organisation as key meetings to take the process forward. One group chose to undertake the continence benchmark and the other chose the privacy and dignity benchmark. See Figure 11.6.

The continence benchmark was enormous and had major issues, and with hindsight was probably not the best one to start with. However, the outcomes of the process enabled me to review and modify the format. The main issues identified in the continence benchmark were first a disparity between the training available for staff and the actual training required and secondly the need for rationalised patient documentation. The continence team were keen to implement a care pathway. However, there was reluctance from ward staff who saw it as a lengthy process. Through the benchmarking process the ward teams and the continence service are now piloting the pathway and are beginning to see a change in the standards of care provided.

Essence of Care is not a panacea for the improvement of care; there are blocks which need to be overcome. Time is a major factor; being in a rural area means that getting to a meeting takes time and incurs cost, and time is also needed to complete the benchmark. Motivation is another issue and, although I have spent time with staff explaining the benefits of the tool, many perceive it as yet another piece of work to be done on top of an already busy schedule. Staff

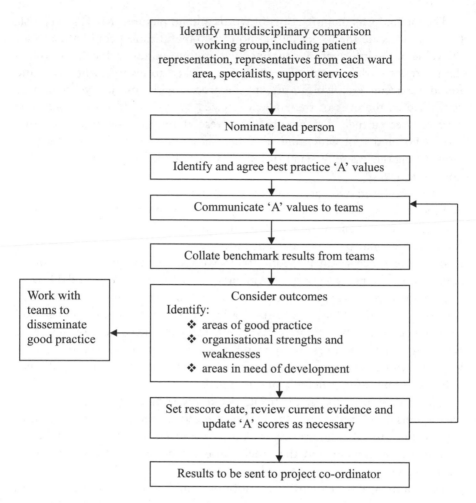

Figure 11.4 Benchmarking process – comparison group action

are often unable to see that a release of time may be one positive outcome if care is rationalised, systems reviewed and outmoded care discarded.

Although Essence of Care has been included in the organisation's risk management and clinical governance strategies, it is still perceived as a nursing tool. However, within the draft ninth benchmark is a very useful tool which I plan to use as an organisation assessment tool to ensure that Essence of Care is embedded within all organisational processes. I am hopeful that this document will make the transition from draft to formal document. It covers the following areas:

- consultation and patient involvement
- clinical risk management

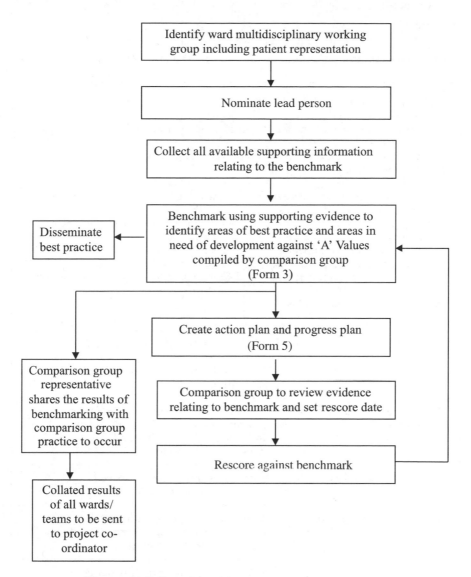

Figure 11.5 Benchmarking process – ward action

■ clinical audit
■ research and effectiveness
■ use of information about the patient experience
■ staffing and staff management
■ education, training and continuing personal and professional development
■ strategic capacity.

Carole Annetts, Project Manager, North Dorset PCT and South and West Dorset PCT, 2003

Standard 4

PRIVACY AND DIGNITY

Privacy = Freedom from intrusion   Dignity = Being worthy of respect

Agreed Patient–Client Focused Outcome
Patients/clients benefit from care that is focused upon respect for the individual
Indicators/information that highlights concerns which may trigger the need for benchmarking activity:

Patient/client satisfaction surveys Complaints figures and analysis Patient/client diary analysis Audit results of related policies/ standards, e.g. environmental audits, accommodation audits, pastoral care audits, interpreter usage Patient's Charter/Guide audits Risk assessments	Educational audits/student placement feedback Litigation/Clinical Negligence Scheme for Trusts Professional concerns Media reports Commission for Health Improvements reports

FACTOR	BENCHMARK OF BEST PRACTICE
1. Attitudes and behaviours	Patients/clients *feel that they matter* all of the time
2. Personal world/personal identity	Patients/clients experience care in an environment that *actively encompasses* individual values, beliefs and personal relationships
3. Personal boundaries/space	Patients'/clients' personal space is *actively promoted by all staff*
4. Communicating with patients/clients	Communication between patients/clients takes place in a *manner which respects their individuality*
5. Privacy of patient – confidentiality of client information	Patient/client information is *shared to enable care*, with their *consent*
6. Privacy, dignity and modesty	Patients'/clients' care *actively promotes their privacy and dignity, and protects their modesty*
7. Availability of an area for complete privacy	Patients/clients/carers *can access* an area that safely provides privacy

Figure 11.6 Essence of Care – privacy and dignity standard
Source: DoH, 2001

Factor 1: Attitudes and behaviours

Patients/ clients experience *deliberate* negative and offensive attitude and behaviour	Patients/clients experience *thoughtless* behaviour and careless insensitive attitude	Patients/clients *experience a sensitive, empathetic attitude on an ad hoc basis* (at certain incidents/events)		Patients/clients feel that they *matter* all of the time
E	D	C	B	A

Statements to stimulate comparison group discussion around best practice:
State how effective leadership is assured
Describe how good attitudes and behaviour are promoted and assured (including consideration of non-verbal behaviour and body language)
State how these issues (including attitudes and behaviour towards minority groups, e.g. black and minority ethnic communities) are addressed with individual staff, e.g. induction programmes, preceptorship, Individual Performance Review/Appraisal
State the philosophy/strategies that support practice (e.g. mission statements)
State how patient/client views are sought and used e.g. focus groups, surveys, partnership strategies, feedback advocacy arrangements
State what policies are in place to address specific ethnic/cultural/religious/ spiritual/linguistic, age-related and particular needs
State the process for monitoring, feedback and actioning of complaints
State how partnerships with others will support the promotion of good attitudes and behaviours.

Factor 2: Personal world/personal identity

Patients'/ clients' individual values, beliefs and personal relationships are *never explored*	Patients'/clients' individual values, beliefs and personal relationships *are considered but not acted upon*	Patients/clients *experience care* from individual practitioners that is relevant, sensitive and responsive to individual values, beliefs and personal relationships		Patients/clients experience care in an environment that *actively encompasses* respect for individual values, beliefs and personal relationships
E	D	C	B	A

Figure 11.6 (*continued*)

Personal World: 'To look at a patient holistically: not only have they got physical needs, but social, spiritual and emotional needs, and they live in the context of who they are, their family, their lifestyle. All of that is going to affect how they respond to the illness they have.' (Liane Jones: *Handle with Care: a year in the life of 12 nurses*, 1995)

Statements to stimulate comparison group discussion around best practice:
State how stereotype views are challenged
State how the valuing of diversities is demonstrated
State how individuals needs and choices are ascertained and continuously reviewed
State education and training available to increase staff awareness
State what policies are in use regarding values and beliefs, e.g. religious, cultural, sexual, age and special needs equality

Factor 3: Personal boundaries/space

Patients'/ clients' personal boundaries are *deliberately invaded*	Patients'/clients' personal boundaries are *thoughtlessly invaded*	Patients'/clients' personal boundaries/space is *respected*	Patients'/clients' personal space is *actively promoted* by all staff
E	D C	B	A

(Link specifically to Privacy and Dignity – Factors 6 & 7)
Personal Space: Patient/client sets boundaries for psychological, physical, emotional and spiritual contact.

Statements to stimulate comparison group discussion around beat practice:
State how the name the patient/client wants to be called is agreed
State how the acceptability of personal contact (touch) is identified with individual patients/clients
State how the patient's/client's personal boundaries are identified and communicated to others (including the use of patient's own language)
State how personal space is respected and protected for individuals
State the philosophy of care and what policies and procedures, education and training are in place to prevent disturbing, interrupting patients, e.g. knocking before entering, sign on closed curtains requesting practitioners/professionals and staff seek permission of patient before entering

Figure 11.6 (*continued*)

State how privacy is effectively maintained, e.g. curtains, screens, walls, rooms, use of blankets, appropriate clothing, appropriate positioning of patient, etc.

State the provision of single-sex facilities, access to separate toilet and washing facilities, age-specific facilities

State how clinical risk is handled in relation to privacy

State how privacy is achieved at times when the presence of others is required

State what type of clothing is available for patients who cannot wear their own clothes, how is their modesty protected

State what policies are in place for patients to have access to their own clothes

State how modesty is achieved for those in transit to differing care environments

State policies in place for chaperoning of patients. State evidence of audit

Describe how the use of policies and procedures and evidence-based guidelines are audited

Factor 4: Communicating with patients/clients

Patient/clients are *communicated at*	Patients/clients are *communicated with* but the means of communication *fails to take into account their individual needs*	Communication between staff and patients/clients takes place in a *manner which respects their individuality*
E	D C B	A

Communicated at: Talked at, talked over, assumptions made re the patient's level of understanding
Communicated with: Listened to, individual needs and views taken into account, respected as a person demonstrates caring and concern, correct pace and level and means, e.g. format verbal, signed, translated
Manner: How the communication takes place
Pace and level: Speed, repetition and explanation to ensure understanding

Statements to stimulate comparison group discussion around best practice:
State how patients'/clients' views and needs ascertained and recorded
State how special needs are met (e.g. ethnic/cultural needs, sensory and physical disability, age-related needs)
State access to translation and interpretation and how the quality is maintained

Figure 11.6 (*continued*)

State how information is adapted to meet the needs of individual patients
State the education, training and ongoing reflection opportunities that are in place to develop and enhance communication skills (including verbal and non-verbal communication and the use of interpreters) and state what records maintained

Factor 5: Privacy of patient – confidentiality of client information

Patients' /clients' information enters the public domain without their consent	Patients'/clients' information is shared *to enable care*, but without their consent	Patients'/clients' information is shared to enable care, *with* their consent
E	D	C	B	A

Note: this includes 'careless talk'
See benchmark on Record-Keeping for issues re written records, e.g. storage and access to documentation

Statements to stimulate comparison group discussion around best practice:
State how patient/client consent is sought to ensure informed and special measures to overcome communication barriers, e.g. use of trained interpreters
State how confidentiality is assured, e.g. policies in use
State the precautions that are taken to prevent information being shared e.g. telephone calls being overheard, computer screens being viewed, white-boards being read
State how confidentially is covered in multidisciplinary training and education, including induction programmes, preceptorship, supervision and PDPs
State procedures for sending/receiving patient information, e.g. handover procedures, consultant and/or teaching rounds, admissions procedures, telephone calls, calling patients in outpatients, breaking bad news, etc.
State evidence of audit of complaints and how matters of confidentiality are addressed

Factor 6: Privacy/dignity/modesty

Patients'/ clients' privacy, dignity and modesty are *not considered*	Patients'/clients' privacy, dignity arid modesty *is considered at times of care*/treatment interventions	Patient'/clients' privacy, dignity and modesty is considered at times of care/treatment *and on request*	Patients'/clients care *actively promotes* their privacy and dignity and *protects* their modesty
E	D	C	B	A

Figure 11.6 (*continued*)

Privacy: Freedom from intrusion
Dignity: Being worthy of respect
Modes: Not being embarrassed

Statements to stimulate comparison group discussion around best practice:
State the philosophy and strategies that exist to actively promote privacy and dignity and to protect patients'/clients' dignity
Describe the training, education and ongoing review of professional practice in relation to the promotion of patients'/clients' privacy and dignity and protection of their modesty (including supervision, appraisal and PDPs and awareness of specific needs)
Describe how patients are protected from unwanted public view, e.g. curtains, screens, walls, clothes/covers, etc.
State what type of clothing is available for patients who cannot wear their own clothes, how is their modesty protected
State what policies are in place for patients to have access to their own clothes
Describe how privacy in access to a telephone is achieved

Factor 7: *Availability of an area for privacy*

Patients/clients are *denied* access to any area which offers privacy	Patients/clients have access to an area that provides privacy when receiving care or treatment	Patients/clients can access an area that safely provides privacy

E	D	C	B	A

Access includes physical facilities, e.g. quiet room, access to gardens, for patients and relatives, but should be conducive to different needs, e.g. if patient on ITU, child protection.
Privacy includes comfort and soundproofing, etc.

Statements to stimulate comparison group discussion around best practice:
State how an area is created (in patients'/clients' homes as well as health service settings)
State how and when patients/clients are informed of the availability of 'quiet' and/or private space, e.g. at orientation, in leaflet, at admission, etc.
State the barriers that exist that restrict the provision of an area of privacy
State the areas available
State how clinical risk is handled in relation to complete privacy

Figure 11.6 (*continued*)
Source: DoH, 2001

Since Carol Annetts wrote of her experience implementing Essence of Care, a new Essence of Care Benchmarking Framework has been published (DoH, 2003) and a National Education Forum for the Essence of Care has been set up under the leadership of John Badham, Director of Essence of Care Clinical Governance Support Team at the Department of Health. This has simplified the process of benchmarking which is now more user-friendly.

Quality Circles

Quality circles are a useful method of solving problems and may result in an improvement in the quality of care. Quality circles were launched in Japan in 1962 as part of an overall quality assurance system. In 1974, quality circles were introduced in America by Lockheed, and four years later, in 1978, Rolls-Royce of Derby became the first British company to introduce them. It was not until 1982 that the National Society of Quality Circles was formed in the UK. In North Warwickshire Health Authority, quality circles were implemented following the 1982 restructuring of the National Health Service, in order to gain greater staff involvement and participation.

A quality circle is a group of five to eight volunteers working in the same area who meet regularly to identify, select and solve problems. The solution to the problem is then implemented and monitored to establish if the problem has been solved.

How a Quality Circle Works

As can be seen from Figure 11.7, a quality circle starts by brainstorming a list of problems. Inevitably, the group will identify a large number of problems, which then have to be sorted into those that can be dealt with, those for which help is needed and those that are really difficult, if not impossible.

The next stage is the selection of the problem. Out of the list of problems, there will appear a general theme, and the group select problems that will give them quick results. In this way, they will maintain the purpose and enthusiasm of the group as well as demonstrating their effectiveness.

The group then analyse the problem that has been selected, decide what facts are needed to solve the problem, and collect, record and interpret data about the problem. Solutions to the problem are discussed in consultation with all concerned, a number of options are established, based on facts, and a solution is produced. The group then prepare a presentation for management, outlining the solution.

The chosen solution to the problem is planned and implemented. The situation is monitored to ensure that the problem is solved and that the desired

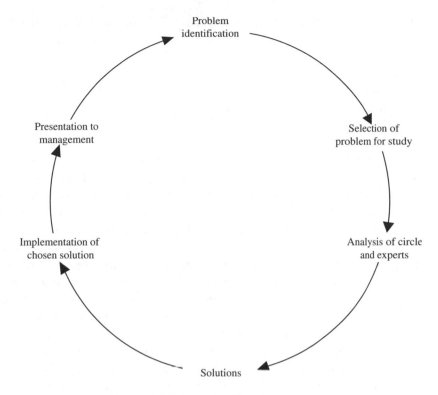

Figure 11.7 The quality circle

effect is maintained. The final stage is the presentation to management demonstrating an improvement in service and the recorded facts.

Members of the circle come from all disciplines and grades of staff who are working in the same clinical area. The only qualification needed to be a member of a circle is the desire to solve problems that will lead to an improvement in the quality of patient care, commitment and plenty of enthusiasm.

Meetings are usually held weekly or fortnightly and last for a set period of time, usually one hour even if all the business is not finished. Sometimes there is work for the members to do outside the meeting, such as researching solutions to the problem and gathering information. Minutes of the meeting are recorded and circulated to all members of the circle and to any other interested parties who may be able to help solve the problem. These minutes serve two purposes: first as a record of the meeting and second as a record of the group's progress towards a solution to the problem.

This may all sound very simple but there is much more to a quality circle than a group of people who simply get together and solve a problem. There is a need for commitment on behalf of the management to the work of a circle. There are also cost implications, as training is required for the various roles that people take in order to develop an active and productive quality circle. The key roles are:

- co-ordinator
- facilitator
- leader
- recorder.

The training for both the facilitators and the leaders is vital to the success of the quality circle programme. There are several training packages and books on the subject, some of which I have listed in the References (see, in particular, Robson, 1984). However, there has been limited success using quality circles. This is not due to the failure of the concept, which is excellent, but related to problems including lack of continuous senior strategic management involvement, lack of close working between departments, and the fact that the concept is based on the notion that problems do occur and, possibly most important, not based around the customer or user of the service. This has led to many organisations focusing on improving customer services. Professor Ishikawa (1985) recognised that training is the firm foundation on which to base total cultural change required by TQM. After the introductory sessions, training had to be related to individual, identified training needs.

In Japan, businesses reviewed the way they operated and then went on to achieve the competitive edge based on producing better goods at better prices than their competitors in the West.

Advantages of Quality Circles

- they offer an opportunity for members to be more involved in decision-making
- members learn valuable problem-solving and presentation skills
- quality circles develop the team concept
- they encourage multidisciplinary interaction and promotes greater understanding of other people's roles in the organisation.

Disadvantages of Quality Circles

- there are cost implications in both time and resources. Inadequate training and lack of commitment from management will mean that the quality circle will fail
- they sound simple but in fact need careful thought and in-depth understanding of the principles

Organisation-wide Measurement of Quality

Quality assurance should not be seen as a task or a technique; it is a philosophy or way of doing something which is part of every aspect of the working life of an organisation. An organisation, which has quality at its heart, is one that continually strives for excellence.

Total Quality Management (TQM)/Continuous Quality Improvement (CQI)

The terms Total Quality Management (TQM) and Continuous Quality Improvement (CQI) are synonymous and are often known as CQI when used in a healthcare setting. Clinical governance is a continuous quality improvement framework and there are many similarities with the TQM/CQI systems that were implemented in healthcare in the USA and later in Europe and the UK during the 1990s. The concept of TQM was developed in the USA during World War II by Dr W. Edwards Deming (1982) and J. M. Juran (1980). They were working in the armaments industry and recognised that putting quality first could reduce costs and improve productivity and that over 85 per cent of quality failures normally come from systems under the direct control of management.

However, TQM in the health service in the UK, although successful in some sites, has not been entirely successful, possibly owing to difficulty in translating some of the lessons learned in the USA and Canada to a healthcare system in the UK that is essentially different. See also Chapter 1.

The TQM approach is about putting the needs of the patient at the centre of every activity of the organisation with the support and involvement of management. TQM is a method of managing quality issues throughout every aspect of an organisation, ensuring that all the staff get it right first time, every time and do not pass on errors and mistakes to someone else in the organisation. TQM has been applied all over the world in manufacturing and service industries. It involves everyone in every department becoming organised as far as quality is concerned. Mistakes, errors and poor practice may be serious in a manufacturing organisation but in the healthcare setting they can be devastating and at times life-threatening. The cost of poor-quality care is often greater than the cost of good-quality care. When treatment does not go as planned, the patient develops complications, stays in hospital longer and requires additional treatment, therapy and care. The patient suffers unnecessary pain, discomfort and inconvenience, and there is a knock-on effect on the waiting list, which will leave another patient in pain for longer than anticipated.

In 1990 the Department of Health selected 23 sites as a demonstration of a managed approach to quality, or TQM. The sites ranged from departments within units, to hospitals, to entire districts and they were part-funded by the Department of Health. Some common themes which helped define a total quality NHS emerged from the demonstration and included:

- actively seeking patients' views and building organisations around their needs
- encouraging staff to respond positively to patients' needs and suggestions
- top management and professional commitment to quality
- creating a culture which encourages wide involvement and devolves responsibility to front-line staff
- systematic training for staff to equip them with the skills they need to participate in change
- effective communications
- continuous improvement based on systematic measurement.

Quality has always been an essential aspect of the delivery of professional clinical care but TQM moved the focus from quality practised within the professions to quality within the organisation as a whole. The key principles and strategies of TQM include:

- customer focus
- teamwork; breaking down professional barriers
- better management of resources.

The Concept of TQM

Every organisation requires processes for ensuring that the service it provides is needed by the consumer and is of an acceptable standard. In a Department of Trade and Industry publication in 1989 John Oakland outlined the TQM processes (Oakland, 1989).

He said that the organisation should:

- focus on the needs and expectations of its market and its consumers
- achieve top-quality performance in all areas of its activity (products, services and internal processes)
- install and operate procedures, simple and complex, necessary for the achievement of top-quality performance
- critically and continuously examine processes to reduce and remove non-productive activities, inefficiencies and waste
- develop and monitor measures of performance, set standards against which this performance is measured and set required improvements
- understand and develop an effective communication strategy

- develop a non-hierarchical team approach to problem-solving and delegating responsibility for change
- develop good procedures for communication and feedback to staff at any level of good work
- continuously review the above processes to develop a culture for never-ending improvement.

Perhaps the key issue is the ownership and commitment to quality of care and service by all staff, at all levels of the organisation. Historically staff within the health service have been committed to delivering quality care and have worked hard to improve the care they give and the service they deliver. The main difference is that instead of having pockets of enthusiasm within the organisation, the whole organisation is part of a structured system of quality that is managed systematically. TQM should encourage every member of staff to be an active cog in the quality wheel, to be loyal to the hospital and department and support staff to deliver higher quality and cost-effective care and services.

Three TQM Managerial Processes

TQM consists of three managerial processes which create continuous improvements in the performance of an organisation. These are:

- *quality leadership*: clear plans to support and develop quality and the resources to meet the goals in terms of manpower, capital expenditure, an explicit strategy and policy commitment to 'getting it right first time'
- *hospital-wide approach*: all the quality initiatives, processes and actions must be implemented throughout the hospital
- *continuous measurement, training and development*: training and development specific to the area in which the staff are working is related to the job. There is continuous measurement of quality.

The Juran Institute identified practice that made top companies and institutions highly successful. These management processes and systems are known as TQM. According to the Juran Institute, TQM succeeds because it leads to:

- delighted patients, purchasers and other customers
- satisfied professionals and employees
- optimal outcomes and health status of populations
- increased revenue
- reduced costs.

Source: www.juran.com

The Essential Components That Make Up TQM

- it is cheaper to prevent failure rather than correct problems. It is also more positive than accepting that the problem is just part of life
- senior managers are seen to lead from the front
- everyone has responsibility for quality
- everyone gets it right first time, every time
- the cost of quality is addressed and accounted for
- quality is the priority in all departments and services
- there is a drive for continuous improvement. All results achieved are reviewed as part of a process of continuous improvement.

TQM is essentially about achieving quality through the involvement of people, who are seen as assets to be nurtured, developed and encouraged to take responsibility for their actions and are recognised as an important part of the culture of TQM.

TQM is built around the key 'customers' who are the patients, their families, the purchasers, the users such as the consultants, the medical staff, the nursing staff and the support staff.

Quality Improvement Process

Philip B. Crosby is an American with a background in quality control. He was the quality manager on the first Pershing missile programme in the USA and then moved on to ITT, where he became the corporate vice-president and quality director. Crosby's approach to TQM is through the development of the quality improvement process (QIP), which is the organised effort to address a performance deficiency or issue in a process. The essentials to a successful project are:

- the involvement of a group of people
- recognition of the project by the organisation
- process analysis
- data and facts.

In his book, *Quality without Tears*, Crosby (1984) identified 14 steps in the QIP:

1. Establish management commitment to make clear where management stands on quality.
2. Form quality improvement team to run the quality improvement process.

3. Establish quality measurement to provide details of non-conformance in a way that permits objective evaluation and correction.
4. Evaluate the cost of quality to identify where quality improvement will be profitable using the measures in steps.
5. Raise quality awareness to provide a method of raising the personal concern felt by all employees about providing a quality service.
6. Take corrective action to provide a systematic method of resolving problems forever.
7. Undertake zero defects planning to examine the various activities in preparation for the continuing phases of the QIP.
8. Provide education to train supervisors and managers in the steps of a QIP, so that in turn they can train others.
9. Hold a Zero Defects Day, an event which lets every individual realise, through personal experience, that there has been a change.
10. Encourage goal-setting to turn intentions into action, by encouraging individuals to establish improvement goals for themselves and their work groups.
11. Encourage obstacle reporting to achieve error-cause removal to give individuals a means of communicating to management the situations that make it difficult to improve.
12. Provide recognition to appreciate those who participate.
13. Establish quality councils to bring together appropriate people to share quality management information on a regular basis.
14. Do it all over again to make sure the quality process never ends.

Steps 1 and 2 address the cultural aspects of the organisation. The first step involves management accepting responsibility for achieving quality. When this is linked to Step 2 – the formation of quality improvement teams – a commitment has been made to achieving that goal. Crosby specifically requires multidisciplinary teams, which means that managers, professionals and other staff must break out of their 'comfort zones' and relinquish some of the 'expert' and 'position' power (Handy, 1985) that goes with the functional organisation.

Steps 3 and 4 are quantitative, establishing quality measurements and evaluating the cost of quality. Step 4 is not possible without Step 3, as measurement is a necessary precursor to evaluation. These steps provide the baseline for the fifth more qualitative step of raising quality awareness and confirming the need for a multidisciplinary approach. Step 6 is to take action to correct problems, standards that have not been achieved and concerns reported by staff about clinical practice or actual poor practice or service provision. Once Step 6 is in place, the trust can then be seen to have established a baseline from which to form quality improvement, and continuous quality improvement should then result. However, Crosby adds an additional process of 'zero defects', which makes up Step 7. Crosby's QIP was developed in industry where the concept of zero defects is perhaps more achievable than in a healthcare setting. When the product is a patient there are more variables and so the focus of this step when applied to healthcare might be the timely reporting of standards not met, the reporting of near misses, accidents and incidents, and a positive approach that analyses the 'defects' and draws up action plans to ensure that they do not happen again and that the quality of care is improved.

Step 8 involves the training of managers and senior staff in the QIP so that they can pass on this training to their staff, thus ensuring a good understanding of the process and encouraging staff involvement. Step 9 is the celebration of achievements through a Zero Defects Day. Crosby also sees this event as a new beginning in the QIP.

Step 10 encourages the setting of goals with appropriate timescales. In Step 11 staff are encouraged to advise managers and quality assurance team leaders about problems they have with equipment or services that prevent them from meeting quality standards. Step 12 provides Crosby with an opportunity to recognise and acknowledge the contribution of the staff to the programme. However, he makes it quite clear that any reward must be in the form of badges, certificates and awards and never financial.

The establishment of quality councils in Step 13 is seen as 'embedding' quality into the culture and the final step, 14, is to do it all over again which Crosby (1979; 1984) describes as a constant reminder that quality improvement never stops.

The steps of the QIP, as set out above, include four phases of a problem-solving approach:

- project definition and organisation
- diagnostic journey
- remedial journey
- holding the gains.

This problem-solving approach may be broken down into 12 steps:

1. List the problems in order of priority:
   - problems may come from the group's brainstorming session, patient-satisfaction surveys, complaints, national reports, results of audit, and so on
   - priorities may arise from data analysis, policy decisions, research, and so on.
2. Define the project and the team:
   - the project is a problem that is to be solved
   - the team is composed of representatives from all sections of the organisation on whom the problem impacts

- the project definition must be objective
- the scope of the project must match the scope of the team.

3. Analyse the symptoms:
   - a symptom is an indication that a problem exists; it is not the cause of the problem. The benefits of analysing the symptoms are that it helps to clarify the problem, focuses effort, establishes the habit of collecting data and leads to a common understanding of the problem.

4. Formulate theories of causes:
   - problems can be caused by the staff, patients, equipment, supplies, procedures and protocols, and inaccurate data or bias measurements
   - establish the views of the different members of the team as to the cause of the problem.

5. Test the theories:
   - a theory is an unproven assertion about a cause
   - the collection and analysis of data will confirm or rule out the theory.

6. Identify the root causes:
   - list all the possible causes and narrow them down to specific causes.

7. Consider alternative solutions:
   - produce a wide range of solutions gathered from the different group members
   - be creative and innovative in your quest for a solution.

8. Design solutions and controls:
   - evaluate the solutions and rank them in order
   - solution selection will depend on cost, time for implementation, potential resistance, impact on other processes, and so on
   - solutions and controls must be designed together with feedback systems and training plans.

9. Address resistance to change:
   - identify the causes of the resistance
   - there are two aspects to process changes: technical and social. Technically sound solutions will fail if the social impact is not addressed through training and support.

10. Implement solutions and controls:
    - apply the prime solution and evaluate the results through a pilot study
    - revise the solution as necessary.

11. Check performance:
    - the implementation of the solution does not guarantee improvement. There is a need to review performance through the collection of data and analysis.

12. Monitor control systems:
    - maintain controls and seek continuous improvement
    - reward and recognise the group
    - consider ways to replicate the project in other similar problem areas.

Common difficulties when carrying out the above steps are:

- missing out a step in the process
- lack of time, analysis skills or objectivity
- implementing the changes before the solutions have been thoroughly evaluated and tested through a pilot study.

John Oakland

John Oakland, the author of *Total Quality Management* (1993) is considered to be the British authority on TQM (for more information, see Chapter 1).

Oakland (1993) believes that quality starts at the top, with quality parameters inherent in every organisational decision. He emphasises seven key characteristics of TQM:

1. Quality is meeting the customer's requirements. This first characteristic stresses that quality is defined by the customer and not by the supplier of the service or – in health service terms – the user of the service and not the provider.
2. Most quality problems are interdepartmental. Oakland emphasises the importance of the quality chain and the fact that most problems occur in the interaction between process steps.
3. Quality control is monitoring, finding and eliminating causes of quality problems.
4. Quality assurance rests on prevention, management systems, effective audit and review. Characteristics 3 and 4 move the focus away from blame and criticism and towards improving performance.
5. Quality must be managed; it does not just happen. Quality must be inherent in management thinking and become part of the everyday practice of the organisation.
6. There should be a focus on prevention, not cure. This goes back to the 'get it right first time, every time' philosophy. Correct policies, procedures and processes result in an acceptable standard of care.
7. Reliability is an extension of quality and enables us to 'delight the customer'. It is perhaps easier to delight the customer in industry when talking about a car or a domestic appliance. However, the patient or the user of the service can be satisfied with the standard of care or service provided.

Although Oakland's model is an industrial model, the characteristics can be applied to a healthcare setting, leading to an organisation that is driven by top management committed to the provision of a high-quality service, created through reliable, consistent organisational processes.

Hugh Koch

Hugh Koch is also an expert on TQM (see also Chapter 1) and has an adapted approach. In his model of TQM Koch (1991) identifies some key components. First, the services must be:

■ accessible
■ effective
■ acceptable
■ appropriate.

Secondly, the services must be organised with the appropriate quality input for:

■ clear management commitment, leadership and capabilities
■ optimum teamwork and recognition of staff value
■ implementation of quality techniques, clinical audit, standards setting, information/monitoring and communications
■ monitoring and identification of performance against contract specification and reduction of 'non-conformance'.

His model considers the quality of the service at four levels:

■ hospital
■ directorate
■ speciality/clinical area
■ individual members of staff.

Koch identifies a number of difficulties in the application of the concepts to TQM (Koch, 1991) which are not dissimilar to those above and include:

■ a lack of top management commitment and vision
■ the 'flavour of the month' attitude of staff
■ the hospital community service culture and management style
■ poor appreciation of TQM concepts, principles and practices
■ lack of structure for TQM activities
■ ineffective leadership.

Accreditation

Accreditation is 'a system of external peer review for determining compliance with a set of standards' (Scrivens, 1995). Accreditation involves the review of an organisation's performance by an external body against measured and explicit standards and agreed criteria, culminating in a report of the results of the organisation.

Accreditation has its roots in the USA as far back as 1913 when the American College of Surgeons stated 'that those institutions having the highest ideals may have proper recognition before the profession'. (Roberts et al., 1987). The American College of Surgeons officially transferred its Hospital Standardisation Programme to the Joint Commission on Accreditation of Hospitals (JCAH). JCAH published *Standards for Hospital Accreditation* in 1953. In the USA, accreditation is linked with funding; if standards fall below predetermined levels, then the hospital organisation is in jeopardy of losing federal or state funding. The hospital accreditation programmes demand evidence that a hospital has systems of quality assurance. Medical audits were developed into medical record audits, which examined in detail the records post-discharge. Today, these systems are often computerised and some of these hospitals employ a team of people to examine the records and report their findings to a quality assurance committee (JCAHO, 2002). In 1987 the Joint Commission on Accreditation of Hospitals (USA) changed its name to the Joint Commission on Accreditation of Healthcare Organisations (JCAHO). The change reflected an expanded scope of activities. The Agenda for Change was launched, with a set of initiatives designed to place the primary emphasis of the accreditation process on actual organisation performance.

In 1979 the Netherlands set up their system of accreditation (Reerink, 1987). In 1987 New Zealand set up their Joint Commission on Accreditation for Hospitals, as did Australia. (Darby and Cane, 1987) In 1989 in the UK the King's Fund Centre established a project steering group which looked critically at existing systems for setting and monitoring national standards, principally those models of accreditation used in the USA, Canada and Australia. The Australian system was considered to be the most appropriate on which to build its own model, with reference to the Canadian system as appropriate. The King's Fund Organisational Audit was established, with the development of national standards for acute hospitals. (Sale, 2000). In 1991 the King's Fund Organisational Audit launched the programme on a fee-paying basis, with clients recruited from the NHS and independent sector; developed and revised programmes for primary care, health authorities, and community, mental health and learning disabilities services, and developed standards for nursing and residential care homes. The King's Fund Organisational Audit was relaunched as the Health Quality Service in 1998, the concept of performance indicators was piloted, and standards and an assessment programme for primary care groups initiated. The Health Quality Service (HQS) gained accreditation from the UK Accreditation Service as an ISO9002 certification body, allowing an organisation to pursue ISO9002 in addition to HQS accreditation by working with the same programme. A new accreditation programme was introduced for acute hospitals, and community mental health, learning disability and specialist palliative care services; a new programme for hospice care was launched, and a revised programme developed for primary care teams Other accreditation schemes include:

■ *Investors in People*: a scheme that sets a standard of good practice for the training and development of staff to achieve business goals which are not specific to health service organisations. It also provides a basis for continuous improvement for the staff and the organisation. The process requires a portfolio of evidence against 24 indicators and an inspection by two assessors.

■ *The Charter Mark*: an award for public-sector organisations who must show measurable and demonstrable improvements in the quality of service across a range of topics. The organisation must have plans for at least one innovative improvement to the quality of the service. It requires continued submissions over a three-year period but there are no on-site inspections.

■ *ISO 9000 (formerly BS5750)*: this scheme focuses on sets of procedures to ensure accountability and a systematic review of the organisation's services against national standards not specific to the health service. There must be systems in place for feedback to users of the service and an inspection is carried out.

Monitoring performance and publishing the results gives the general public, the user of the service, a more objective indication of how well an NHS trust is performing, and is certainly preferable to the lack of information that was available in the past. Star ratings are motivating for staff, but if the ratings are lower than expected or if the staff feel that they have worked hard and deserve a higher rating it can have a demotivating effect and a 'why bother' attitude is the result. The number of inspections from various external bodies has grown to an enormous number over the past few years and the preparation for these should not be underestimated. Whether or not this approach has improved patient care is a debate that continues.

Conclusion

The systems of organisational quality assurance are the precursors of clinical governance, which is simply a continuous quality assurance framework with the patient as the focus and centre of the system. The next chapter is about the tools for measuring the quality of care and it is important to remember that when these audit tools were introduced into UK healthcare organisations this was often undertaken by a small group of quality assurance enthusiasts and not on an organisation-wide basis. In the UK it was the nursing profession that implemented systems of standard-setting in the 1980s, which led to the start of a systematic approach to monitoring the quality of care in the UK. At the start of the standard-setting project in 1986 there was considerable apathy and lack of support from clinical and management colleagues for the nurses who were developing standards and ways of monitoring them. The arrival of clinical governance and the clear lines of responsibility and accountability for the quality of clinical care is a very positive step forward in assuring the quality of care for patients.

Tools for Measuring the Quality of Care

12

Chapter Contents:

- Qualpacs
- Phaneuf's nursing audit
- monitor
- the advantages and disadvantages of 'off-the-shelf' tools
- setting and monitoring standards.

This chapter starts with a review of a selection of 'off-the-shelf' audit tools. There are some audit tools that have been tried and tested both in the USA and across Europe. If you are planning to develop your own audit tool or need to measure a particular aspect of care, part or all of some of these tools may be useful. They set out an approach which has resulted in a valid measurement tool. Three of the most commonly used tools, Qualpacs (Wandelt and Ager, 1974), Phaneuf's Nursing Audit (Phaneuf, 1976) and Monitor (Goldstone et al., 1983). Other nursing audit tools are briefly described in the appendix. It is important to remember that when these audit tools were introduced into UK healthcare organisations they were often used by a small group of quality assurance enthusiasts and were not an organisation-wide activity. In the UK it was the nursing profession that implemented systems of standard-setting in the 1980s and led the start of a systematic approach to monitoring the quality of care in the UK. At the time there was considerable apathy and lack of support from clinical and management colleagues when implementing Monitor and at the start of the standard-setting initiative. The arrival of clinical governance and the quality of clinical care is clearly the responsibility of the NHS Trust Chief Executive, a designated senior clinician, and the quality assurance agenda the responsibility of the board.

Qualpacs

The Quality Patient Care Scale (Qualpacs) is an American tool, being the result of the combined work of two professors, Wandelt and Ager, and their faculty members at Wayne State University College of Nursing (Wandelt and Ager, 1974). Many of the items are derived from the Slater Nursing Performance Rating Scale (Wandelt and Stewart, 1975). The Slater scale evaluates the competence of the nurse while he/she is giving patient care by observing and measuring his/her performance against predetermined standards within the scale. Qualpacs, on the other hand, measures the quality of care received by the patients from the nursing staff of a ward or unit.

Qualpacs uses a method of concurrent review that is designed to evaluate the process of care at the time it is being provided, including a review of the records, a patient interview (asking the patient to comment on certain aspects of his/her care), direct observation of the patient's behaviours related to predetermined criteria, a staff interview (asking the staff to comment on specific aspects of patient care) and staff observation of nursing behaviours related to predetermined criteria. The first audits of nursing care were in the USA and early examples included Stewart, Abdellah, and Slater. See appendix for more details.

Using Qualpacs

Qualpacs is used to evaluate the direct and indirect interaction of nursing staff with patients. It contains 68 items that are divided into the following six categories:

- psychosocial: individual (15 items)
- psychosocial: group (8 items)
- physical (15 items)
- general (15 items)
- communication (8 items)
- professional implications (7 items).

The Qualpacs for the first of the six categories is shown in Table 12.1.

For each item a list of clues is provided to clarify exactly how the item should be interpreted. Taking the first item in the psychosocial: individual section, 'Patient receives nurse's full attention', the clues suggested by Wandelt and Ager are:

- patient is appropriately responded to verbally and non-verbally, without being asked to repeat phrases
- staff assume positions that will aid in observation and communication with patient
- conversation of staff is restricted to patient who is receiving care
- the infant is looked at and talked to as he/she receives a bottle feed

Table 12.1 Quality Patient Care Scale (Qualpacs) (Wandelt and Ager, 1974)

Date:

Patient (name or no.): Rater (name or no.):

INTERACTIONS RECORD: AM/PM

No: ☐☐☐☐☐☐☐☐☐☐☐☐
Time: ☐☐☐☐☐☐☐☐☐☐☐☐

	5	4	3	2	1	0	0	
PSYCHOSOCIAL : INDIVIDUAL — Actions directed toward meeting psychosocial needs of individual patients:	Item number	Best care	Between	Average care	Between	Poorest care	Not applicable	Not observed	Mean score
1. Patient receives nurse's full attention ★D	1	×		×		×			11–12
	5		× (6)		1			12	3
2. Patient is given an opportunity to explain his feelings ★D	2	×	×	×	×				13–14
				×	×				19 3.2
3. Patient is approached in a kind, gentle and friendly manner ★D	3	×		×		×			15–16
				×					12 3
4. Patient's inappropriate behaviour is responded to in a therapeutic manner ★D	4	×		×	×				17–18
				×					13 3.3
5. Appropriate action is taken in response to anticipated or manifest patient anxiety or distress ★D/★I	5	×		×	×	×			19–20
			×					14	2.8
6. Patient receives explanation and verbal reassurance when needed ★D	6	×		×	×				21–22
				×					10 3.3
7. Patient receives attention from nurse with neither becoming involved in a non-therapeutic way ★D	7	×		×	×				23–24
			×					13	3.3
8. Patient is given consideration as a member of a family and society ★D	8			×		×			25–26
									4 2
9. Patient receives attention for his spiritual needs ★D/★I	9			×	×		×		27–28
									8 2.7
10. The rejecting or demanding patient continues to receive acceptance ★D/★I	10			×		×			29–30
				×					9 3
11. Patient receives care that communicates worth and dignity of man ★D	11		×	×	×				31–32
					×				11 2.8
12. The healthy aspects of the patient's personality are utilised ★D/★I	12			×	×		×		33–34
				×					11 2.8
13. An atmosphere of trust, acceptance and respect is created rather than one of power, prestige and authority ★D	13		×	×		×			35–36
			×					9	3
14. Appropriate topics for conversation are chosen ★D	14			×	×	×			37–38
				×					11 2.8
15. The unconscious or non-oriented patient is cared for with the same respectful manner as the conscious patient ★D	15			×	×		×		39–40
				×				11	2.8
AREA 1 MEAN									41–42–43

Key: ★D = direct care observation is appropriate
★D/I = direct or indirect observation is appropriate

Notes: In total there are 15 items to rate for the psychosocial : individual and this continues with a further 8 items for the psychosocial group. Once all the scoring is completed the total of each item is added together using 5 for best, 3 for average and 1 for poorest care. This gives the total score per item. The number is recorded above and to the left of the diagonal line in the 'mean score' column. This total is then divided by the number of entries made against that item and the number recorded below the diagonal line. The total mean score gives an overall measurement of the quality of care as observed by the trained observers. This score is calculated by adding all the item means together and dividing this figure by the number of items which received a score. 'Not applicable' and 'Not observed' receive a zero score. The same calculation can be made to calculate the score over the whole area. For example, for psychosocial add all the mean scores for each item together and divide this by the total number of items that received a score. See an example of the totals in Figure 12.2.

■ questions are asked which encourage the patient to express feelings
■ evidence is given by staff of anticipation of projected needs of the patient.

These clues may be modified to suit the particular situation and do not affect the scale as it is the items which are scored, not the clues.

The items listed can be either directly observed or indirectly gathered from the staff, the patients and/or the records. Most of the items require direct observation of the behaviour, although a few may be implied from charts and other sources. Nursing care delivered to the patient is evaluated regardless of the skill level of the nurse providing the care. The observation scoring time is usually three and a half to four hours, which includes one hour for preparation, two hours for direct observation and one hour spent rating the direct observation period.

The information is gathered by specially trained, non-participant nurse observers, through direct observation and indirect means. The role of the non-participant observer is to evaluate the care that the patient receives – they must not communicate, verbally or non-verbally, with patients, relatives or members of staff, nor must they contribute or intervene in patient care, as this would alter the care received by the patient. Observers should only intervene if the patient is at risk. The criteria used by these observers are that care is safe, adequate and therapeutic. To reduce the risk of observer bias, it is recommended that at least two observers should watch the same incident. The assessors use their own judgement as to whether they observe just one patient or a small group of patients at a time.

Prior to the evaluation of a ward, the person who requested the assessment is responsible for ensuring that all the nursing staff are fully aware of and understand what is involved. All patients, relatives and visitors must also be informed, and permission sought from those selected for the evaluation. The patients selected are those who are representative of those being cared for in that particular ward.

The Process of the Evaluation

The evaluation starts with a verbal report from the nurse who is responsible for the selected patient. The observers then read the patient's records and draw up their own plan of care for each patient, using information available and their professional judgement. This enables them to identify actions that they would expect to see during the observation period. The observer then takes up his/her position so that it is possible to both observe and hear the selected patient, and begins the two hour non-participation observation period.

The nurse-observer rates the quality of care that the patient receives as 'best care' (5 points), 'between' (4 points), 'average care' (3 points), 'between'

(2 points) and 'poorest care' (1 point). Items may also be deemed 'not applicable' or 'not observed', since this system was designed to evaluate nursing care currently being received by the patient. These items are rated zero.

Within one aspect of nursing care, several items in different sections may be observed concurrently. The observer notes all these and places an X in the appropriate column and subsection for each interaction observed. The number of each item and the commencing time of each interaction is recorded at the top of the scale. The interaction is considered to be completed when there is an interruption or break in the communication between the patient and the nurse. It may be considered more useful to identify the grade of nurse from which care is received, so instead of an X the letters S for sister, R for registered nurse and L for learner may be used. Various symbols are acceptable, but the names of the nurses are not recorded on the form. The observer may also add a number to the symbol, indicating the number of interactions, such as L6 or S3 – this allows a more detailed analysis of the content of the interactions.

At the end of the observation period, the observer looks for indirect evidence of care by reviewing the selected patient's records and charts, which are also scored. As before, the symbol X is used if there is no evidence of the level of the nurse. Many of the items will not have received scores, so the assessor must decide if the item was relevant to the patient's care; if not, then the column 'not applicable' is marked with an 'X'. If the item is considered essential for that patient's care, then the observer, in discussion with the nurse and with reference to the records, must decide if the omission was reasonable. For example, it might be considered reasonable if the item was scheduled for later in the day in order to meet the patient's needs, in which case an 'X' is marked in the 'not observed' column. If the item of care was needed by the patient, and expected by the observer but not given, then X is marked in the 'poorest care' column.

Scoring Qualpacs

Table 12.2 demonstrates how the total scores are calculated and recorded.

When the scale has been checked, every item should have at least one symbol against it. The mean score of each item is established as follows:

■ every entry against an item is awarded a value. These figures are added together and give a total score for the item
■ this figure is entered above the line in the column headed 'mean score'
■ this total score is then divided by the number of entries made against that item and the figure entered below the line.

Items rated 'not applicable' or 'not observed' receive no score. All 68 items are scored in this way.

Table 12.2 Final Qualpacs Scores

PROFESSIONAL IMPLICATIONS Care given to patient reflects initiative and responsibility indicative of professional expectations	Item No.	5 Best care	4 Be-tween	3 Av. care	2 Be-tween	1 Poorest care	0 Not Applic-able	0 Not ob-served	Mean Score	
62. Decisions that are made by staff reflect knowledge of facts and good judgement ★D/★I	62									78–79
63. Evidence (spoken, behavioural, recorded) is given by staff of insight into deeper problems and needs of the patient ★D/★I	63									11–12
64. Changes in care and care plans reflect continuous evaluation of results of nursing care	64									13–14
65. Staff are reliable: follow through with responsibilities for the patient's whereabouts ★D	65									15–16
66. Assigned staff keep informed of the patient's condition and whereabouts ★D	66									17–18
67. Care given the patient reflects flexibility in rules and regulations as indicated by individual patient needs ★D/★I	67									19–20
68. Organisation and management of nursing activities reflect due consideration for patient needs ★D/★I	68								21–22	
AREA VI MEAN										23–24–25

FINAL QUALPACS SCORE

Area I		Area IV		Sum of item means	140	
Area II		Area V		Number of items rated	48	
Area III		Area VI	2.9	Mean of items means	2.9	26–27–28
		TOTAL				

Key: ★D indicates that direct observation is appropriate
★D/★I indicates that either direct or indirect observation is appropriate

The total mean score gives the overall measurement of the quality of care and is found by:

- adding together the mean scores for all the items
- dividing this total by the number of items that received a score, again excluding those rated 'not applicable' or 'not observed'. These figures are recorded at the end of the scale.

The mean score for each of the areas can be worked out in the same way by:

- adding together the mean scores for all the items within an area
- dividing this total by the number of items that received a score. These figures are recorded at the end of each subsection.

It is important to note that it is not arithmetically correct to use the mean scores of the area subsections to calculate the total mean score. This can only be done by adding the means of all the items together, and dividing this number by the number of items scored.

Finally, the results are discussed and analysed before a report is sent to the person who requested the evaluation. This will include the overall mean score, the assessor's impression of the care, points for improvement, suggestions and recommendations for change, and the scores for the subsections, with examples of how good and bad scores were awarded.

Qualpacs is a concurrent audit tool which looks at care as it is delivered through a review of the patient's records, patient and staff views and observation of staff so it has the advantage that the auditors observe both verbal and non-verbal behaviours of patients, carers, nurses, therapists and medical staff. It also has the advantage over tools like Monitor that focus on the documentation of care and the nursing process.

Advantages of Qualpacs

- it has been subjected to rigorous testing by researchers in the USA, and there is documented evidence of its reliability, validity and discriminatory ability
- it has been used in this country, in particular at the Nursing Development Unit, Oxford
- use of direct observation provides data that cannot be collected by other means. For example, observation of verbal and non-verbal behaviours provides information on interaction between nurses, patients, their families and other professionals. It is not possible to evaluate this type of interaction by reviewing charts and records – it has to be seen or observed

- it uses more than one method of concurrent review
- it provides nurses with an evaluation of their own performance, which can lead to a greater awareness and change in practice, and so improve patient care
- it provides positive feedback for the nursing team.

Disadvantages of Qualpacs

- the content represents American values, although many of the implied values in the items on the scale may match your own values
- it requires highly skilled and trained observers
- it is time-consuming
- observer bias can occur during direct observation, for example by giving a rating that is either too negative or too positive, and being influenced by one's own expectations and attitudes
- it has been criticised for being subjective and reliant on professional judgement, although most nurses seem to agree on what constitutes good or bad care
- the scoring system is time-consuming and quite complicated.

Phaneuf's Nursing Audit

The nursing audit by Phaneuf is a retrospective appraisal of the nursing process as reflected in the patient's records. There are two methods of auditing records: concurrent and retrospective. A retrospective audit is the evaluation of patient care following the discharge of the patient, focusing on the documentation of nursing care given. This type of audit is based on the assumption that what has been written down has been done effectively, or that 'good' documentation reflects 'good' care, which is not necessarily the case.

This audit was devised around the following seven functions of nursing, as listed by Lesnik and Anderson (1955) in their book *Nursing Practice and the Law:*

- the application and execution of the physician's legal orders
- the observation of symptoms and reactions
- the supervision of the patients
- the supervision of those participating in care
- reporting and recording
- the application and execution of nursing procedures and techniques
- the promotion of physical and emotional health by direction and teaching.

Six of these functions are independent nursing functions, including emotional aspects and teaching, while the seventh is the application of the physician's legal orders. From these seven functions, Phaneuf developed 50 components to help auditors to evaluate the quality of nursing care. These 50 components are stated in terms of actions by the nurses in relation to the patient, in the form of questions to be answered by the auditors when they review the records.

Audit Committee

Before carrying out an audit, an audit committee is formed, comprising a minimum of five members who are interested in quality assurance, clinically competent and able to work together in a group. It is recommended that each member should review no more than ten patients each month and that the auditor should have the ability to carry out an audit in about 15 minutes. If there are fewer than 50 discharges per month, then all the records may be audited; if there are large numbers of records to be audited, then an auditor may select 10 per cent of discharges.

Training for auditors includes the following:

■ a detailed discussion of the seven components
■ a group discussion to see how the group rates the care received using the notes of a patient who has been discharge. These should be anonymous and should reflect a total period of care not exceeding two weeks in length
■ each individual auditor then undertakes the same exercise as above. This is followed by a meeting of the whole committee which compares and discusses its findings, and finally reaches a consensus of opinion on each of the components.

Carrying out the Audit

The audit comprises two parts.

Part I: this applies to the setting, of which there are two separate formats: one for a hospital setting and one for the community – see Table 12.3 for an example of a hospital or nursing home audit. Phaneuf (1976) states that this part does not need to be completed by a nurse; it is acceptable for a member of the clerical staff to fill in the details, as it does not require professional judgement. The items in this part are not scored but are necessary for information and reference.

Part II: this is the section where all 50 components, developed into questions from the seven nursing functions, are audited. The audit form has three boxes to the right of each component, as indicated in Table 12.4. The score is clearly

Table 12.3 Phaneuf's nursing audit: Part I – Hospital or nursing home audit

Data must be held in STRICT confidence and MUST NOT BE FILED with patient's record

All entries to be completed by trained clerk

1. Name of patient: 2. Sex   3. Age   4. Admission   5. Discharge
   (LAST) (FIRST)   date   date

6. Nursing agency: 7. Floor   8. Medical   Private □   Ward □   OPD/Clinic □
                                supervision

9. Complete diagnosis(es):

10. Admitted by   Physician   MD not hospital   Clinic/OPD   11. Via emergency
    referral from: on staff □   affiliated □   □   □

12. Patient discharged   Self-care □   Family care □   PHN agency □   Other   Died □   Unknown □
    to: specify:

13. If patient   MD   MD promptly   Family   Family   14. If patient
    died: present   notified   present   promptly   Catholic
                 □   □   □   notified   Last rites given:
                                                      □   YES □   NO □

15. All nursing entries signed by   16. Nursing entries show whether make by
    name and dated: professional, practical, student nurse, or other:
    YES □   NO □   YES □   NO □

17. Patient's clothing, valuables and other personal items   YES □   NO □
    were accounted for in accordance with policy:

	YES	NO
18. Operative and other patient or family consent forms completed as required by policy		
19. A. Were there any accidents or other special incidents?		
B. If yes, chart indicates report was submitted to administration		
C. Or, report is part of chart		
20. A. Kardex in use		
B. If yes, Kardex becomes part of permanent chart		
21. Nursing care plan is recorded in the chart		
22. A. Nursing admission entry shows assessment of patient's condition physical emotional		
B. Nursing discharge entry shows assessment of patient's condition physical emotional		

Source: Phaneuf, 1976

Table 12.4 Phaneuf's nursing audit – Part II –
Audit of all seven nursing functions

All entries to be completed by a member of the Nursing Audit Committee
(Please check in box of choice; DO NOT obscure number in box)

Name of patient:

	(LAST)	(FIRST)			

I	APPLICATION AND EXECUTION OF PHYSICIAN'S LEGAL ORDERS	YES	NO	UNCERTAIN	TOTALS
	1. Medical diagnosis complete	7	0	3	
	2. Orders complete	7	0	3	
	3. Orders current	7	0	3	
	4. Orders promptly executed	7	0	3	
	5. Evidence that nurse understood cause and effect	7	0	3	
	6. Evidence that nurse took health history into account	7	0	3	
	(42) TOTALS		0		

II	OBSERVATIONS OF SYMPTOMS AND REACTIONS				
	7. Related to course of above disease(s) in general	7	0	3	
	8. Related to course of above disease(s) in patient	7	0	3	
	9. Related to complications due to therapy (each medication and each procedure)	7	0	3	
	10. Vital signs	7	0	3	
	11. Patient to his condition	7	0	3	
	12. Patient to his course of disease(s)	5	0	2	
	(40) TOTALS		0		

III	SUPERVISION OF PATIENT				
	13. Evidence that initial nursing diagnosis was made	4	0	1	
	14. Safety of patient	4	0	1	
	15. Security of patient	4	0	1	
	16. Adaptation (support of patient in reaction to condition and care)	4	0	1	
	17. Continuing assessment of patient's condition and capacity	4	0	1	
	18. Nursing plans changed in accordance with assessment	4	0	1	
	19. Interaction with family and with others considered	4	0	1	
	(28) TOTALS		0		

IV	SUPERVISION OF THOSE PARTICIPATING IN CARE (EXCEPT THE PHYSICIAN)				
	20. Care taught to patient, family, or others, nursing personnel	5	0	2	
	21. Physical, emotional, mental capacity to learn considered	5	0	2	
	22. Continuity of supervision to those taught	5	0	2	
	23. Support of those giving care	5	0	2	
	(20) TOTALS		0		

V	REPORTING AND RECORDING				
	24. Facts on which further care depended were recorded	4	0	1	
	25. Essential facts reported to physician	4	0	1	
	26. Reporting of facts included evaluation thereof	4	0	1	
	27. Patient or family alerted as to what to report to physician	4	0	1	
	28. Record permitted continuity of intramural and extramural care	4	0	1	
	(20) TOTALS		0		

Table 12.4 (*continued*)

		YES	NO	UNCERTAIN	TOTALS	DOES NOT APPLY
VI	APPLICATION AND EXECUTION OF NURSING PROCEDURES AND TECHNIQUES					
	29. Administration and/or supervision of medications	2	0	05		2
	30. Personal care (bathing, oral hygiene, skin, nail care, shampoo)	2	0	05		2
	31. Nutrition (including special diets)	2	0	05		2
	32. Fluid balance plus electrolytes	2	0	05		2
	33. Elimination	2	0	05		2
	34. Rest and sleep	2	0	05		2
	35. Physical activity	2	0	05		2
	36. Irrigations (including enemas)	2	0	05		2
	37. Dressings and bandages	2	0	05		2
	38. Formal exercise programme	2	0	05		2
	39. Rehabilitation (other than formal exercise)	2	0	05		2
	40. Prevention of complications and infections	2	0	05		2
	41. Recreation, diversion	2	0	05		2
	42. Clinical procedures – urinalysis, B/P	2	0	05		2
	43. Special treatments (care of tracheotomy, use of oxygen, colostomy of catheter care, etc.)	2	0	05		2
	44. Procedures and techniques taught to patient	2	0	05		2
	(32) TOTALS		0			
VII	PROMOTION OF PHYSICAL AND EMOTIONAL HEALTH BY DIRECTION AND TEACHING					
	45. Plans for medical emergency evident	3	0	1		3
	46. Emotional support to patient	3	0	1		3
	47. Emotional support to family	3	0	1		3
	48. Teaching promotion and maintenance of health	3	0	1		3
	49. Evaluation of need for additional resources (spiritual, social service, homemaker service, physical or occupational therapy)	3	0	1		3
	50. Action taken in regard to needs identified	3	0	1		3
	(18) TOTALS		0			

TOTAL SCORE
FINAL SCORE

Note: Record reflects the service as:
Excellent (161–200)
Good (121–160)
Incomplete (81–120)
Poor (41–80)
Unsafe (0–40)
Source: Phaneuf, 1976

indicated and the auditor must enter 'yes', 'no' or 'uncertain' against each component. Uncertainty applies when the auditor is unsure as to whether there is enough evidence to state that the component has been adhered to, although it is clear that it has been considered. In Sections I–V every component is considered to be applicable, while in Sections VI and VII there is a 'does not apply' box. The audit committee will decide in advance which criteria they will accept for meeting the requirements of each component concerned. The final score is obtained by multiplying the total of the individual component scores by a value determined by the 'does not apply' responses. The final score is rated as follows:

- 161–200: excellent
- 121–160: good
- 81–120: incomplete
- 41–80: poor
- 0–40: unsafe

Advantages of Phaneuf's nursing audit

- it can be used as a method of measurement in all areas of nursing
- the seven functions are easily understood
- the scoring system is fairly simple
- the results are easily understood
- it assesses the work of all those involved in recording care
- it may be a useful tool as part of a quality assurance programme in areas where accurate records of care are kept.

Disadvantages of Phaneuf's nursing audit

- it appraises the outcomes of the nursing process, so it is not so useful in areas where the nursing process has not been implemented
- it is designed for a country that has a very different culture to that to the UK. It has not been adapted to take account of British nursing, politics, policies and procedures. This tool was devised over 20 years ago in the USA
- it is time-consuming
- it requires a team of trained auditors
- it deals with a large amount of information
- it only evaluates record-keeping; it only serves to improve documentation, not nursing care (Hegyvary and Haussman, 1975)
- the main area of criticism is the assumption that what is done is documented and what is documented is done (Meyers et al.)

■ Jelinek et al. argue that nurses soon learn how to document in a way that favourably influences the audit results, without necessarily changing the delivery of nursing.

Monitor

Monitor, an anglicised version of the Rush Medicus methodology, was produced by North-West Region and Newcastle-upon-Tyne Polytechnic. The Rush Medicus instrument was developed by the Rush Presbyterian St Luke's Medical Centre and the Medicus Systems Corporation of Chicago from 1972 and was completed in 1975. This system evolved from research in two main areas:

1. The development of a 'conceptual framework' stating what is being measured. As this constitutes a patient-centred approach, the nursing process and patient needs were the identified components.
2. The identification of criteria for evaluating the quality of care within this framework.

Within the system, there are a series of objectives and sub-objectives, which represent the structure of the nursing process (see Table 12.5).

At the same time as the development of this system, criteria were developed and tested to measure each of the subobjectives within the six main objectives. These criteria are written so that a 'yes' or 'no' response indicates the quality of care and, where appropriate, 'not applicable' may be applied. Each item is written in such a way as to minimise ambiguity and to ensure reliable interpretations and responses from the observers carrying out the study. Looking through the criteria, it is clear that they are relevant to almost any situation of patient care. This system is computerised and involves a simple dependency rating system, which enables the computer to select 30–50 criteria at random for each patient according to his/her dependency rating. In order to test the criteria, information is gained from the following sources:

■ questioning patients
■ questioning nurses
■ observing patients
■ observing nurses
■ observing the patient's environment
■ observing the general environment
■ examining records
■ the observer making inferences.

Table 12.5 Rush Medicus – objectives

1.0 *The plan of nursing care is formulated*
   1.1 The condition of the patient is assessed on admission.
   1.2 Data relevant to hospital care are ascertained on admission.
   1.3 The current condition of the patient is assessed.
   1.4 The written plan of nursing care is formulated.
   1.5 The plan of nursing care is co-ordinated with the medical plan of care.

2.0 *The physical needs of the patient are met*
   2.1 The patient is protected from accident and injury.
   2.2 The need for physical comfort and rest is met.
   2.3 The need for physical hygiene is met.
   2.4 The need for a supply of oxygen is met.
   2.5 The need for activity is met.
   2.6 The need for nutrition and fluid balance is met.
   2.7 The need for elimination is met.
   2.8 The need for skin care is met.
   2.9 The patient is protected from infection.

3.0 *The physical, emotional and social needs of the patient are met*
   3.1 The patient is orientated to hospital facilities on admission.
   3.2 The patient is extended social courtesy by the nursing staff.
   3.3 The patient's privacy and civil rights are honoured.
   3.4 The need for psychological, emotional wellbeing is met.
   3.5 The patient is taught measures of health maintenance and prevention of illness.
   3.6 The patient's family is included in the nursing care process.

4.0 *Achievement of nursing care objectives is evaluated*
   4.1 Records document the care provided for the patient.
   4.2 The patient's response to care and treatment is evaluated.

5.0 *Unit procedures are followed for the protection of all patients*
   5.1 Isolation and infection control procedures are followed.
   5.2 The unit is prepared for emergency situations.

6.0 *The delivery of nursing care is facilitated by administrative and managerial services*
   6.1 Nursing reporting follows prescribed standards.
   6.2 Nursing management is provided.
   6.3 Clerical services are provided.
   6.4 Environmental and support services are provided.

Rush Medicus developed a method for evaluating the quality of nursing care for medical, surgical and paediatric patients, including the relevant intensive care units. Evaluation is through the production of two indexes. The first is an average score of the quality of patient care and the second is a score for the unit environment. Management scoring is on a scale of 0–100, where a higher score indicates a better quality of care. The score obtained by the unit is an indicator of the quality of care rather than a measure of all aspects of the quality of care.

In the UK, Ball et al. (1983) successfully adapted the Rush Medicus methodology, resulting in the development of the monitoring tool, Monitor. The original version was designed for use on acute surgical and medical wards. However, more recent versions have been developed for use in geriatric wards and district nursing, followed by a version for psychiatric and paediatric wards in 1987. The midwifery and health-visiting versions were published by Leeds Polytechnic in 1989.

Monitor has a patient-orientated approach and two main concepts: individualised patient care and the patient's needs. Linked with these concepts is the monitoring of the support services who influence the delivery of good standards of patient care.

Monitor is based on a master list of 455 questions about patient care. Only 80–150 are directed at the care of any one patient and they are grouped into four sections:

- assessment and planning
- physical care
- non-physical care
- evaluation.

For typical questions, see Table 12.6.

Monitor follows the structure of the nursing process but the authors state that the clinical area being assessed does not have to be using this approach to patient care in order to use Monitor.

Table 12.6 Typical questions representing the different sections of the Monitor patient questionaire

---

ASSESSMENT AND PLANNING
- Is there a statement written within 24 hours of admission on the condition of the skin?
- Do the nursing orders or care plan include attention to the patient's need for discharge teaching?

PHYSICAL CARE
- Has the patient received attention to complaints of nausea and vomiting?
- Is adequate equipment for oral hygiene available?

NON-PHYSICAL CARE
- Do the nursing staff call the patient by the name he prefers?
- Are special procedures or studies explained to the patient?

EVALUATION
- Do records document the effect of the administration of 'as required' medication?
- Do records document the patient's response to teaching?

Source: Ball et al., 1983

Patients are classified into dependency groups according to the following factors:

- personal care
- feeding
- mobility
- nursing attention (frequency of nursing requirements)
- others (including incontinence, preparation for surgery, severe behavioural problems).

There are four levels of dependency:

- Category I – minimal care
- Category II – average care
- Category III – above-average care
- Category IV – maximum care.

The definitions of these levels of dependency are defined in Table 12.7.

There are four different questionnaires, each appropriate to a specific dependency category of patients. The criteria are presented as questions and the information is gained from a variety of sources – by asking the nurse or the patient, consulting records, and observing both the environment and the patient (see Table 12.8). The questions are answered by trained assessors with a ' yes', ' no', or 'not applicable' or ' not available'. The scoring system is 1 for 'yes' and 0 for 'no' – the 'not applicable/available' answers are deleted. The total score is given as the percentage of 'yes' responses obtained. The closer the score is to 100 per cent, the better the standard of care being delivered.

Most of the questions can be answered 'yes', 'no', or 'not applicable' or 'not available'. In some questions, the 'yes' answer is further divided into 'yes, always', 'yes, complete', and so on. All these variations of 'yes' count as a full 'yes' and score one. There is also 'yes, sometimes', 'yes in part' and 'yes incomplete', and so on. All of these variations score a half point. The answer 'no' does not score a point. Answers such as 'not applicable' or 'not available' are marked X. To obtain the per cent index for each section, and consequently the whole tool, which is an index of the quality of care of the patient, the assessor:

- deducts the number of inapplicable responses from the total number of questions to get the number of applicable answers
- adds together all the 'yes' answers as described to obtain the total score
- divides the total score by the number of applicable responses and multiplies by 100 to give the percentage.

Table 12.7 Definition of categories of dependency

CATEGORY I – MINIMAL CARE
Patient is physically capable of caring for himself but requires minimal nursing supervision and may require treatments and/or monitoring (e.g., B.P., T.P.R., clinical observations) by nursing staff.

CATEGORY II – AVERAGE CARE
Patient requires an average or moderate amount of nursing care, including some nursing supervision and encouragement. The patient may require some assistance with personal care needs as well as monitoring and treatments. Some examples would include:

- a patient past the acute stage of his disease or surgery
- a 3–4 day post-op cholecystectomy
- a diabetic patient for reassessment
- an independent patient requiring extensive investigative procedure

CATEGORY III – ABOVE-AVERAGE CARE
Patient requires a greater than average amount of nursing care, including nursing supervision, encouragement and almost complete assistance to meet personal care needs. The patient usually requires medical support and sometimes the use of special equipment. Some examples would be:

- a patient after the acute phase of CVA (residual paralysis)
- a first day post-op radical mastectomy or cholecystectomy
- a debilitated, dependent elderly person
- a newly diagnosed diabetic requiring extensive health teaching and support from nursing staff.

CATEGORY IV – MAXIMUM CARE
Patient requires very frequent to continuous nursing care along with close supervision by medical personnel and/or health team members, and/or support from technical equipment. Some examples would include:

- a quadriplegic in early rehabilitative stages
- a severely burned patient
- a comatose patient

Source: Ball et al., 1983

There is a software programme, which will calculate and print out the scores for patients, groups and wards. These results are then discussed with the charge nurse or sister and an action plan is developed to improve patient care. Ward scores can be compared within a trust or across trusts as part of benchmarking.

Advantages of Monitor

- using this tool involves the systematic collection of information related to the clinical area including documenting systems, management systems, the environment, the delivery of care and outcomes

Table 12.8 Extracts from the Monitor assessment form for dependency one patients

Source of information		Patient's code or initials:							

2. Nursing Staff Courtesy towards Patients

Ask Patient e. DO STAFF SEEK PATIENT'S PARTICIPATION DURING ROUNDS?
To patient: When doctors and nurses come to see you in a group, do they include you in their discussion

No	✓					
Yes, sometimes						
Yes, always						
Not applicable/ Not available						
52						
SCORE	0					

3. Patient's Privacy and Civil Rights

Records a. IS WRITTEN CONSENT OBTAINED BEFORE SPECIAL PROCEDURES ARE UNDERTAKEN?
Includes all procedures for which written consent must be given, e.g. surgery, lumbar puncture, etc.

No						
Yes	✓					
Not applicable/ Not available						
53						
SCORE	1					

Ask nurse b. IS THE NURSE AWARE OF WHAT THE PATIENT HAS BEEN TOLD ABOUT HIS/ HER ILLNESS?
To nurse: Has Mr/Mrs ... been told anything about his/her illness? Code 'no' If nurse is unsure or does not know

No						
Yes	✓					
Not aplicable/ Not available						
54						
SCORE	1					

Ask patient c. ARE SPECIAL PROCEDURES OR STUDIES EXPLAINED TO PATIENT
To patient: Have you had any special tests or procedures while you have been in hospital? If 'no' code 'not applicable/not available'. If 'yes' ask 'Were they explained to you before they were done?'

'Were the results of the tests explained to you?' Code 'yes fully' if yes to both. Code 'yes in part' if yes to only one.

No						
Yes in part						
Yes fully	✓					
Not applicable						
Not available						
55						
SCORE	1					

Source: Ball et al., 1984, p. c14

- it gives feedback to ward staff about the quality of care
- it helps staff to improve their performance
- it gives an indication of patient satisfaction
- it can compare performance with other wards and/or trusts
- it measures the effectiveness of the nursing process
- it provides information that can be used to facilitate future planning in areas such as training and the development of nursing.

Disadvantages of Monitor

- it requires a team of trained observers to monitor the ward or unit. This activity has resource and cost implications for the service
- it requires the purchase of several copies of the document
- the criteria measured are preset and therefore not owned by the staff whose performance is being measured
- a clear statement of its philosophy of nursing is lacking
- there are problems of observer reliability and subjective interpretation which may well be reduced if the observers have extensive training.

The Advantages and Disadvantages of 'Off-the-Shelf' Tools

Advantages

- 'off-the-shelf' tools are easy to use as they have already been developed, tried and tested and are therefore ready for immediate use
- the development of an audit tool can be a long process requiring a great deal of time in order to perfect it. The tools mentioned above give a broad picture of a ward predominately using criteria-based tools on the nursing process format
- they act as a baseline measure over time and, given that the study could be carried out annually within the same framework, they should act as a reliable indicator of change in care standards
- these tools are replicable in the same and in different areas
- they require an assessor who may be a staff nurse or the nurse in charge and can therefore find this a valuable learning experience
- as the tools are easy to implement, the data collected can be collated on software without difficulty

Disadvantages

- 'off the shelf' tools generally tend to focus on documentation, although Qualpacs does depend more on observational skills
- the focus of the tools tend to be non-specific, as they cover a wide range of topics and criteria
- areas that choose to undertake a study often feel anxious and threatened by having assessors – usually known to them – observing and checking documentation over a number of days
- regardless of preparation, most staff still admit to feeling nervous about these types of study.

Setting and Monitoring Standards

Background

In the late 1980s and the 1990s a large number of single discipline and some multidiscipline standards were written in the UK. Some of the standards were excellent and there is evidence that the use of standards improved patient care. Standards have been written as part of a standard-setting exercise by individual wards and departments and by whole services, directorates and hospitals, but they have also been written and validated as part of audit tools such as Monitor. Monitor is described in detail earlier in this chapter and contains a series of standards against which to measure the quality of care. The Audit Commission, when auditing a specific service, develops an audit guide based around a series of well-developed, evidence-based standards against which an auditor can measure a trust and compare the results of one trust against another. To review a service or a particular aspect of care, evidence-based standards can be drawn up to form an audit tool. An example of this would be an audit tool developed to measure how well staff dispose of sharps as part of an infection control audit. It is essential for any audit to be well researched and is evidence-based and to set out what is considered to be best practice. Part of an example of an audit tool is shown in Table 12.9.

The standard is developed and the criteria that allow the standard to be monitored become the audit tool. In order to develop these tools, it is essential to have a working knowledge of how to set and monitor standards. In Chapter 1 some of the key concepts, theories and principles were discussed and, in particular, the structure, process and outcome criteria approach to setting standards as described by Avedis Donabedian (1969). The following framework is the approach that was adapted by the Royal College of Nursing (RCN, 1980; 1981) as the Dynamic Standard Setting System (DYSSY), based on Donabedian's work. Although this framework has been used to set

Table 12.9 Part of an audit tool to measure the quality of infection control on a ward (the safe use and disposal of sharps)

Observe	Yes	No
1. Sharps are not passed directly from hand to hand		
2. Handling of sharps is kept to a minimum		
3. Needles are not broken prior to disposal		
4. Needles are not bent prior to disposal		
5. Needles and syringes are not disassembled prior to disposal		
6. Needles are not recapped		
7. Sharps are discarded into a sharps container		
8. Sharps containers are not filled above the mark on the container		
9. Containers in public areas are not placed on the floor		

standards in nursing, it has also been used successfully by staff from the professions allied to medicine, and by multidisciplinary teams. It is very simple, straightforward and could be adapted to set standards anywhere.

Setting and monitoring standards of care and quality assurance are separate issues, although you may hear people discuss them as though they were the same. For example, it may be stated that standards are poor, implying that quality is poor, and this leads to the misconception that standards and quality assurance are one and the same, but this is not the case. A standard is an instrument with which to measure the quality of care as part of quality assurance.

What are Standards of Care?

Standards are valid, acceptable definitions of the quality of care. Standards cannot be valid unless they contain criteria to enable care to be measured and evaluated in terms of effectiveness and quality. Standards written without criteria can be likened to using a ruler without any measurements marked upon it, and then attempting a scale drawing; the 'measurements' would be an estimate and therefore inaccurate and variable.

The Quality Assurance Cycle and Standards

It is important to understand where standards fit into the quality assurance cycle (see Figure 1.4). Professionals have often stated that 'it is very difficult to describe care in measurable terms', and standards will help professionals to achieve this.

1. *Describing standards*: it is helpful to start by writing a philosophy of care. This is really a statement about beliefs held to help and care for patients or clients, and an answer to questions such as Why are we here? – What do we believe we are doing? From this will come the objectives – what is hoped to be achieved. Once the philosophy and the objectives have been written, it will become clear what standards need to be written. If a specific audit tool is being developed, then first develop the objectives of the audit, and the standards to measure these objectives will become apparent. So the first step is to describe what must be done in measurable terms and then to identify standards and criteria in order to establish the quality of service.

2. *Measuring standards*: it is not possible to measure the quality of care unless it has been accurately described in measurable terms. Once the standard has been measured, the results should be reviewed, criteria not achieved should be identified and interpretations made about compliance with the standard.

3. *Taking action*: this is the last and most important step. It compares what should be with what is and then take action to ensure that the quality of care is assured. Then the cycle starts again to ensure that improvements were made.

Terminology Used in Standard-Setting

A standard statement

A standard statement is a professionally agreed level of performance, appropriate to the population addressed, which reflects what is acceptable, achievable, observable, and measurable. The first part of the statement, 'A standard statement is professionally agreed', means that a group of professionals or members of the healthcare team get together and in discussion agree a standard, taking into account research findings and changes in practice.

Table 12.10 A standard for measuring the quality of environmental hygiene

Topic:	Hospital-acquired infection
Sub Topic:	Hospital environmental hygiene
Care Group:	In-patients
Standard Statement:	The hospital environment within which the patient is cared for minimise the opportunity of the patient acquiring a hospital-acquired Infection and to acceptable to patients, visitors and staff.

Structure	Process	Outcome
Staff educated and trained in the prevention of hospital-acquired infection	Staff ensure that: 1. The hospital environment is clean	■ The hospital environment is: ☐ visibly clean ☐ free from dust ☐ free from soilage.
Policies regarding prevention of hospital-acquired infection	2. Equipment is cleaned by staff as per agreed procedure between usage by patients, i.e. commodes, bath hoists, IV pumps and stands, etc.	■ The patient/visitor/staff states that the environment is clean
Statutory requirements – disposal of waste, soiled and infected linen, food hygiene and pest control		■ Monitoring – random audits at least monthly of the environment
Infection control nurses	3. Staff wash their hands before and after contact with patients	■ Review of infection rates
Staff skills and knowledge		■ The patient states that the equipment is clean
Hospital acquired infection rate recorded and reported annually	Staff receive training and education related to preventing infection control	■ Commodes cleaned by nurses between usage by patients
	Hospital-acquired infections are reported to the infection control nurse	■ Bath hoists cleaned by nurses between usage by patients
		■ Bed washed down between patients
		■ Bed space cleaned between patients
		■ IV pumps cleaned between patients
		■ IV stands cleaned between patients
		■ Hospital-acquired infection rates are reduced.

Evidence Base
1. Hempshall P. and Thomson M. Grime watch. *Nursing Times* 1998; **16(94)** 37: 66–69.
2. National Audit Office. The Management and Control of Hospital-acquired Infection in Acute NHS Trusts in England. HC 230 Session 1999–00. London: The Stationery Office. 1999; 117.
3. Pratt R. J., Pellowe C., Loveday H. P., Robinson N. *epic phase 1: The Development of National Evidence-based Guidelines for Preventing Hospital-acquired Infections in England – Standard Principles: Technical Report.* London: Thames Valley University; 2000; 191. Available from (Internet): *http://www.epic.tvu.ac.uk*
4. Dance S.J. Mopping up hospital infection. *Journal of Hospital Infection* 1999; **43**: 85–100.
5. Garner J.S., Favero M.S. CDC Guideline for Handwashing and Hospital Environmental Control, 1985. Infection Control 1986; 7: 231–235.
6. Working Party for Standards for Environmental Cleanliness in Hospitals. *Standards for Environmental Cleanliness in Hospitals.* ICNA & Association of Domestic Management. 1999; 68.
7. NHS estates. Standards for environmental cleanliness in hospitals. London: The Stationery Office. 2000; 35.
8. Expert Advisory group on AIDS and the Advisory group on Hepatitis. *Guidance for clinical health care workers: Protection against infection with bloodborne viruses.* London: Department of Health 1998; 46.
9. Microbiology Advisory Committee. *Decontamination of equipment, linen or other surfaces contaminated with Hepatitis B and/or human immunodeficiency viruses.* HC (91) 33 London: Department of Health 1991; 6.
10. National Health Service Executive. *Controls Assurance Standard Infection control.* Leeds: Department of Health; 1999; 21.
11. National Health Service Executive. *Guidelines for Implementing Controls Assurance in the NHS (Guidance for Directors).* Leeds: Department of Health 1999; 36.
12. National Health Service Executive. *A First Class Service: Quality in the new NHS.* Leeds: Department of Health; 1998; 86.

The first and vital step in standard-setting is the beginning of the provision of continuity of care for the patient. The discussions about 'what we do' and 'who does it' prior to setting the standard are very valuable. These discussions may identify duplication of effort by professionals, differences in the way care is given and a debate on what should be done, how and when it should be done, and by whom.

The standard statement should include the indicators of quality, for example 'the hospital environment within which the patient is cared for minimises the opportunity for the patient to acquire a hospital-acquired infection. This statement could be strengthened by an indicator of quality and the additional words 'and is acceptable to patients, visitors and staff'. The second part of the statement, 'which relates to a level of performance', means establishing what you are trying to achieve for your patients/clients within your resources, and reaching the desired outcome. 'Appropriate to the population addressed' refers to the care group for which the standard is written, taking into account the patient's/client's and relatives' needs, negotiating care with patients/clients, and developing shared plans of care. The standard may be written for children or patients admitted for surgery, and so on. See Table 12.10.

Criteria

Criteria may be defined as descriptive statements of performance, behaviours, circumstances or clinical status that represent a satisfactory, positive or excellent state of affairs.

A criterion is a variable, or item, that is selected as a relevant indicator of the quality of care. Criteria make the standard work because they are detailed indicators of the standard and must be specific to the area or type of patient. Criteria must be:

- *measurable*: illustrating the standard and providing local measures
- *specific*: giving a clear description of behaviours/action/situation/resources desired or required
- *relevant*: items that you can identify as being necessary in order to achieve a set level of performance; there may be numerous criteria that you can think of, but you have to learn to be selective and pick out only those criteria that are the relevant indicators of quality of care and which must be met in order to achieve a set level of performance
- *clearly understandable*: they should each contain only one major theme or thought
- *clearly and simply stated*: so as to avoid being misunderstood
- *achievable*: it is important to avoid unrealistic expectations in either performance or results

■ *clinically sound*: they must be selected by practitioners who are clinically up to date, and base their knowledge on sound research or evidence.
■ *reviewed periodically*: to ensure that they are reflective of good practice based on current research
■ *reflective of all aspects of the patient or client status*: physiological, psychological and social.

In summary, a criterion must be:

■ a detailed indicator of the standard
■ specific to the area and type of patient or client
■ measurable.

Think of the standard as a tape measure or ruler and the criteria as the measurement marks. The criteria allow you to measure the standard; they make it possible to measure the standard statement.

There are three types of criteria:

■ structure
■ process
■ outcome.

When thinking about and writing a standard, it is easier to start with the outcome and work backwards, working on the theory that if you know what you want to achieve, it is easier to establish what you need to do to get there.

Outcome criteria
Outcome criteria describe the effect of the care – the results expected in order to achieve the standard in terms of behaviours, responses, levels of knowledge and health status; in other words, what is expected and desirable described in a specific and measurable form (see Table 12.9).
Consider the following statements:

■ the professional can state ... (For example, 'Please explain the procedure for cleaning equipment by staff before and after use by a patient')
■ the patient can state ... (For example, 'Did the staff treating you wash their hands prior to contact with you?' – 'yes' or 'no')
■ there is documented evidence ... (This evidence may be found in the patient's records, nursing records, on charts, etc. For example, the infection rate has reduced)
■ the professional observed ... (This will include the observation of patient behaviour, staff behaviour, the environment. For example, the professional or the assessor of the standard observes that the ward environment is clean.)

One of the reasons for developing the outcome criteria into immediately measurable criteria is to ensure that standards are measured all the time as part of the evaluation of care. Many professionals see the measurement of standards as 'someone else's responsibility', rather than part of patient or client care. Outcomes that are not being achieved need to be corrected immediately, not left for quarterly or six-monthly formal monitoring.

Monitoring outcomes

Outcome criteria can be very broad, for example 'the hospital environment is clean'. This outcome requires a monitoring tool in order to measure what aspects of the hospital environment are clean. An alternative is to state the outcome criteria as shown in Table 12.10 and simply add on 'yes' or 'no' columns in the outcome column. Monitoring should be carried out using the criteria marked with a bullet point through observation of activity and asking the patients and carers.

The standard is measured for all patients in the hospital all the time as part of the process of care. Any outcome criteria that are not achieved are investigated and corrected at the time, thus ensuring good-quality care.

Process criteria

Process criteria (see Table 12.10) describe what action must take place in order to achieve the outcome that has already been set:

- assessment techniques and procedures
- methods of delivery of care
- methods of intervention
- methods of patient, client, relative/carer education
- methods of giving information
- methods of documenting
- how resources are used
- evaluation of the competence of staff carrying out the care.

The following headings indicate the areas to include in process criteria – what must be done to meet the standard statement and the outcome:

- the professional assesses ... (For example, the patient's needs)
- the professional includes in the plan ... (For example, the patient's care plan)
- the professional does ... (For example, follows set policies, procedures, guidelines, pathways)
- the professional ensures ... (For example, infections, accidents and incidents are reported; equipment is clean; documentation is completed, and so on)

- the professional reviews ... (For example, reviews the plan of care, that policies and procedures are current, and so on)
- the professional and the patient or client ... (For example, negotiates the plan for discharge from hospital, plans the patient's care together, and so on).

Structure criteria

Structure criteria may be seen as a 'shopping list' of requirements; the items of service which must be provided in order to achieve the standard (see Table 12.10), such as:

- the physical environment and buildings
- ancillary and support services
- equipment
- staff: numbers, skill-mix, training, expertise
- information: agreed policies and procedures, rules and regulations, protocols, guidelines, research and evidence
- organisational system.

In summary, criteria state:

- what is needed to meet the standard
- what must be done to meet the standard
- the expected results or outcome.

It is important to remember that the criteria describe the activities to be performed, whereas the standard states the level at which they are to be performed. The criteria are like the strings on a puppet, making the standard come alive. By following this process, patient or client care can be measured by comparing actual practice against the stated criteria and then checking to see if the activity has met the agreed standard.

Checking Standards

Once the standard has been written, check that the criteria:

- describe the desired quality of performance
- have been agreed
- are clearly written (not open to misinterpretation)
- contain only one major thought
- are measurable
- are concise
- are specific

■ are achievable
■ are clinically sound
■ are evidence-based.

Monitoring Standards

There are two approaches to monitoring standards:

■ retrospective evaluation
■ concurrent evaluation.

Retrospective evaluation involves all assessment methods that occur after the patient or client has been discharged. Concurrent evaluation involves assessment that takes place while the patient or client is still receiving care. Table 12.11 lists the approaches used to assess the quality of care. The use of concurrent evaluation is perhaps more valuable, as it gives staff the opportunity to correct any negative outcomes while the patient is still in their care.

Approaches to monitoring standards

Type 1: as discussed earlier, the process of monitoring standards may be made simpler and more effective by writing the outcome criteria in a form that requires a 'yes' or 'no' answer. Remember that each outcome criterion must contain only one question or theme. The patient states that he is satisfied with the standard of cleanliness of the hospital and the equipment used. The patient may feel that the hospital environment is clean but that the equipment that the

---

Table 12.11 Retrospective and concurrent evaluation of care

At the end of an episode of care	As care is being given
Retrospective evaluation of the quality of nursing care may be affected by: ■ Post-care patient interview ■ Post-care patient questionnaire ■ Post-care staff conference ■ Audit of the records	Concurrent evaluation may be affected by: ■ Assessment of the outcome ■ Patient interview ■ Conference between patient, staff and relatives ■ Direct observation of care ■ Measurement of the competency of the nurse ■ Audit of the records

staff use is not always clean. This is difficult to measure and the patient should be asked two specific questions:

- is the environment always clean?
- is the equipment used always clean?

Type 2: an alternative approach is to take criteria from structure, process and outcome and turn them into a list of questions. Each question is used as an indicator which requires a 'yes' or 'no' answer. The total number of 'yes' answers may be added together to calculate a score and demonstrate whether or not the standard has been achieved.

Retrospective Monitoring

Retrospective monitoring involves all assessment mechanisms carried out after the patient has been discharged. These include:

- *closed-chart auditing*, which is the review of the patient's records and identification of strengths and deficits of care. This can be achieved by a structured audit of the patient's records
- *post-care patient interview*, which is carried out when the patient has left the hospital or care has ceased in the home. It involves inviting the patient and/or family members to meet to discuss experiences. This may be un- structured, semi-structured or structured using a checklist or questionnaire
- *post-care questionnaires*, which should be completed by the patient on discharge. They are usually designed to measure patient satisfaction
- *review of data collected* such as hospital-acquired infection rates, accidents and incidents, complaints and so on.

Concurrent Monitoring

Concurrent monitoring involves all assessments performed while the patient is receiving care. These include:

- *open-chart auditing*, which is the review of the patient's charts and records against pre-set criteria. As the patient is still receiving care, this process gives staff immediate feedback
- *patient interview or observation*, which involves talking to the patient about certain aspects of care, conducting a bedside audit or observing the patient's behaviour to pre-set criteria

- *staff interview or observation*, which involves talking to and observing nursing behaviour related to pre-set criteria
- *group conferences*, which involve the patient and/or family in joint discussion with staff about the care being received. This leads to problems being discussed and improved plans agreed.

The various types of measurement need to be discussed by the group and the most appropriate method selected.

The Final Stage

The final stage in standard-setting is to compare current practice with the standard and to act on the monitoring result. If the standard has not been achieved, you need to check why:

- is it an achievable standard?
- is the standard realistic?

If the answer to these questions is 'no', then review and revise the standard. However, if it is achievable, then develop an action plan to ensure that practice meets the standard.

As demonstrated in Figure 1.5, the measurement of standards is not 'quality assured'. Quality assurance only occurs when gaps have been identified following measurement, and action has been taken to ensure that standards are achieved, gaps are closed and the cycle begins again.

Summary of Points on Standard-Setting

It is important to remember that standards at local level are written by those who deliver the care. The very process of setting standards leads to discussion about practice: who does what and how. Any team of professionals will comprise people who were trained at different times, have different professional backgrounds and have varying levels of experience and competence.

Talking about practice gives everyone a chance to share experience and expertise, and this alone improves the quality of care. In order to have an agreed standard, there must be consensus of opinion, which inevitably leads to improved continuity of care.

Continuity of care, practising according to research findings and keeping up to date can be a potential problem, particularly for professionals working in isolation, and the process of setting standards is a very useful method of promoting good-quality care that is evidence-based.

Monitoring standards is like taking a snapshot of the quality of care to establish the standard of care. If the standard is poor or there are problems, then there may be a need to develop and set up a clinical audit around the problem area in order to make a thorough investigation and to identify and implement the solutions. Whilst the monitoring of standards may be seen as a snapshot of activity, the process of clinical audit should be viewed as a detailed portrait. Table 12.9 demonstrates what a written standard might look like. When using this methodology to develop an audit tool, the criteria may be taken from the structure, process and/or outcome criteria.

Advantages of Setting Standards

- standards are written and monitored by staff in clinical areas or at organisational level
- standards are written and monitored by the multidisciplinary team in order to monitor the quality of patient care
- standards reflect the philosophy and values of those who have written them
- standards are dynamic and change in response to changes in practice, resources and research findings
- the very process of setting standards gives a group of clinical staff the chance to discuss and review their practice
- once standards have been set, they can be incorporated into ward, department, unit and health authority targets
- written standards can be used to monitor care, assess the level of service provided, identify deficiencies, communicate expectations and introduce new knowledge
- there is no need for a team of trained observers to monitor standards.

Disadvantages of Setting Standards

- problems can arise from badly written or poorly articulated standards or standards that have no evidence base and do not reflect best practice
- staff may be unfamiliar with measurement techniques and the development of measurement tools by staff may lead to unreliability
- there are a large number of standards that have been set at national level as part of the NSFs and so on, and as standard-setting is time-consuming it is possibly no longer necessary to write many local standards
- researching the evidence is time-consuming and requires critical-appraisal skills

- to set standards effectively, an individual who has experience of setting and measuring standards is required to facilitate the activity at least to start with
- teaching staff how to set and monitor standards has resource implications.

Conclusion

Advantages of Criteria-Based Audits

- criteria-based audits are useful when staff feel that a problem might exist but they are unsure of the scale of the problem or the reason for its existence
- valid, comprehensive and easy-to-use audit criteria are formulated after a study of research-based information, reading other audit tools and formulating questionnnaires
- staff at ward level are fully included in the whole change process and therefore feel less threatened by the audit. It also assists in the implementation of the action plan.

Disadvantages of Criteria-based Audits

- the methods used to formulate a criteria-based audit are not methodologically pure and it could be argued that the results obtained can only be specific for that area
- if they were to be transferable, the tool would need to be piloted further and tested by a number of assessors to prove its validity
- only when there is a very clear idea of what is being measured will they be of use and avoid the trap of being general and non-specific.

The principles set out in this chapter have been included to give some insight into a variety of tools that have been tried and tested in the quest for monitoring the quality of care. Today it is not enough to introduce a system of setting and monitoring standards, to use Monitor or to develop a clinical audit. To be effective, a combination of methodologies to monitor the quality of care is essential as part of a systematic framework for clinical governance.

One difference between the 'off-the-shelf' tools and clinical governance is that the clinical governance framework includes all staff from all disciplines, with no single profession taking responsibility for quality improvement. However, the most important difference is that 'off-the-shelf' tools audited the care received by patients but their involvement was often passive. In clinical governance this is not the case; patient and public involvement is paramount to the success of the clinical governance framework.

The successful implementation of clinical governance and continuous quality improvement by its nature will necessitate change and the next chapter looks at the management of this change.

Skills to Support Clinical Governance – The Management of Change

13

Chapter Contents:

- background
- definitions of change
- theories and models
- change methodology.

Having a broad knowledge of clinical governance and quality assurance techniques and approaches is an excellent start to the implementation of clinical governance in practice. But how does all this theory become reality? Whatever approach is used to assure and improve the quality of care, there is bound to be a need for change to either existing views or to approaches to the delivery of a service or practice. Techniques such as working with groups, facilitator training, project management and empowerment are all essentials tools to be used in the process of change and these are included in detail in the following chapters. The management of change is an essential skill to ensure that clinical governance becomes a sustained reality: 'Clinical governance is about assuring sustainable continuous quality improvement' (NHS Executive 1999). Such quality improvement inevitably requires change.

Background

Since the founding of the NHS in 1948 there have been reorganisations and changes to meet the changing need of the populace and improved care to meet the patient's needs, for example the implementation of special care units, general management, the purchaser–provider split, resource management, the creation of trusts, GP fundholding and other changes too numerous to mention. Much of this change has been driven by:

- health policy
- raising patient and carer expectations through the Patient's Charter

- the increasingly ageing population and the resulting increase in high-dependency patients and those with multiple needs
- demographic changes
- advances in health technology
- lack of public confidence in the NHS because of media coverage of poor practice and an increase in the number of complaints going to litigation.

The breadth and complexity of these developments require the skilful management of change. This chapter sets out to explore some change models that have been successfully used in the NHS and through a worked example of a management of change methodology. This is about successfully implementing change through an organisation and then expanding on the principles of change as applied to a ward or department. It concludes with a worked example of change management.

Definitions of Change

There are numerous definitions that surround 'change', one of which describes change as ' the process of moving from one system to another' (Gillies, 1988), which perhaps encompasses the elements of the change process requiring the consideration of input, throughput and output linking the present situation with the anticipated changed situation. There are some common characteristics of change in the healthcare environment:

- change is vital if patient care is to avoid becoming stagnant
- change is a process and not an event
- change is normal and constant
- the pace of change has increased and is likely to increase in response to health policy, demographic changes and advances in health technology
- change can be reactive to external circumstances and pressures
- change can be 'top down', instigated by management and 'bottom up', instigated from those people directly involved in the impact of change
- change can be a continuous series of small changes or a radical 'one off' change shift from current to new practice
- the impact of change is not predictable and often needs adjustment in the light of experience and experimentation
- there is a relationship between change and the culture of the organisation.

Theories and Models

Any change process involves a series of identifiable stages. Some models are more complex than others but all the examples below have clearly defined steps. This chapter does not set out to give a critique of these models but simply provides a small sample of those models that might be useful in managing change in a health service environment either clinical or non-clinical.

Bennis et al. (1998) identify three strategies that can be used in the process of change:

- empirical rational
- normative re-educative
- power coercive.

The empirical rational strategies are based on the notion that people are rational and act according to self-interest. The model is based, therefore, on the expectation that individuals will adopt change if they can accept that it is justified and that they will benefit from that change.

Normative re-education strategy is based on the idea that people act according to their commitment to sociocultural norms. Attitudes and values, intelligence and rationality are taken into account in this strategy.

Power coercive strategy is the acceptance by less powerful people of the leadership of the powerful. Conflict is part of the strategy. The conflict theory of social change states that most organisational change is the result of dissatisfaction, frustration or some other form of conflict. The resolution of this conflict leads to change within the organisation. However, the authors also point out that the efforts of change may, and often do, lead to conflict with other groups who have no difficulty with the present systems and therefore no desire to change.

Rogers's Model

Rogers (1979) identifies five stages through which the individual has to move: awareness, interest, evaluation, trial and adaptation. The awareness stage leads to an 'unfreezing' phase in the form of interest, and evaluation of this leads on to the trial or 'moving' phase and then on to the adaptation or 'refreezing' phase when the adaptation is either accepted or rejected.

This theory is underpinned by the individual's need to be interested in the innovation and to be committed to making the change happen. However, Rogers believes that enabling change is not just about education and that, having changed the knowledge base of an individual, he/she can either adopt or reject the change. Adopting the change will mean the implementation of the change in their practice and the testing of the change to ensure that it is best practice (Rogers, 1983).

Fretwell's Model

Fretwell (1985) developed a demographic model of change, which facilitates teams through the change process and includes:

- research findings
- insight
- consultation (which links with controlled anxiety and teamwork)
- support
- praise
- peer groups
- teamwork
- the control of anxiety
- creativity
- progress.

Open Systems Model

This model attempts to address the whole change cycle, and according to Beckhard and Harris (1987) there are four key steps:

- identifying what is driving change, its power and the control you have over this
- describing how the future will be, which may involve setting goals or standards to be achieved
- assessing the current situation or setting a baseline compared to future objectives: what is against what will be
- defining what is required to move from the present to the future position, including the management of this process.

These steps do not have to be taken in the order set out above, as demand may require each to be given simultaneous attention in order to arrive at a solution.

Lewin's Forcefield Theory

Lewin (1953) sets out three stages of the change process:

- unfreezing
- moving to a new level
- refreezing.

Unfreezing: this stage recognises that for change to come about, the individual or the team need to become aware of the problem or catalyst for change, to recognise the need for change and to believe that there is room for improvement. Lewin suggests that there is a need to understand what driving and restraining forces exist and that unfreezing only exists when the driving forces are increased and the restraining forces decreased.

Moving to a new level: this step involves the exploration and examination of change, the clarification of the problem and the start of acceptance and adjustment to the changes being implemented. It is also at this stage that key roles and responsibilities emerge and the planning of action for change takes place.

Refreezing: refreezing occurs after the change has been accepted by the group or organisation when individuals take on new roles and responsibilities and there is evidence of integration and stabilisation of change in everyday practice.

Hinings's Model

Hinings's model (Hinings, 1983) has five stages:

1. *Diagnosis*: the starting point and the identification of what change is required or desired.
2. *Identifying resistance*: not everyone involved in the process will necessarily be in favour of the proposed change and their resistance must be identified so that the issues can be addressed.
3. *Allocating responsibility*: this step is about developing commitment to the planned change and involves giving people leadership roles in managing the change process. This in turn strengthens their commitment to change and helps them to motivate others to implement change.
4. *Developing and implementing strategies*: this stage is concerned with the implementation of the planned change.
5. *Monitoring*: this is the final part of the process. Monitoring must be carried out in observable and measurable terms, followed by an assessment of whether or not the planned change has been achieved. Results of monitoring may take the group back to any stage already mentioned: for example, monitoring may identify resistance not previously identified, which would take the group back to Stage 2.

Hinings's model and indeed all models and theories of change developed by researchers and academics have one thing in common: the emphasis on the interrelationships and interactivity between the different stages that can be distinguished and labelled. Organisations and organisational change are not that simple and it is not possible to follow a linear series of activities as listed by the authors of these models. Hinings recognised that the five stages should not be seen as free-standing, rather that planned change must be an interactive process. The stages set out should be seen as a series of steps that are flexible and can be taken forwards and sideways as well as backwards. In the quest for change some steps may be repeated, some may be omitted and some may even merge into each other.

Perhaps one of the most powerful methods of change is Total Quality Management (TQM). TQM in healthcare is often known as continuous quality improvement (CQI), which by its very name suggests a system of continuous planned change. Some of the changes will be radical and extensive, perhaps of whole services, while others will be small continuous steps to the improvement of quality in a combination of 'top down' and 'bottom up' change initiatives. See Chapter 11 for more information on TQM.

Change Methodology

The following methodology (see Figure 13.1) is based on the principles of change adapted for use in a trust and taken from a compilation of a number of well-documented methodologies from the business world and the health service. The change methodology was developed to guide organisations through the tasks and activities required to achieve successful change across a whole organisation or indeed on a smaller scale in a ward or department. This change methodology may be used for process improvement efforts focused on:

- improving quality
- reducing waiting times
- lowering costs
- organisational developments such as restructuring, job design, and training to provide new capabilities.

Designed to be flexibly applied, the change methodology is essentially a practical framework that addresses four key issues:

- what needs to be done
- when it should be done
- how should it be done
- how changes are implemented successfully.

The methodology includes four stages necessary to assess the need for change and implement the changes required to improve performance or care.

1. *Assess (assessment of the current situation)*: this is the stage:
   - when the identification of change drivers takes place. These include reorganisation, changes in management and changes in practice
   - which includes an assessment of the current environment and the readiness for change of the organisation, and the identification of issues and opportunities for improvement
   - at which to validate strategies, assess current performance, and analyse issues and opportunities (see Figure 13.1).
2. *Envision*: at this stage there is development of the vision, and performance measures and targets, in other words:
   - what is to be achieved
   - the design of a target environment capable of achieving the vision and overall performance measures and targets
   - the development of a change implementation plan.
3. *Implement*: this is the stage of the implementation of new processes, systems, structure, skills, culture, technologies and facilities through one of several concurrent implementation projects (see Figure 13.1).
4. *Evaluate*: this is the final stage where interim performance improvement levels are achieved, continuous improvement capability is in place and in use, and there is an evaluation of the change that has taken place (see Figure 13.1).

During all four stages it is important to keep managers, clinicians and all those immediately involved in the project well-informed of the stages reached in the project and of the progress of the group so a system of 'deliverables' and 'interim outputs' may be used to support good communication. Deliverables include:

- evaluation reports
- a target environment design
- a change plan
- an implementation change report
- a continuous improvement plan.

Interim outputs are usually internal project team documents that support and mark the progress towards the deliverables.

In addition to project stages, phases and tasks that result in work products and deliverables, the change methodology includes activities used to facilitate the transition to a new working environment such as managing communications, securing commitment to change, and building teams and transferring skills. This is the approach that would be used by a project team to undertake and implement organisational change on a large scale, but the same principles apply for a project that requires change in a single ward or department or in a group of staff working together.

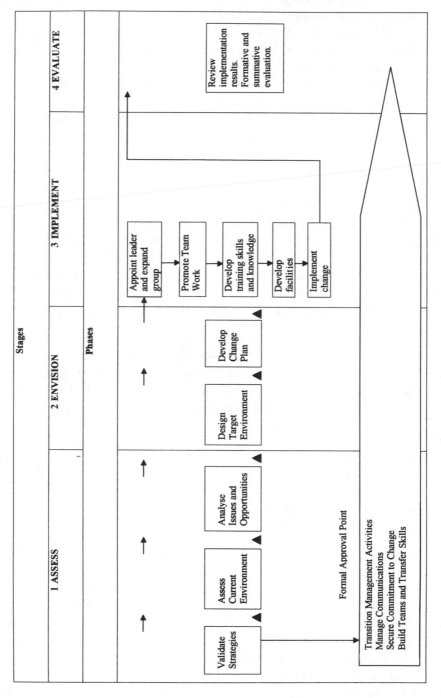

Figure 13.1 Change methodology – stages and phases

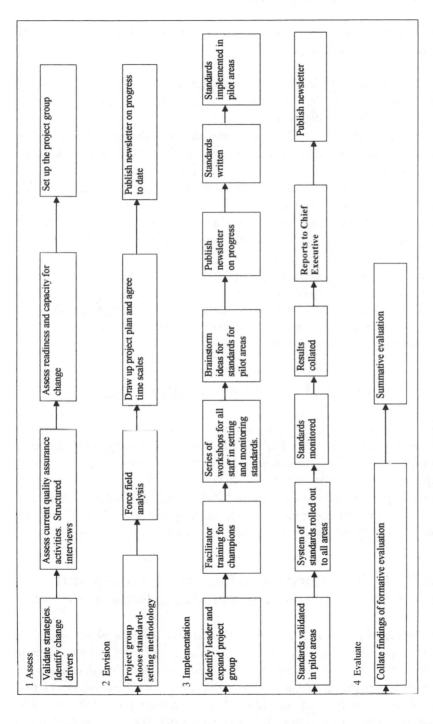

Figure 13.2 Change methodology flow chart – implementation of a system of setting and monitoring standards across an acute general hospital

Summary of Change Methodology

The change methodology provides a practical framework for addressing the four primary issues in change projects:

1. *What needs to be done*: the change methodology defines a comprehensive set of activities useful in achieving change and guides the reader in selecting certain tasks for specific projects.
2. *When it should be done*: the change methodology defines the sequence in which activities are to be completed and identifies their interrelationships and dependencies.
3. *How it should be done*: the change methodology provides instruction on activities and techniques including:
   - assessment of current environment and performance
   - design of target environment performance measures and targets and change implementation plan
   - development of the project group
   - choice of leadership of the group.
4. *How changes are implemented successfully*: the change methodology provides information on the evaluation of the change project, performance review and communication of the results.

Worked Example of the Change Methodology

In order to demonstrate a worked example of the methodology it is necessary to take each stage as set out in Figure 13.2, to expand on each of the identified activities and to link the activities with examples of change within a healthcare setting – starting with assessment, which is Stage 1. Within this section there are three major activities to be addressed, which include validating strategies, assessing the current environment and assessing the group's readiness for change. Each of these activities is broken down into specific actions.

Case Study: Implementing a System of Setting and Monitoring Standards across an Acute General Hospital

The background to this change plan is that the project took place before the introduction of clinical governance. The hospital in question had no system in place for monitoring the quality of care and the chief executive decided that a systematic approach was needed. An external expert was brought in to set up and implement a system that would result in a regular report to the board on the quality of care in the hospital. It was agreed that the place to start was a system of setting and monitoring standards for all disciplines and departments. Some standards would be multidisciplinary and others single-discipline and, once this system was in place, the hospital would move on to addressing the implementation of other quality assurance initiatives including clinical audit, integrated care pathways, and so on. The flow chart set out in Figure 13.2 shows the process of implementing a system for the setting and monitoring of standards across a hospital. The theory of change methodology which follows can be applied to Figure 13.2.

1. Assess (assessment of the current situation)

Validate strategies and identify change drivers
This includes identifying the change drivers or levers, reviewing the mission statement and undertaking a SWOT analysis. The four stages are set out in Figure 13.2 and the process starts with the validation of strategies, which requires the group to identify the change drivers.

- *change drivers/levers*: the group start by identifying the change drivers or the levers for change, for example:
  - □ events that drive the need for change such as untoward incidents, complaints, and changes in healthcare and Government policy
  - □ a change in management or restructuring requiring changes in the way services are provided
  - □ shortfalls in performance, for example waiting lists
  - □ changes in practice
  - □ financial pressures
  - □ the results of a visit by the Healthcare Commission which has led to the identification of areas that require change or improvement
  - □ the publication of guidelines, evidence or recommendations by NICE
  - □ recent research
  - □ the requirements of a National Service Framework.
- *mission statement*: the group must take time to become familiar with the trust's mission statement. A mission statement usually contains no more than three sentences and the priority of each of the statements is the order in which they are written. These statements provide a check for each stage of the change programme to ensure that staff are working within the agreed mission or vision of the trust directorate or department. The accident and emergency department, for example, may exist to provide the highest quality of care for the largest number of patients seeking emergency treatment, while maintaining professional standards and minimising waiting times. Therefore any changes must be seen to fit within the boundaries of this vision. If the proposed change is about introducing nurses with advanced training to work as nurse practitioners then the first step is to consider if such an innovation would compromise the mission statement.

■ *strengths, weaknesses, opportunities and threats (SWOT)*: the group meet to carry out a SWOT analysis of the organisation, ward or department:
  □ what are the strengths of the organisation, ward or department compared with other similar areas? What does it do well?
  □ what are the weaknesses of the organisation, ward or department compared with other similar areas? What areas of care or service could be improved upon?
  □ what are the opportunities for the organisation, ward or department in its environment? What could it do to improve the service /care?
  □ what are the threats to the organisation, ward or department? What potential threats might there be?

Assess the current environment/define the present state:
It is essential to have a clear understanding of the possible knock-on effect that one part of the system will have on another: for example, if changes are made to the running of the supplies department these may well affect the smooth running and the delivery of care to patients in the accident and emergency department.

The current environment can be assessed through environment or process mapping, which is a technique that can be used to establish the total environment that affects, and is affected by, the system that the group wants to change. See Chapter 8 for more information on process mapping. The system consists of formal and informal structures, the goals, cultural norms, behaviours, skills and beliefs of individual members, and the interaction between these. The group may think that they know where change is needed and be tempted to impose change but most change agents fail because they have not undertaken a thorough diagnosis or analysis of all aspects of the existing situation.

Assess readiness for change
Identify and list the key people and their readiness and capability for the proposed change (see Figure 13.3).

If capability is low, then the group will need to spend less time working with the individual. It is inefficient to spend time on an individual who has no further potential as a resource, demonstrating low capability to further the process of change; it is more efficient to focus on those with medium-to-high readiness and capability. This approach shows where the effort should be directed. This is a useful exercise prior to getting the group together to manage the process of change.

Analyse issues and opportunities
Carry out an analysis of the information gathered in the steps outlined above in the 'establish the current situation' stage: this will support the baseline for the implementation of change. For example, what quality assurance activities

The Principles of Change Stage 1: Evaluate – assess readiness for change						

Readiness/capability charting

Key Players	Readiness			Capability		
	High	Medium	Low	High	Medium	Low
Doctor 1	0-----------X			0X		
Doctor 2	0X			0X		
Manager	X	0			0X	
Nurse 1	0-----------X				0X	
Nurse 2			0X			0X
Physiotherapist		0-----------X		0----------------------X		
Receptionist	0-----------------------X			0X		

X = current level
0 = potential level

Figure 13.3 A readiness and capability chart for use in Stage 1 – assess readiness for change
Source: Broome, 1998

exist within the organisation? Who has set standards? Who has the skills to set standards? Is there any enthusiasm for standard-setting? With the answers to these questions, set up the project group.

Summary
During this stage the following tasks have been completed:
■ the mission statement and strategies have been validated
■ readiness and capability for change has been assessed
■ process mapping has been completed
■ the information gathering has been analysed
■ the project group has been set up.

2. Envision

Envision the future environment with standards as a system for monitoring the quality of care
Design the target environment: describe the desired future state, develop several scenarios and visualise the change.

In order to plan change, the group must have some idea of what the future situation will look like. This vision gives the group something to aim for or aspire to. This vision may be arrived at through techniques such as brainstorming, which is outlined in detail in Chapter 16. The vision may be imposed from external sources such as reducing waiting times or implementing a National Service Framework or it may be an innovative change to improve patient care by a team within a directorate. Beckhard and Harris (1987) suggest two steps in scenario planning: first, agree on an ideal end state, what life will look like after the change process is completed, for example in July 2005; secondly, select a midpoint and identify a specific date for this, for example July 2004. Then visualise the scenario and the actual conditions that will exist by that date in behavioural terms. This sets the agenda for change.

Diagnosis

This involves making some key decisions. Broom (1998) suggests the following questions to help with this stage:

- what types of changes are needed? Are these attitudes, behaviour, policies or practice?
- which systems and parts of the organisation are involved and what are the boundaries/domains which will have to be managed?
- establish the system's readiness for change. What are the forces for and against change? How realistic is change? Is it really possible or are you wasting your time?
- determine your own resources in helping the change effort:
  - □ what is your motivation?
  - □ why do others want to change?
  - □ are there career benefits?
  - □ will patient care improve?
- what level of energy do key people bring to the project?
  - □ are they ready?
  - □ are they capable?
- which system is most vulnerable to change?
  - □ what is the linkage with other parts of the hospital/system?
  - □ can you use a domino effect?

Forcefield analysis

Forcefield analysis is a technique to identify those forces which assist or obstruct the implementation of change. To undertake a forcefield analysis, take a piece of paper and describe the planned change in a simple sentence and then list the driving forces which support the change on the left-hand side of the paper and the restraining forces on the right-hand side. Establish which of the restraining forces pose the greatest threat to change and highlight them for specific action in the change plan. Then determine which of the driving forces represent the best levers for implementing change and highlight them for action. It is important to maximise the driving forces, but breaking down the barriers to change of the restraining forces is generally more effective than promoting the favourable ones.

Shared vision: Communication

The vision may be the restructuring of a service or the streamlining of a service but in all cases the vision must be grounded in reality through the development of performance measures and targets. Achieving the vision requires the organisation, ward, department or group to change, and people do not change until they are motivated to change. More often than not, the vision encompasses the need to satisfy the users of a service such as the patients, carers, staff, and so on. Performance measurement of user satisfaction should, therefore, be part of the vision.

Undertake a literature search and review the resulting information to establish if the change planned has previously been undertaken, either in part or in its totality. Use this information to inform the change plan.

Setting targets is also important: for example, if the proposed change is to set up a discharge lounge for surgical patients, then one of the targets might be to reduce cancellations for booked surgery, because patients can be discharged to a comfortable, supervised lounge first thing in the morning instead of occupying a bed on the ward until they are able to leave the ward. Benchmarking against other trusts on many aspects of the health service can be useful and provide motivation to be the best.

If the vision is to introduce a nurse practitioner into an accident and emergency department, then one of the targets will be to reduce waiting times for the minor injury patients that the nurse practitioner will treat. However, this will potentially have a knock-on effect on the waiting times for all patients attending the department.

The vision must be shared, involving people meeting together to share their concerns about an organisation and agreeing as a group to resolve some of the problems. Sharing ideas leads to a shared vision, which can give drive and encouragement to the group through the process of change. One of the key issues is to develop and communicate a vision of the future together with a credible and honest analysis why change is required.

Developing the change plan

In order to determine what needs to occur to move from the current situation to the vision or future scenario, the change plan must:

- define and communicate objectives and responsibilities
- identify who will lead the project
- set out how goals are to be achieved in priority order and the processes to get there
- include objectives and a timetable that are realistic and agreed by the group

■ set out a series of logical steps to achieve change with dates
■ set out the tools and techniques to be used, preferably ones that are proven and valid
■ be clear about resources including time, access to expertise and organisational commitment to the plan
■ involve patients if the change is clinically based
■ demonstrate flexibility and adaptability to take into account any changes which may occur
■ include a period for testing how the changes will be achieved
■ have a monitoring system to check how new change is affecting the whole organisation.

To develop the monitoring system, the group need to consider what data must be collected to test the process of change, whether the method of collection will be concurrent or retrospective, who will collect the data, how much is requested, who will analyse it and by what method.

Publish newsletter on progress to date
Everyone receives the same message through regular publication of a newsletter. This keeps everyone up to date.

Summary
During this stage the following tasks have been completed:
■ the target environment has been designed
■ the desired future state has been described
■ several scenarios have been developed
■ the change has been visualised
■ the change actions have been identified
■ the change plan has been developed
■ newsletter published.

3. Implement

The change plan is implemented through the development of new processes, systems, structures, skills, culture, information technology and facilities. Successful implementation requires a detailed assessment of resources in terms of people, time and materials.

Identify a leader and expand the project group
To implement the change plan the group need to:

■ appoint a project manager or someone to take the lead
■ develop project teams from different levels of the organisation, including people with different skills, people who are natural leaders, those already

committed to the proposed change, those already assessed as capable of making the change happen, those who will take responsibility for actions and manage the change, and people who will build commitment.

Leadership of the process of change

There are many distinguished writers on the subject of leadership. However, Mintzberg (1973) suggests a range of group roles that leaders may adopt which seem particularly relevant to the process of change and includes the:

- figurehead role: ceremonial public-speaking role
- group leader role: resolving operational problems
- liaison role: being a representative for the group
- information role
- spokesperson role: representing your profession externally
- entrepreneurial role: innovating and encouraging change
- resource allocator: deciding who does what
- disturbance handler: dealing with conflict
- negotiator and conciliator.

Burns (1978) suggests that there are two leadership styles: transformational and transactional. These leadership styles are distinguished by different characteristics.

Transformational leadership is a style that works on vision and builds on common commitment. A transformational leader:

- empowers
- inspires by vision and ideals
- mixes home and work
- has a long-term focus
- challenges
- rewards informally and personally
- is emotional and turbulent
- simplifies.

Transactional leaders, on the other hand, are more conforming, explicit and orderly. A transactional leader:

- bargains
- is task-centred
- separates home and work
- has short- or medium-term focus
- coaches sheltered learning
- rewards formally
- is comfortable and orderly
- complicates.

Turrell (1986) suggests that the transformational leader is more effective at large visionary changes of new or renewing organisations and that the transactional leader is best at the systematic work of a leader at the consolidation stage. Leadership skills need to match the demands of each situation and area of change. In Chapters 14 and 16 there is more detailed information on working with groups and group leadership. See also Chapter 6 for more on clinical governance and leadership.

There are a few more key factors to consider if the change is taking place within a healthcare setting:

- if change is taking place in a clinical situation that involves the medical staff, it may be advantageous to enlist a local clinician to lead the change plan. The advantages are that a senior clinician will have professional status and local influence with his/her colleagues, which may ease the process of change
- alternatively, a manager might be more appropriate as they have responsibility for local services, and understand local priorities and resources. They are also knowledgeable about monitoring the effectiveness of the service and often have experience in the management of change
- choose a leader who has a good understanding of the process of change in the NHS
- choose a leader with a sound knowledge of the local situation and who is familiar with local policies and politics.

Facilitator training for champions

Having chosen the right leader, it is then important to have the right team to implement the change plan. The different aspects of the work are likely to require a range of skills and experiences. Building on the specific skills of the existing group is important; for example, some one with facilitation skills will ensure that time set aside for reflection is used to maximum effect. A facilitator will also ensure that the learning from the process is recorded and disseminated to other people and used for future projects as appropriate. Some other skills required might include education and training, critical appraisal, auditing, facilitating, information technology, budgeting, public relations and project management. Good teamworking is essential and this is discussed in more detail in Chapter 14. Training a group of people as champions is an excellent approach to extending knowledge and skills across an organisation. Develop a training programme to give the champions the skills to support, facilitate and encourage staff to set standards successfully.

As part of the process of change, there is a need to change the behaviour of some of the staff and, in particular, overcome resistance to change. As Bowman suggests (1986), people often resist new ideas and are opposed to change if they feel threatened or uncertain, if they are inconvenienced, if their work environment, content or relationships change or if they feel change is being imposed on them. Other issues include lack of information and understanding of what is expected of them, and fear of an increased workload without the resources to support the additional activity. Towell and Harries (1979) suggest that offering information and support, ensuring effective communication and involving people in formulating and implementing any change activity will help to enhance its acceptance.

Rosabeth Moss Kanter (1984) suggests some interesting solutions to resistance to change through negotiation, manipulation and coercion:

- wait – they might eventually go away
- wear them down – keep pushing and arguing, be persistent
- appeal to a higher authority – you had better agree because he does
- invite them in – have them join the party
- send emissaries – get friends in whom they believe to talk to them
- display support – have 'your' people present and active at key meetings
- reduce the stakes – alter parts of the proposal that are particularly damaging
- warn them off – let them know that senior management are on your side
- remember that only afterwards does an innovation look like the right thing to have done all along.

Series of workshops for all staff in setting and monitoring standards
Increasing the knowledge base leads to ideas for standards for pilot areas (see Figure 13.2).

Plant (1987) suggests a very positive and workable approach through six activities that are fundamental to the implementation of change:

- *helping individuals or groups face up to change*: it is important that the people involved in any change accept and understand the reason for the introduction of a new idea or a new way of carrying out a procedure. Once people have evidence that change is likely to improve an aspect of care or a service, they are more likely to accept it. As Rogers and Shoemaker (1971) suggest, if the people involved in the proposed change can see that the new ideas are superior to the old ones, that they fit in with existing values, and that they are easily understood, relevant to them and can be pretested for success, then they are more likely to accept them
- *communicating*: there should be systems of communication from the top down, the bottom up and across the organisation. Every one involved in the change plan must fully understand their role and responsibilities and be supported in this. The management style and the ethos of the organisation needs to be open and blame free so that staff feel able to question decisions and be part of the decision making process. Communication can be

achieved through regular meetings at local level and on a wider level part of team briefing. It can also be achieved through the development of a newsletter that is published on a regular bases and distributed to all those involved in the change and to the wider organisation. The production of reports on progress, again for use at local level as a progress report and a more formal level as a report to the Trust Board

▪ *gaining commitment to change*: in every organisation there are individuals who respond to the idea of change in a positive way; they will adapt to the new process or approach at the beginning of the change plan and will continue to support and develop the process of change through to its conclusion. These people are sometimes known as opinion leaders or product champions. People like this should be identified early in the process of change and encouraged to support and develop other members of the organisation, who are not quite so sure of the need for change. These champions or opinion leaders often come from within the organisation and they bring with them knowledge of the organisation. However, it is sometimes thought to be more beneficial to bring in someone from outside, someone who has undertaken a similar process within an other organisation and therefore brings independent expertise. The key to success is to welcome and value everyone's opinions, new ideas and contributions so that they feel valued and want to be part of the change process

▪ *early involvement*: involve all staff that are part of the team or service in which the change is proposed. This includes all staff, the clinicians, the managers and the support staff; be very careful not to leave anyone out. Invite them all to initial meetings, workshops, presentations, discussions, communications, and so on. Anyone who is left out will feel undervalued and marginalised and, as a result, will resist and prove to be a problem

▪ *turning perceptions of threats into opportunities*: organisations that encourage staff to be open, creative and innovative will be more successful in the process of change and encounter less resistance from their staff

▪ *avoiding over-organising*: it is important to have a systematic approach to the implementation of change but not one that is so inflexible that it cannot be changed in the light of changing circumstances or when suggestions and contributions are made by the staff.

These six activities sit very comfortably within the ethos of clinical governance and a culture that supports continuous quality improvement.

Training and development
During this stage, new processes, approaches, knowledge and skills may well be required to support staff in the process of change. Training needs must be identified and relevant programmes offered to staff to support them. Resistance to change often comes from a fear of the unknown, of not having the right

skills and knowledge to do something differently. Training and education will support staff in learning new and improved approaches to delivery of care.

Monitoring progress: this involves keeping the change plan under review. There may be a need to adjust timescales when the plan moves more quickly or more slowly than anticipated. Communicate with the group and all those affected by the change through clear, simple and consistent messages, which keep people informed as the plan progresses. Identify a small number of key benefits of the change and promote these to all those involved and those working in related areas which might benefit from a similar change plan.

Undertake a review of implementation results to:

- ensure objectives and goals were met
- ensure deadlines were met
- ensure all project requirements were addressed
- resolve all questions and issues
- establish if resistance to change was overcome and commitment to change achieved
- evaluate change project results
- gain management approval of change results.

Publish newsletter on progress (see Figure 13.2)

Standards written (see Figure 13.2)
As a result of the change processes, the group writes and sets standards which are implemented within the pilot wards to ensure that they are valid measurements of the quality of care.

Action (see Figure 13.2)
Once the standards have been tested in a pilot situation, the results are reviewed by the group, changes made and standards altered to ensure that they are robust enough to be true indicators of the quality of patient care on the pilot wards. Once the group is sure that the standards are valid then the standards will be rolled out to all the wards through the champions, supported by continuing education through workshops and facilitation to ensure that the staff on all wards are knowledgeable about standards and committed to the process of monitoring standards.

Once the monitoring results are collated, then a report in written which is sent to the Chief Executive of the Clinical Governance Committee and finally to the board.

Finally, the results of the project are published in the newsletter so that all staff have a picture of the standards project in all areas of the trust or healthcare organisation.

Summary

During this stage the following tasks have been completed:

- a leader has been chosen
- the group has been expanded to match the skills required to implement the change plan
- the plan has been implemented
- the staff has been supported with training and development
- the progress of the plan has been monitored
- changes to the plan have been made as necessary
- progress has been communicated.

4. Evaluate

There are two types of evaluation of the process of change: formative and summative. Formative evaluation is the process of evaluating the change plan as the plan develops; it is a continuous process making changes in response to the evaluation of the process. Summative evaluation, on the other hand, is more commonly done at the completion of a project. It examines the outcomes against the identified goals and compares what happened with what was planned. Any change that has been through the process of change as outlined above should be subject to a post-implementation review, which should:

- objectively assess the change against the objectives and measure and compare the benefits of the change by reviewing the results of benchmarking, targets that have been met, the results of audits, the costs, and so on
- subjectively assess the effectiveness of the change and the methods of implementation through discussion with those involved in the new practice or process. This information may be gathered through one-to-one interviews and from a wider audience through questionnaires
- share all the results with everyone who was involved in the change
- provide a report on the process and the results. This will help other groups who intend to look at similar areas of change.

Summary

During this stage the following tasks have been completed:

- a formative evaluation has been collated and reported
- a summative evaluation has been completed
- reports have been completed
- the results have been disseminated.

There are a variety of techniques to support the management of change and, as they can be used for other areas such as working with groups, developing integrated care pathways and implementing and sustaining a dynamic approach to clinical governance, they have been included in Chapter 16. The techniques that are particularly relevant to this chapter and that could be used at the various stages of the change methodology are:

- the structured interview – for establishing the current situation
- brainstorming and activity diagrams – for generating solutions
- a forcefield analysis – for planning and implementation (see earlier in this chapter and a block schedule or Gantt chart [p. 284]).

Conclusion

There are a few key points to remember about the process of change and these are (King's Fund, 1999):

- change is a complex non-linear process; it is unlikely to move forward in a logical sequence
- change requires time and resources to support activity
- change requires flexibility to respond to the unexpected
- change requires good communication to ensure that those involved and affected by the change have a clear understanding of the proposed actions and the progress of the project.

The process of change is managed through working parties, groups and teams and through effective leadership. Working with and facilitating groups require specific skills and the next chapter addresses these issues.

Skills to Support Clinical Governance – Working with and Facilitating Groups

14

Chapter Contents:

- facilitation
- adult learning
- group dynamics
- group roles
- process consultation.

Facilitation

As described in the previous chapter, organisations and trusts are changing rapidly and this involves everyone at every level, whether it be radical change on a wide scale such as the implementation of clinical governance, changing the delivery of a service in response to one of the National Service Frameworks or the development and implementation of an integrated care pathway for a specific service such as caring for patients with breast cancer. As a result, there are numerous groups and teams set up for a variety of purposes including the coordination of interdependent work, the integration of multifunctional and multidisciplinary expertise, the sharing of information, decision-making, problem-solving and plans for change.

These groups may be large or small, temporary or permanent, within a department or across a whole directorate. They may be called committees, steering groups, project teams, planning groups, working groups, and so on.

However, whatever the group is called and whatever its reason for existence, it will benefit from a better understanding of how groups work and of facilitation.

According to the *Oxford English Dictionary*, to facilitate means to promote or render easier. Justice and Jamieson (1999) define facilitation as a neutral process (with respect to the content and participants) which enables groups to succeed, and which focuses on:

- what needs to be accomplished?
- who needs to be involved?
- the design, flow and sequences of tasks
- communication patterns, effectiveness and completeness
- appropriate methods of participation and the use of resources
- group energy, momentum and capability
- the physical and psychological environment.

There are three phases of facilitation:

- preparation
- group work
- follow-up.

Each of these phases has intended outcomes and primary tasks as set out in Table 14.1.

Facilitating a group involves establishing informal, relaxed relationships. This in turn means developing a cohesive group which is effective in managing process issues. It is about enabling and not teaching. The methods used must support the development of effective group processes, remembering that the group itself is a vehicle for individual learning. There should be flexibility in developing plans, leaving room for them to be adapted in response to changing circumstances and demands. To achieve all this, the effective facilitator must have a good knowledge of the use and application of group theories, and some basic skills, which include:

- contracting
- designing structure activities and processes
- listening, paraphrasing, observing, clarifying and elaborating
- interpreting verbal and non-verbal behaviour
- confronting others
- managing differences
- collaborating with others
- project management
- meeting with management
- logistics management.

Table 14.1 Facilitation phases

Preparation	Group work	Follow-up
Outcomes	**Outcomes**	**Outcomes**
1. Group organised	1. Meeting purposes and	1. Meeting record/
2. Membership	outcomes achieved	outputs produced and
determined	2. Participants worked	distributed
3. Purposes made clear	well together	2. Results of group work
4. Roles clarified	3. Participants satisfied	communicated to
5. Logistics planned	with progress	members, sponsors
6. Facilitation work	4. Meeting design	and stakeholders
contract clear	effectively	3. Approvals of results
7. Group, work,	implemented	obtained and
participants and	5. Facilitation capacity of	announced
context understood	group enhanced	4. Next steps carried out
8. Agenda determined	6. Next steps clear	5. Need for further group
and communicated	7. Effective group task	work determined
	and maintenance	
	behaviours observed	
Primary Tasks	**Primary Tasks**	**Primary Tasks**
1. Establishing the	1. Creating a foundation	1. Preparing the meeting
contract for facilitation	for working together	record/outputs
2. Collecting information	2. Managing data	2. Informing and
on context, work, and	generation	communicating with
participants	3. Managing analysis and	others
3. Clarifying the group	interpretation of the	3. Obtaining approvals of
charter	data	group work
4. Analysing	4. Managing decision-	4. Monitoring interim/
stakeholders	making	implementation work
5. Selecting group	5. Managing group	5. Identifying further
members and group	dynamics	needs for group work
leader	6. Evaluating group	
6. Building agendas for	process and progress	
meetings	7. Closing group	
7. Publishing agenda and	sessions	
disseminating		
information		
8. Attending to meeting		
logistics		

Source: Justice and Jamieson, 1999

One of the challenges faced by a facilitator is the ability to detach himself/ herself from and to give up the control of the results of the group's work. However, the personal characteristics of an effective facilitator might include being:

■ serene – calm and centred
■ confident
■ assertive

- open
- flexible
- optimistic
- results-orientated.

Facilitating a group involves methods that utilise the group as a vehicle for change and requires effective processes from within the group. Stewart (1999) suggests that the following behaviours displayed by the facilitator will reinforce this and influence the group:

- being an effective communicator and addressing contributions to the whole group by sharing eye contact with all members
- being a good listener and attending to whoever speaks by active listening behaviour such as looking, maintaining eye contact and reflecting
- valuing all group members and their contributions equally by acknowledging, responding to and welcoming all contributions
- being willing to share leadership and influence within the group by, for example, encouraging group members with particular expertise to provide direction
- adopting consensus-decision-making procedures by, for example, requiring the group to decide criteria for the composition of subgroups or syndicates
- being flexible and open to alternative views and ideas by, for example, negotiating content and methods and not adhering strictly to a planned programme
- being open and honest with the group by practising self-disclosure in terms of feelings and personal doubts
- engaging overall in authentic behaviour in relating to and with the group.

Some of these behaviours may be more significant than others and some may not be relevant at all within the context of the group. However, at the beginning of the life of the group the facilitator is the natural leader and should be a model for behaviour to be emulated by the group. Justice and Jamieson (1999), advocate that there are basic areas of knowledge that are essential to facilitation:

- the principles of adult learning
- group dynamics and decision-making processes
- understanding process consultation.

Adult Learning

Within the context of this book it is not possible to go into detail of how adults learn. Indeed, this would be a book in itself and there are many authors who have researched and written on this subject with much greater knowledge than I. However, there are some key considerations about adults requiring learning which need to be taken into account when designing or planning a session as a facilitator:

- learning occurs best when it is motivated, not coerced or forced. The motivation comes from the knowledge that the work of the group is understood and agreed with, that there is a clear reason for the work to be undertaken and that the work is relevant to the organisation or trust
- learning occurs best when it is conducted as a partnership
- adults need to stay engaged and use their senses, experience, knowledge and skills. They need to be listening, talking, doing, watching, moving or reading
- adults learn best when they can see the whole picture, which parts they need to know, where they are going and where they have been so new ideas, new skills and new ways of thinking all need constant reinforcement
- learning occurs when an adult's attention and energy are engaged and focused and that is not possible if they are suffering discomfort; the physical surroundings must be comfortable and the psychological environment should feel safe. An open environment will encourage the group to express their ideas without fear of disapproval, ridicule or attack.

It is important for the facilitator to keep these points in mind when preparing to facilitate a group or indeed when looking for reasons why a group appears hostile or unwilling to participate.

Group Dynamics

Numerous experts have published studies about the dynamics of groups. The intention of the information in this chapter is to give anyone, either setting up or working within a group, some insight into how groups work in order to help their group work effectively. In an organisation like an NHS trust, groups of all kinds are part of everyday life and so it is important to have some knowledge of how groups work. This chapter only skims the surface of this important subject, but experts such as Charles Handy (1985) and Peter Drucker (1977) give comprehensive and detailed information on the workings of groups.

Group dynamics is the social process by which people interact and behave in a group environment. It involves the influences of power, personality and behaviour upon the group process. Essentially there are two types of groups: the formal group, which is set up to undertake a specific task or tackle a problem, and the informal group which comes together as a natural response to a common interest.

The size of the group can vary from two people to many hundreds, but a working group should be kept to the optimum number for encouraging interaction and debate. Larger groups are likely to increase the possibility of conflict owing to the lack of opportunity for the development of social relationships within the group, the lack of opportunity for individual development and the wider variety of opinions and views held by the group. On the positive side, larger groups offer a much wider knowledge base and greater experience and expertise, which, it could be argued, increase the quality and quantity of the achievement of the task. Larger groups also give a wider representation of legitimate interests in groups such as working parties and committees. It is generally accepted that in a training setting a group of twenty is considered the maximum number for effective working. Others suggest that twelve to fifteen is a more manageable size of group, with enough people to generate a variety of views and opinions but also small enough to allow members to contribute to the work of the group. When setting standards in groups as a facilitator, I found that a group of eight to ten people proved to be the most productive. The group was small enough to form a cohesive group quickly, with everyone working together and contributing in a very short space of time.

It is essential to consider the knowledge, experience and skills required when forming a group to ensure that the group is able to complete the task. However, a group is more than a collection of individual personalities with different needs, influences and characteristics. Theories of group behaviour suggest that there are three characteristics inherent in groups:

- individuals are aware of each other
- there is some level of social interaction between members
- the group has a common objective.

These characteristics could be true of any group, for example a queue of people waiting in a shop to be served. However, this queue of people would probably not see themselves as a group; they may be in the queue because they have the same individual objective but they do not have a common objective. The task in hand cannot be achieved by an individual but it requires a group to achieve the common objective. A group may therefore be defined as any collection of people who perceive themselves to be a group, and the first step in becoming a group is to accept and identify with a common objective.

One theory of group dynamics makes a distinction between the content and the process of the group. The content of the group is the purpose or task of the group, whereas the process is how the group achieves its purpose or task such as by planning, allocating work, making decisions and solving problems, which is similar to the concept of process consultancy. Process consultation is discussed later in this chapter as part of the skills of the facilitator. Group processes are about how the individual members of the group interact and work together to complete the task. It is not uncommon for the group to concentrate on the content and task at the expense of the process. However, the quality of the process is very important as poor-quality processes lead to poor-quality decisions and therefore a poor resolution of the task.

Key Process Issues

All the issues listed below critically affect the quality of the group processes and this in turn affects the quality of the outcome of the group's task. An effective group will be aware of these process issues and manage them so as to ensure good-quality processes. The key process issues include:

1. *Participation*: this is about the level of participation by all members of the group, identifying who is participating and who is not, and identifying the reasons for non-participation and overcoming these.
2. *Communication*: good communication within the group is essential but is it really happening? Through observation of the group it may become evident that when one member speaks not everyone listens and that there may be others in the group carrying on a conversation at the same time. Do the speakers address the whole group or just one or two members of the group? Looking for and identifying the communication patterns within a group can be very enlightening and demonstrate weaknesses in the group.
3. *Information-Sharing*: if the group is to be effective then the whole group must share all information. However, withholding information can be seen as a way of retaining power. This needs to be resolved.
4. *Leadership Style*: all groups require leadership and for some groups this will be a senior manager or another natural leader from within the hierarchy of the organisation. If there is no formal or natural leader, then the leadership may be undertaken by some or all of the group. There are different styles of leadership. An autocratic style is unlikely to bring out the best in a group as the strong control and lack of involvement of others in making decisions would not be a favourable basis on which to develop a cohesive, problem-solving, decision-making group. The laissez-faire leader is unlikely to bring the members of a group together to enable them to make decisions and complete the task. On the other hand, a democratic style encourages shared leadership and decision-making and facilitates the work of the group. See also Chapters 6, 13 and 16, and Table 6.1.
5. *Influence*: the question here is who influences the group and why, and does the influence shift? Is it the person who speaks first or the one who speaks loudest who influences the group's thinking or is the group influenced, on a more rational basis, by members of the group? For example, does the group listen to members of the group with particular skills and/or experience,

which influences the group's thinking. For a group to be effective, influence must shift on a rotational basis acknowledging the knowledge, expertise and experience of all group members.

6. *Decision-making*: there are two process issues in decision-making. The first is fairly common and that is when the group does not recognise decision points. This means that the group goes on debating and discussing an issue long after the decision should and could have been made. This unproductive work continues because the group is not skilled at recognising the decision points. The second issue involves not making a decision by using 'avoidance behaviour', usually because the group is not comfortable making a difficult decision. There is no right or wrong way of making decisions, but the group have to work out a process to support their decision-making. Decision-making is a crucial part of all group work and is discussed in more detail further on in this chapter.

7. *Feelings*: the last process issue concerns feelings and how the group cope with the feelings of other members, for example when members of the group express negative feelings of anger and frustration or positive feelings of enjoyment, pride and pleasure. Indeed, do individuals feel free to express their feelings in a group? In every group at some point there will inevitably be conflict, a difference of opinion, and sometimes this is seen as negative so the group suppresses it, which can be very unproductive. However, conflict can be seen as a positive force and an open expression and resolution can be healthy and lead to positive outcomes for the group.

The processes described above outline the collective behaviours of individual members of the group in the way that they work together. These behaviours support two separate but related functions: task functions, which contribute to the work of the group, and maintenance functions, which build and develop group cohesiveness.

Task Functions

Task functions help the group define and complete its work and reach its goals and desired outcomes. They include:

- initiating, proposing or suggesting
- building on or elaborating
- co-ordinating or integrating
- seeking information and opinions
- giving information or opinions
- clarifying
- questioning

- disagreeing or challenging
- testing for understanding
- orientating the group to its task
- testing for consensus
- summarising
- recording or capturing content.

Maintenance Functions

Maintenance functions are about keeping the group together, maintaining functional relationships and strengthening the group's ability to perform and include:

- motivating
- gate-keeping by attempting to keep communication flowing: helping people stay included and participating by inviting others to express their views and opinions; checking understanding and agreement; requesting advice and contributions from others
- building trust through accepting the judgement of others, delegating tasks and agreeing to follow another's lead
- harmonising by reconciling differences and reducing group tensions
- encouraging
- compromising by admitting errors and looking for alternatives
- setting standards by reminding members of the group's norms (social standards and acceptable behaviours), rules and roles
- being a good listener
- observing the process and providing feedback on process issues.

Effective Group Practices

- members do not ignore or ridicule seriously intended contributions
- members check to make sure they know what a speaker means by a contribution before they agree or disagree
- each member speaks only for himself/herself and lets others speak for themselves
- all contributions are viewed as belonging to the group to be used or not used as the group decides
- all members participate, but in different and complementary ways
- whenever the group sees it is having trouble getting work done, it tries to find out why

- people support what they help to create. The group makes decisions together openly rather than by default
- the group attempts to make consensus decisions. However, when a majority decision is made, members accept it and work together, even if they may not have agreed with the majority
- the group brings conflict into the open and deals with it.

Group Development

According to Tuckman (1965) a group's growth is:

- sequential – the stages occur in a specifically stated order
- developmental – issues and concerns in each stage must be resolved in order for the group to move on to the next stage
- thematic – each stage is characterised by two dominant themes, one reflecting task dimension and one reflecting the relationship dimension.

Tuckman's theory of group development is popular and widely used, and describes the four stages of forming, storming, norming and performing.

1. *Forming*: at this stage of development the group has just come together so members are often dependent on an individual, such as a leader or someone outside the group, to provide structure in the way that the members of the group relate to each other. This is the point at which the group begins to look at the reasons why the group was set up, the task in hand and the clarification and setting of goals and objectives.

   At this initial stage the group:

   - is task-orientated, as it clarifies and sets goals and objectives
   - needs plenty of information
   - works on relationship issues: resolving dependency; making leadership roles clear; getting to know one another.

   The issues that concern the group at this stage are questions such as 'What', 'Why' and 'How'.
2. *Storming*: this stage is also known as the counter-dependent stage as the group encounters conflict by challenging formal authority, testing the limits and sorting out an acceptable, 'pecking order' among those of equal status within the group. Issues that arise include the identification of roles and responsibilities, operational rules and procedures and the individual recognition of each member's skills and abilities.

   Excessive storming can lead to anxiety and tension, whereas suppressed storming may lead to resentment and bitterness. Sometimes the group has difficulty getting through this stage, particularly if there are problems clarifying the task, agreeing the mission or deciding how to go forward as a group. Lack of skills, ability or aptitude can also contribute to the group's inability to go beyond this stage. Conflict resolution may be the goal, but conflict management is just as important because, as new situations develop, the group may briefly return to this stage.

At this second stage the group:

■ is involved in resistance to task demands and hostility in relationships
■ challenges the group's leadership; the leader at this stage must provide clarification about the role
■ indentifes roles and responsibilities, operational rules and procedures and the individual need for recognition of skills and abilities
■ flexes its muscles in search of identity.

The issues that concern the group at this stage are based around leadership, power and questions such as 'Who is in charge'?, 'Who is included'? and 'How will the group operate?' Also differences about the answers to the 'What?', 'How?', 'Who?' and 'When?' questions.

3. *Norming*: this is the start of the group's most productive work towards achieving the task. The group starts to resolve the issues that are creating conflict and begins to develop its social agreements. It has established its own identity which separates it from other groups. The members of the group begin to recognise their interdependence, develop cohesion and agree on the group norms that will help them function effectively in their quest to complete their task. They now work together exchanging and sharing ideas and information, exploring options and discussing possible actions, and giving and receiving feedback.

At this third stage the group is:

■ characterised by co-operation
■ cohesive
■ communicating
■ team-building to increase group identity and increase shared responsibility.

The issues that concern the group at this stage are that it has created a working climate, resolved issues, established agreement on roles, leadership, work methods, timescales and operating norms and is ready to perform.

4. *Performing*: from the third stage the group will move naturally to the fourth and final stage which is performing. The group has sorted out its social structure and understands its goals, tasks and individual roles and moves towards completing the task. There is mutual trust within the group, which is demonstrated through the use of pairs, small groups and individuals carrying out tasks for the group and feeding back their results. The group becomes independent and tends to rely on its own resources.

The group is now efficient and effective at problem-solving and at this stage it is beneficial to encourage continued development for the group to stimulate new problems for their problem-solving skills.

At this fourth stage the group:

- encourages co-operation
- is functioning efficiently to achieve the group goals and complete the task
- assumes roles that are necessary to achieve goals, learning independence with dependence.

The issues that concern the group at this stage are based around achieving goals and completing the task.

Although the stages are sequential it is important to recognise that the actual work to achieve the group's goals and the task does get done throughout all four stages. The stages are necessary as a group cannot expect to go from norming to performing and be successful in achieving its goals. There is no time limit on the stages; the group will move from one stage to the next as it progresses. Some groups will move through stages 1 and 2 in a matter of hours, while others may take days, weeks, months or years. Indeed, they may never progress beyond stages 1 or 2. The time limits are likely to be driven by timescales set for the group by outside influences: for example, targets to be met, or changes to be implemented by a given time as part of a trust-wide strategy. It is important to remember that whenever a member of the group leaves and is replaced, the group must return to stage 1 of its development.

Group Roles

Belbin (1981) has made a study of the best characteristics in a team and developed a list of eight roles that are needed for a fully effective group (see Table 14.2):

Decision-making

This is a critical part of the work of a group striving towards the solution of a problem or completion of its task. The facilitator or the leader should offer the group a variety of approaches to support its decision-making and listed below are some of those approaches:

1. *Individual*: this is when the leader of the group makes the decision, often when the group is in conflict and cannot agree or when the group is

Table 14.2 Personality types for the effective team

Chairman/team leader	Stable, dominant, extrovert Concentrates on objectives Does not originate ideas Focuses people on what they do best
Plant	Dominant, high IQ, introvert A 'scatterer of seeds', originates ideas Misses out on detail Trustful but easily offended
Resource investigator	Stable, dominant, extrovert Sociable Contacts with outside world Salesman/diplomat/liaison officer Not original thinker
Shaper	Anxious, dominant, extrovert Emotional, impulsive Quick to challenge and respond to challenge Unites ideas, objectives and possibilities Competitive Intolerant of woolliness and vagueness
Company worker	Stable, controlled Practical organiser Can be inflexible but likely to adapt to established systems Not an innovator
Monitor evaluation	High IQ, stable, introvert Measured analyses not innovation Unambitious and lacking enthusiasm Solid, dependable
Team worker	Stable, extrovert, low dominance Concerned with individual's needs Builds on others' ideas Cools things down
Finisher	Anxious, introvert Worries over what will go wrong Permanent sense of urgency Preoccupied with order Concerned with 'following through'

Source: Belbin, 1976

required to make a decision quickly. The individual decision may be appropriate when one member of the group has more expertise than all the others and the group agree to follow the expert's lead. Some members of the group may feel marginalised by this approach and it can lead to resentment, but this approach is quick, simple and clear.

2. *Consultative*: the leader makes the decision after listening to the views of all members of the group. This may be appropriate when the leader is an

expert in the area in which the decision is being made. Alternatively, the leader is keen to listen to alternative ideas but either does not want to or cannot invest time in the discussion, or wishes to retain control of the group in order to get the decision made. Again this may lead to resentment amongst those members of the group who feel that their input has been rejected and the group loses the interaction of different ideas and options. However, this can be a quick and effective approach to getting a decision made.

3. *Consultative consensus*: the leader seeks consensus from the group but continues to keep control of the decision. This approach takes time and the group may not have enough time to spend on this approach. It also combines the individual and consultative approaches which requires strong facilitation and leadership skills if the group is not to feel that it has been manipulated into a decision. However, the result of this approach is that it can bring about a decision when the group has reached the point where a decision is not possible. Consensus of the group to the decision provides more support for the implementation of the decision.

   This approach is useful when one person has particular knowledge and skills to support the decision or he/she has some responsibility for the implementation of that decision.

4. *Modified consensus*: the group reach a point where they all either agree with the decision or can at least live with it. This is an appropriate method when group agreement is critical, or the group is the team who will implement the decision. This method is democratic and participative and will result in commitment to the decision. However, it is time-consuming and may result in compromise, which does not necessarily result in a good-quality decision.

5. *Absolute consensus*: everyone in the group agrees that the decision is the right one and that it will result in improvement to a current situation. The group supports the decision it has made but using this approach does not always end in a positive result; as many as two out of three times a group will fail to get a decision using this method. This is an appropriate method if the group is making decisions around clinical procedures and it has adequate time in which to debate and agree the decision.

6. *Voting*: the group takes a vote on the alternative proposals and the majority vote becomes the group's decision. This is effective as long as it is seen by the group as fair. It is useful when the group cannot agree on a decision and it is sometimes the only solution to a conflict of views. It is also useful when there is no leader to apply the methods set out above, when no consensus can be reached or when little discussion or debate is required and any choice of decision will probably work. However, this approach creates division as people take sides and in doing so detract from the cohesion of the group.

7. *Process consultation*: this is one of many Organisation Development (OD) methodologies which are used to bring about change in an organisation. Process consultancy, unlike other forms of consultancy, does not provide solutions and answers, but is about developing the ability of the group and decreasing its dependency on the consultant.

Process Consultation

Process consultation was developed by Schein (1969) and is defined as: 'A set of activities on the part of the consultant which help the client to perceive, understand and act upon process events which occur in the client's environment.' Schein also writes 'The process consultant seeks to give the client 'insight' into what is going on around him, and between him, and other people.'

He extends this later by saying, 'as long as organizations are networks of people, there will be processes occurring between them. Therefore it is obvious that the better understood and the better diagnosed these processes are, the greater will be the chances of finding solutions to technical problems which will be accepted and used by members of the organization.'

He describes a number of assumptions underlying process- rather than content-based consulting, including the following:

■ managers are keen to improve their organisation but are not always sure what is wrong and need help in diagnosing the situation. Managers must be involved in this diagnosis so that they see the problems and possibilities for themselves and learn how to respond
■ process consultation concentrates on helping to establish the most effective means of diagnosis and helping relationships by getting people together in various ways to solve the issues.

Processes, as opposed to content, are generally about how individuals, groups and organisations interact and conduct their work. Processes include:

■ communications
■ decision-making
■ problem-solving
■ intergroup co-operation
■ leadership
■ interpersonal relationships.

These processes provide the focus for process consultation. It is useful for a facilitator to have an understanding of process consultation as much of the facilitator's work is concerned with supporting and helping groups to work effectively with processes that will enable the group to complete its task.

The process consultant is someone who is skilled in process observation and analysis, and has an in-depth knowledge and understanding of the psychological and sociological theories which explain human processes. The activities of the process consultant may be divided into two main areas: diagnosis and intervention. Diagnosis is concerned with data collection and intervention is concerned with effecting change. Each of these is interchangeable as diagnosis is a form of intervention and new data is often collected during implementation. Schein sets out some identifiable stages of process consultation and these are:

1. *Establishing contact*: this is the stage when the client or the group first come together to discuss a potential project. The main focus is defining and agreeing the formal and psychological contract. The formal contract is about agreeing timescales, consultancy days, and so on, whereas the psychological contract is concerned with roles and the contributions and expectations of the group.
2. *Selecting setting and method*: at this stage the focus of the work is agreed: who will be involved; the methodology to be used, for example observation, interviews, and so on.
3. *Data-gathering*: the process consultant and the people involved in the project or group apply the agreed diagnostic method and collect and analyse the data.
4. *Intervention*: during this stage the process consultant will be concerned with effecting change and improving the group's ability to manage process issues. This may be achieved through problem-identification workshops, team-building, coaching, individual counselling, agenda-setting workshops, and so on (see the appendix for more information on some of these techniques). At the same time the data-collecting stage will have increased the group's ability to diagnose process problems through its active involvement.
5. *Evaluation*: this stage is about measuring benefits to the group in terms of changes in values, and skills in managing human processes.
6. *Disengagement*: this is the final stage when the group's ability develops, and dependence on the process consultant ceases.

The purpose of process consultation is to help groups of people to manage interaction more effectively. A facilitator is required to take people from being a collection of individuals and to support them in becoming a group, and as the group develops the facilitator may help to resolve problems or difficulties between members of the group before it can move on to complete its task. Listed below are some common techniques to help facilitate a group. Facilitation is a skill and is useful to support many aspects of the clinical governance agenda and therefore relevant to most of the chapters in this book, so for clarity I have included a few techniques in Chapter 16. The tools, techniques and skills with particular relevance to Chapter 16 are:

- using the group memory
- project definition/group charter
- selecting the group leader
- giving and receiving feedback
- interventions skills
- reflective listening
- facilitating group dynamics
- encouraging members of the group to be involved
- problems with groups including:
  - □ an individual who does not want to join in
  - □ a group which does not keep to the agenda
  - □ disruptive behaviour
  - □ an unresponsive or complaining group
  - □ people who dominate the group
  - □ people who interrupt while others are speaking
- brainstorming
- problem-solving
- conflict resolution.

Conclusion

When can the information included above be used in the quest for clinical governance to support continuous quality improvement? In the world of quality assurance, continuous quality improvement and clinical governance there are numerous opportunities to use the knowledge of how groups work and how to facilitate a group or indeed what to look for when choosing someone to facilitate your group. Groups come in all shapes and sizes. There are small groups that set out to undertake clinical audit, patients and staff working groups benchmarking, those reviewing and writing policies and procedures, and groups reviewing and improving a service or aspect of patient care. There are bigger groups in the form of working parties or formal committees. Whatever the size of the group, the same rules apply.

Good facilitation can help a group unlock the solution to a problem or support the new development of a service. A group may be set up to develop the risk management strategy for a trust, in which case it is important to choose the group carefully with people with the right skills and knowledge to develop a strategy; it is possible that such a group would benefit from facilitation to keep the momentum going and support the group in its task. The next chapter is about project management where the project group is essential to the smooth running of a project from its inception to its conclusion.

Skills to Support Clinical Governance – Project Management

15

Chapter Contents:

- project management
- Project Management Body of Knowledge
- worked example of a project
- project teams.

Project Management

Project management and change management really go hand in hand, as the management of change often requires the skills of a project manager. The implementation of clinical governance and the process of continuous quality improvement requires an ongoing need for skilled project management as part of the process of change. This chapter links with the information in Chapters 13 and 14. However, it only provides an overview of the complex world of project management, and writers of books such as *Project Change Management* (Harrington, Conner and Horney, 2000), and *Practical PRINCE2* (Bentley, 2002), which is a guide to using the PRINCE2 methodology, will give the reader a detailed step-by-step guide to project management. PRINCE methodology is the approach to project management that the NHS favours.

It could be said that almost any activity that involves carrying out a non-repetitive task could be called a project. *Collins Modern English Dictionary* (1988) describes a project as 'a proposal, scheme or design, a task requiring considerable or concerned effort'. Project management is the skilful or resourceful application of knowledge, skills, techniques and tools to project activities in order to meet the expectations for the project. It is carefully planned and organised to accomplish a specific and usually 'one-off' effort, for example the development of a crisis-response service in mental health, a restructure of the staffing in theatre to improve efficiency, or the development and implementation of an integrated care pathway. Project management includes:

- developing a project plan, which includes defining project goals and objectives, specifying tasks or how goals will be achieved, identifying what resources are needed and establishing the budgets and timescales for completion
- implementing the project plan and using strict controls to ensure that controls to ensure that all aspects of the plan are completed as planned.

There are usually four major phases, which include a feasibility study, project planning, implementation, and evaluation and support or maintenance.

Project managers can be found in all industries and their numbers have grown rapidly as industry and commerce has realised that much of what it does is project work. The NHS is no exception to this and as an ever-increasing number of projects tumble out of national initiatives such as the NHS Plan, the National Service Frameworks and targets that require service review and change, so project management has become established as a career path. The Modernisation Agency (see Chapter 1) was created in April 2001 to help healthcare staff redesign local health services in accordance with good practice and numerous projects supporting change in the NHS.

Project Management Body of Knowledge

The Project Management Institute in Upper Darby, Pennsylvania is the leader in defining the body of knowledge for project management. This Project Management Body of Knowledge (PMBK) approach to project management is widely accepted (Project Management Institute, Standards Committee, 1996) and it has nine knowledge areas:

- *project integration management* (the processes required to ensure the various elements of the project are co-ordinated):
  - ☐ project plan development – putting together the project plan
  - ☐ project plan execution – carrying out the plan.
- *project scope management* (the processes required to ensure that the project includes all the work that is required to complete the project successfully):
  - ☐ initiation – committing the organisation to beginning the next phase of the project
  - ☐ scope planning – a written statement, the scope of the project, that is the basis for future project decisions
  - ☐ scope definition – dividing the major project deliverables into smaller more manageable parts
  - ☐ scope verification – formal acceptance of the scope of the project.

- *project time management* (the processes require to ensure the project is completed on time):
  - ☐ activity definition – identifying the specific activities that must be undertaken to produce the project deliverables
  - ☐ activity sequencing – identifying and documenting the interactivity of the activities
  - ☐ activity-duration estimating – estimating the time needed to complete the individual activities
  - ☐ schedule development – analysing the activity sequences, timescales and resource requirements to create the project plan
  - ☐ schedule control – controlling the changes to the project plan.
- *project cost management* (the processes to ensure that the project is completed within the approved budget):
  - ☐ resource planning – determining what resources are required, the people, equipment, materials, and so on
  - ☐ cost estimating – developing an estimate of the cost of all the resources required to complete the project
  - ☐ cost budgeting – allocating overall costs to individual items of work
  - ☐ cost control – controlling any changes to the project budget.
- *project quality management* (the processes required to ensure that the project will meet the goals set to secure a successful outcome).
  - ☐ quality planning – identifying the standards that are relevant to the project and determining how the standards will be met
  - ☐ quality assurance – ongoing evaluation of the project's performance to provide confidence that the overall project will meet expected standards
  - ☐ quality control – monitoring specific project results to establish if they comply with the relevant quality standards and identifying approaches to eliminate any unsatisfactory performance.
- *project human resource management* (the processes required to make the most effective use of the people involved in the project team):
  - ☐ organisational planning – identifying, documenting and assigning project roles, responsibilities and reporting relationships
  - ☐ staff acquisition – getting the people required, to complete the project, assigned to them
  - ☐ team development – developing the group and individual skills to meet the project's goals.
- *project communications management* (the processes to ensure timely and appropriate generation, collection, storage and, at completion, disposal of project information):
  - ☐ communications planning – identifying the information needs of the stakeholders, who requires the information and when and how they require it

- ☐ information distribution – providing information to the stakeholders in a preferred and timely manner
- ☐ performance reporting – collecting and disseminating performance information
- ☐ providing status reports and reports on progress measurement and forecast
- ☐ administrative closure – generating, gathering and disseminating information at the end of a stage and/or at the completion of the project.
- *project risk management* (the processes concerned with the identification and analysis of and response to project risk):
  - ☐ risk identification – identifying and documenting risks that are likely to affect the project
  - ☐ risk qualification – evaluating risks and risk interactions to assess the range of possible project outcomes
  - ☐ risk response development – defining enhancement steps for opportunities and response to threats
  - ☐ risk response control – responding to risk over the duration of the project.
- *project procurement management* (the processes required to acquire goods and services from outside the organisation):
  - ☐ procurement planning – determining when and what to procure
  - ☐ solicitation planning – documenting product requirements and identifying potential sources
  - ☐ solicitation – getting quotations, bids, offers or proposals as appropriate
  - ☐ source selection – choosing from among potential suppliers
  - ☐ contract administration – managing the relationship with the suppliers
  - ☐ contract closeout – completing and settling the contract, including the resolution of any unresolved items.

This is a recognised approach to project management but is more commonly used in business or industry. However, most of these key processes can be applied to project management in the health service and an example of such an approach is outlined later in this chapter.

Within healthcare organisations there are complex projects such as mergers, large projects such as service reviews and process re-engineering, and small projects such as developing and implementing an integrated care pathway. In all cases the organisation or the stakeholder requires that the project be completed on time and that it should meet quality objectives and keep within the budget. These requirements form the classic time, quality and cost triangle.

The individual project manager is responsible for defining the process by which a project is initiated, controlled and brought to a successful conclusion. A successful project may be defined in the following terms:

- it was completed on time
- it was completed within budget
- the organisation and the stakeholders are satisfied (stakeholders are people and organisations associated directly or indirectly with a project who stand to lose or gain by actions taken)
- the project team members are satisfied.

Apart from understanding the processes of project management, the tools and the techniques, there are some essential skills required to be a successful project manager and these include:

- communication – the ability to:
  - □ convey complex ideas easily
  - □ articulate clearly what must be accomplished
  - □ keep the team moving towards a common goal
  - □ foster an environment that supports the team in communicating openly and honestly and admitting their own mistakes without losing respect
  - □ listen effectively
  - □ facilitate.
- organisational effectiveness – in order to obtain resources and gain support, the project manager must understand:
  - □ the culture of the trust or organisation
  - □ the dynamics of the trust or organisation
  - □ the individuals with whom they are working
- leadership – the project manager must build authority through effective leadership as he/she does not usually have direct authority within the organisation.
- problem-solving and decision-making – this is a large part of the role of the project manager, Each part of the project will have a set of problems that require resolution using strong problem-solving skills.
- team-building – the project manager must have the skills to build a strong team.
- flexibility and creativity – it requires more than a proven framework to guide the project manager he/she must adapt to the needs of the project using appropriate tools and techniques to assist in the delivery of a successful project.
- trustworthiness – the project manager must gain the trust of the stakeholders involved in the project. The stakeholders need to believe and trust that the project manager will do the right thing on a day-to-day basis to keep the project successful.
- time-management skills.
- expectation management – the project manager must make sure that people know in advance what is required and expected.

- coaching skills.
- mentoring skills (see also Chapter 6).
- the ability to work with people at all levels of the organisation.
- project management cannot be separated from the management of change and therefore the project manager will also be a change agent, change advocate, change facilitator and change target.

Worked Example of a Project

Over the years I have managed numerous projects within healthcare organisations in the NHS and the private sector, and outside the UK. This particular approach uses five stages of project management – initiating, planning, executing, controlling and closing the project – and follows most of the PMBK processes set out above. At the end of each of these stages there is a checklist of activities that should have been completed. Table 15.1 is a worked example of a workload project that was set up to review staffing and skill-mix for an organisation caring for people with learning disabilities, to support the theory with a practical example.

I have chosen workforce planning as the example for the project plan because it is not possible to assure the quality of care, nor can it be said that a trust has clinical governance in place if the organisation does not have the right staff numbers or skills to support good-quality evidence-based care. This is just one element of clinical governance but a very important one to get right.

Steps to Managing a Project

1. Initiating the project

Before the project begins, the initiators of the project establish that there is a need for the project, perhaps through a feasibility study. The organisation gains commitment to the project and authority for the resources to complete the project. The authorisation of the project should be a written agreement from which the project manager can begin the planning stage. The organisation appoints a project manager to the project and initiators of the project produce the aims and objectives in terms of what they want to achieve in deliverables and outcomes. Before the work begins, the project manager spends time making sure that the work is fully understood and checks his/her understanding with the initiators of the project. The project manager defines the

Table 15.1 A worked example of a workload project that was set up to review staffing and skill-mix for an organisation caring for people with learning disabilities

Project schedule following agreement of project plan*

Item of work	Deliverables	Time required	Costs	Responsible person	Timescales (completed by)
1. Select project team	Project team appointed	2 hours	–	Project manager	03/02
2. Meetings with staff involved to give an overview of the project	Project explained and discussed with all staff involved	1 week 6 × 1 hour meetings	–	Project manager	10/02
3. Develop data-gathering tools and documents	Unit profile structured questionnaire	–	£50 photocopying	Project manager	07/02
4. Collect activity data	Baseline activity data	1 week		Project manager and secretary	10/02
5. Set up workshops for project team in the use of data-sampling, dependency and activity methodology Prepare handouts	Workshop design to support project teams with skills and knowledge	2 days	£50 photocoying	Project manager and secretary	12/02
6. Workshop for project team	Project team have skills and knowledge to support the project	1 day	£50 refreshment	Project manager and project team	17/02
7. Set up workshops for staff for support completion of dependency ratings night and day (opportunity to attend 10 half-day workshops)	All staff booked to attend a workshop	6 hours	–	Secretary	24/02
8. Project team members allocated four units each to review	Each project team member has completed the baseline data-gathering exercises	2 weeks	–	Project team and project manager	28/02
9. Analyse baseline data and complete a profile for each unit	Profile of each unit	3 days	–	Project manager and project team	07/03

Table 15.1 (*continued*)

Project schedule following agreement of project plan*

Item of work	Deliverables	Time required	Costs	Responsible person	Timescales (completed by)
10. Discuss and develop dependency-tool documentation	Dependency documentation	2 days	£50 photocopying	Project team, project management and secretary	07/03
11. Feedback results of profiles to unit staff (6 × 1 hour meetings)	Staff agreed profiles are accurate	4 days		Project manager and project team	14/03
12. Run workshops	All staff who will be responsible for allocating a dependency rating for each of patients have attended a workshop to learn this skill	5 days		Project manager, project team and unit staff	04/04
13. Distribute dependency tool to all units	All units have enough dependency-rating sheets and guidelines to cover 2 weeks	4 hours		Secretary	04/04
14. Pilot dependency tool. For 2 starting 07/04	Dependency-scoring system piloted	2 weeks		Project manager, project team and unit staff	21/04
15. Project team undertake activity sampling exercise in each unit	Activity sampling	2 weeks		Project team	21/04
16. Analysis of activity sampling	Activity timings valid	1 week		Project manager and project team	25/04
17. Analysis of returned dependency scoring sheets – all inaccuracies followed up and corrected	Staff complete the scoring sheets accurately	3 weeks		Project manager and project team	21/05
18. Progress report to the steering group	Progress report	1 day		Project manager	02/06

Table 15.1 (*continued*)

Project schedule following agreement of project plan*

Item of work	Deliverables	Time required	Costs	Responsible person	Timescales (completed by)
19. Revisit any units having problems	Staff competent at dependency scoring	2 weeks		Project team	09/05
20. Resample activities if data collected	Timings are accurate	2 weeks		Project team	09/05
21. Commence study 2-week period of recording ratings	Dependency scores for all residents for a 2-week period	2 weeks		Project management, project team and unit staff	12/05– 06/06
22. Project team monitor progress	Accurate completion of dependency scores	2 weeks		Project management and project team	06/06
23. Data input	All dependency scores input in the software system	5 weeks		Data input clerk	12/05– 13/06
24. Analysis of data, review date for inconsistencies, resolve any inconsistencies	Data sheet completed	1 week		Project manager	23/06
25. Feedback initial findings to steering groups	Feedback meeting interim report	$\frac{1}{2}$ day		Project manager	30/06
28. Final report to steering group. Agree the way forward	Final report	$\frac{1}{2}$ day		Project manager	07/07
29. Presentations to staff will identify way forward	Communicate results to all staff	4×2 hour meetings		Project manager and project team	14/07
30. Secure all project information	All project data secured	$\frac{1}{2}$ day		Project manager	15/07

*Project commenced 03/02 – 5 project team members – 20 units to be reviewed

work to ensure that everyone involved in the project has a clear and common understanding of the project. This includes:

- what is to be delivered
- when it is to be completed
- what it will cost

- who will do the work
- how the work will be done
- what benefits there will be.

It is important to get this level of understanding in order to avoid a conflict of views on what the project was intended to do at a later stage. This is sometimes known as project definition or a project charter. See Chapter 16 for more information on project definition/group charter.

Outcomes of the initiating stage:

- there is a document confirming the need for the project, including the deliverables set out in broad terms, the cost of the deliverables and benefits to be obtained by implementing the deliverables
- a project manager has been appointed
- the organisation has authorised the project manager to apply resources to project activities
- the initiators of the project have produced the aims and objectives in terms of what they want to achieve in deliverables and outcomes
- there is written approval for the project to go ahead
- there is an agreed project definition or project charter.

2. Planning the project

Building the project plan: during this stage the project plan is developed and agreed. The project plan is vital to ensure that the project team has a clear picture of what is required to deliver the project. The size of the project will determine the complexity of the plan. Large projects may be easier to develop using a software programme to guide the process such as Microsoft Project. On the other hand, use a simple spreadsheet or just use a piece of paper as for example, in the project set out in Table 15.1.

Scoping the project: first, describe the scope of the project in terms of what work is required to meet the objectives of the project. Take out any work that does not relate to the deliverables; only do what must to done to meet the objectives of the project. Scoping a project is a way of defining the boundaries of a project; it defines what the project will and will not deliver. Once the major areas of work have been identified, then these are divided into sub-divisions of manageable items of work. For example, in the worked project in Table 15.1, the collection of data about the background of the organisation and how the units work is divided into structured interviews with staff and managers, observation of the geography of each unit, completion of self-assessment questionnaires by the staff, and the completion of a unit profile for each unit.

Defining the sequence: make a list of all the activities to be undertaken in order to complete the project successfully and put them into a logical order, ensuring that one part of the project leads naturally on to the next. For example, in the worked example there is no point in implementing the dependency tool until the staff have attended the workshops and have a clear understanding of how to use the tool. If they are asked to complete the data sheets without understanding the correct use of the tool, then the data generated at the end will be flawed.

Defining time and resources: estimate the time required for activities and the resources required. For example, the observation of the geography of each unit is estimated at two hours per unit. The units are all on one site, so the two hours includes an allowance of ten minutes for the members of the project team to get from one unit to the next. If there are 20 units then the total time required is 40 hours to complete this element of the project. This activity will require a team of people or one or two people from the project team to complete the data-collection process, so decisions must be made about how many people are required, the training they will need to fulfil this task effectively, the production of forms, questionnaires, and so on.

This section highlights the issue that some aspects of the project plan will be developed into a subproject plan to support specific activities. For example, the project team will need to develop a schedule of times to meet with staff on the units and observe the surroundings, carry out the interview and identify any issues specific to each unit prior to completing the unit profile.

Identify any agreed timescales. For example, if the project is to be in stages then the agreed completion dates on stages one, two and three and the date for the completion of the project.

Developing the project schedule: there are several ways to document the project schedule, including a Gantt chart, milestone charts or text tables. How to develop a Gantt chart is set out at the end of this chapter under techniques and tools for project management. The example of the project plan in Table 15.1 (a worked example of a workload project that was set up to review staffing and skill-mix for an organisation caring for people with learning disabilities) is using a text-table approach and includes the schedule plus a record of the resources required. The plan has also been developed as a Gantt chart (see Table 15.2).

Table 15.2 Project schedule – Gantt chart

Project Schedule	February				March					April				May				June					July	
	03	10	17	24	03	10	17	24	31	07	14	21	28	05	12	19	26	02	09	16	23	30	07	14
1. Select project team	■																							
2. Meeting overview to staff		■																						
3. Develop tools and documents		■																						
4. Collect activity data		■	■																					
5. Set up workshops for project team																								
6. Workshop for project team			■																					
7. Set up workshops for staff				■																				
8. Project team gather data				■																				
9. Analyse baseline data					■																			
10. Develop dependency documentation						■																		
11. Feedback profiles to staff							■																	
12. Staff workshops									■															
13. Distribute dependency sheets										■														
14. Pilot dependency tool											■													

15. Activity sampling																							
16. Analysis of sampling																							
17. Analysis of dependency sheets																							
18. Progress report to steering group																							
19. Visit units																							
20. Resample activities																							
21. Dependency recording for 2 weeks																							
22. Project team monitors progress																							
23. Data input from study																							
24. Analysis of data																							
25. Feedback to steering group																							
26. First draft report																							
27. Draft report to steering group																							
28. Final report to steering group																							
29. Presentation to staff																							
30. Secure all data																							

Estimating the costs: include in the plan an estimated cost of completing each activity, for example the cost of staff replacement, running workshops, copying of papers, forms, and so on.

Setting a budget or spending plan: develop a cost baseline or time-phased budget for monitoring costs, along with a spending plan setting out how much will be spent on what resources at what time. The level of detail required for this stage of the process will depend on the size and complexity of the project. Large and complex projects, such as mergers or complete service re-engineering, will involve substantial costs and a clearly defined budget and therefore a time-phased budget to monitor the spending. However, small projects such as the development of an integrated care pathway (ICP) will involve little extra cost as the project team will be part of the service implementing the ICP and the only extra cost may be replacement costs associated with staff required to attend meetings, or travel costs to visit sites with similar ICPs. In this case there is no need for a complicated budget and spending plan but a simple record to support activity.

Identifying quality assurance measures: quality is ultimately defined by the initiators of the project, who set the aims and objectives of the project at the start of the process. The goal of the project manager is to meet these requirements. At the start of the project set some indicators which will facilitate the measurement of the quality of the project to ensure that it has achieved what it set out to achieve. For example:

- were the dependency ratings completed during the scheduled week period as per the project plan? Answer yes/no – if no, why not?
- were the unit profiles completed accurately by the project team? Answer yes/no – if no, why not?
- were the dependency rating sheets completed accurately by all staff? Answer yes/no – if no, why not?
- were all the stated project deadlines met? Answer yes/no – if no, why not?
- was the report completed on time? Answer yes/no – if no, why not?

This approach will be adequate for a small-to-medium-size project but a large project such as a merger will require a separate quality assurance plan using the information set out in previous chapters in this book.

Setting up a system for communication and monitoring work progress: effective communication is a critical success factor for managing the expectations of all concerned with the project, but in particular the stakeholders. If the stakeholders are not kept well-informed of the progress of the project, then there is a much greater chance of problems and difficulties occurring owing to differing levels of expectation. To ensure effective communication, it is important to discuss with the stakeholders or initiators of the project the format in which they require the progress of the project to be reported. This is often through a steering group that is set up to monitor the progress of the project, support the project manager and to help when difficulties arise. The frequency of the meetings will depend on the size and length of the project. A complex project that is scheduled to run for more than a year may require monthly meetings, whereas a simpler project may require a meeting halfway through the project and a final meeting at its conclusion.

Other methods of communication may be through a newsletter, which is published at regular intervals during the project, explaining the progress and achievements to date, or a regular written report to the stakeholders or initiators of the project.

Internal communication: internal communication within the project team is just as important, and a simple reporting system is very valuable and particularly useful when there are subgroups working on particular aspects of the project who are producing work of their own. For example, the workload project requires the project team to gather the baseline data for each unit. As they carry out their work, the project manager needs to know which tasks they have completed and which are outstanding. The form set out in Table 15.3 allows the project manager to track the progress of the project team.

The detailed work plan is developed at the start of the project and is prepared by the members of the project team carrying out this aspect of work and agreed by the project manager. The frequency with which the forms are returned to the project manager will depend on the time span of the activity. For example, if the work is to be carried out over a four-week period, then a weekly return of the report will keep the project manager informed of progress.

Setting up a system for managing the documentation: whatever size the project, whether it is large and complicated or small and relatively simple, it is important to give some thought to how the information, data, reports and so on will be stored, whether in electronic or paper form. The data needs to be systematically stored or filed somewhere for both security and easy access. Once the project starts, large amounts of data will begin to pile up on the desk and this is not the time to start thinking about how to organise it all. Organising data is not just about where it will be filed but consideration should be given to a system for managing the numerous versions of project status reports and final reports, from their draft stage to the final report status. For example, the version of the report may be set out in the header or footer of

Table 15.3 A detailed work plan

Detailed Project Plan   Page 1 of
Project ... Workforce Planning – Staff Review – Objective number 7 ....

Project main objective: (use one sheet for each major objective)
To gather all baseline data from the units prior to implementation of the dependency rating system.

Final deadline date ... 28/02 ....

Subtasks of main objectives Break the main objective into a series of tasks and list below	Completion deadline Put in dates for each task	Progress to date Brief outline of progress, explain if not achieved	Work outstanding What needs to be done next, add new tasks	Date
1. Meet with sister or charge nurse to go through the structured interview on units 4, 5, 12 and 14	28/02	Meet with sister/ charge nurse on units 4 and 5. Unable to book a time to visit 12 and 14 – staff not available	Arrange to visit units 12 and 14 on week beginning 24/02	21/02
2. Visit the units, note the geography of the units and observe the delivery of care	28/02	Completed as above	Progress as above	21/02

3. Talk to staff about the design of the unit and identify any areas that cause problems and increase the workload	28/02	Completed as above	Progress as above	21/02
4. Talk to the patients about staffing and any concerns they might have about staff shortages	28/02	Consent forms returned from all units	Visit and talk to patients starting week beginning 24/02	21/02
5. Report on the findings to project manager	28/03	Data for units 4, 5, 6, 10, 11 and 16 gathered	Analyse data from units 4 and 5. Gather data from 12 and 14 by 28/02	21/02
6. Complete unit profile to the project manager	28/03	None to date	Start working out structure of report	21/02

the report, or different coloured paper may be used for different status, for example green for first draft, yellow for second draft, and so on.

Acquiring and organising the staff: more often than not, the project team is identified by the initiators or the stakeholders of the project, so the project manager will need to meet with the project team and identify what skills, knowledge and experience there is in the team and if there are any gaps that need to be filled. The next step is to allocate roles and responsibilities to the team members. Listed at the end of this chapter is an overview of the roles people play in teams. In the project plan, identify who will be carrying out what tasks as shown in Table 15.2.

Risk management: this step is about the identification of any areas of risk and the establishment of ways of managing the risk. Successful project managers try to resolve potential problems before they arise. This is the art of risk management, which is a proactive process that is set up to attempt to eliminate potential problems before they occur. In the worked example in Table 15.1, the biggest risk to the project is the inaccurate completion by the staff of the dependency ratings of the residents. This is likely to occur if the staff do not understand how the dependency tool works and how to complete the form accurately. Some of the staff may be inclined to put in a higher dependency to deliberately 'skew' the figures, hoping that the result will indicate the need for more staff to meet the residents' needs. To avoid this situation, education on the use of the tool is required so that staff are knowledgeable about the system, but also built into the project is a system of scanning the data and identifying where data are inconsistent.

Planning for and acquiring outside resources: in some projects there may be a need to set out the process of procurement and how contactors will be managed. However, in the health service any procurement will go through supplies and will therefore link with the project plan at this stage.

Organising the project plan: this stage is the final organisation of the project plan, ensuring that all the stages set out above have been addressed.

Completing the plan: the plan is completed and agreed by the stakeholders or the initiators of the project, and the project team and the project commences.

Reviewing the plan and revising as necessary: the project manager continues to review the project plan to ensure that it is still accurate and will result in a positive conclusion. If anything changes, then the project manager revisits and reviews the project plan.

Outcomes of the planning stage:

- the project has been scoped
- the sequence of events has been organised
- time and resources have been defined
- the project schedule has been developed
- costs have been estimated
- the budget and spending plan are defined
- quality assurance measures are identified
- the system of communication has been set up
- the system for managing the documentation has been set up
- the roles and responsibilities of the project team and staff have been assigned
- the risks have been identified and plans to manage the risks have been outlined
- the plans for acquired outside resources have been completed
- the the project plan is organised
- the the project plan is completed
- the project plan is reviewed and revised.

3. Executing the project

Effectively this is the stage when the project is started and proceeds to its successful conclusion. Both the internal progress detailed reports and the reports to the steering group and the stakeholders/initiators of the project are started. The project manager assesses the performance of the project team through regular meetings with the team and evaluation of its work and ensures that the project schedule is maintained.

Outcomes of the executing stage:

- work is in progress
- reporting systems have commenced
- an ongoing evaluation of the work has begun.

4. Controlling the project

The role of the project manager is to control and manage the project through:

- ensuring that the schedule is followed and that targets are met as agreed by the right people at the right time and with the predicted results
- keeping track of the progress of the project, particularly where subgroups are working independently through the collection and processing of the

worksheets on a weekly basis, and then feeding back to the subgroup satisfaction or dissatisfaction with the progress
- the production of regular progress reports to the steering group
- making changes to the schedule as required
- sending progress reports to the initiators of the project, the stakeholders and the steering group
- meeting on a regular basis with the steering group to report progress and any problems
- keeping the project plan and schedule up to date
- organising the information, data, reports and so on in preparation for the final presentation and report
- documenting what action was taken to resolve any problems, risks or other untoward incidents which arose
- monitoring the indicators of quality as the project progresses and improving quality where required
- monitoring the cost of the project and ensuring that the budget is not exceeded. If there are unforeseen developments that are taking the project over the budget, these issues then need to be taken to the steering group.

Outcomes of the controlling stage:

- the project is managed
- the project team is working effectively
- quality is monitored
- the project is within budget
- communication is good
- documentation is good
- preparation for the final presentation and/or report has commenced.

5. Closing the project

At this stage the project manager brings the project to a close through a presentation of the project to the steering group and the initiators of the project and/or the stakeholders. This is followed up with a final report. All documentation supporting the project is filed away or stored electronically. If a follow-up or review of the project is required, then this is organised by the project manager.

Outcomes of the closing stage:

- the project was completed on time
- the project was completed within budget
- the aims and objectives were met

- final presentation and/or report was accepted by the initiators and/or stakeholders
- all project information has been stored
- the project was signed off by the initiators.

Once the project is completed, then a review of how well things went or indeed what went wrong is helpful in improving performance for the next time. Some general questions may help with this process:

- were you pleased with the way that the project went?
- what was done really well?
- what was the most frustrating part of the project?
- what did not go well?
- what would you do differently next time?
- were the steering group and the initiators of the project supportive?
- did you meet your objectives?

Project Teams

Part of the role of the project manager is working with, developing and supporting the project team. Critchley and Casey (1984) outline the characteristics of a functioning team:

- people care for each other
- people are open and truthful
- decisions are made by consensus
- there is strong team commitment
- conflict is dealt with and feelings are expressed.

They also suggest that there are some tasks that are suitable for a team to address and some where the use of a team is simply a luxury inasmuch as one person could manage the task. However, a project team is essential if the task carries a high degree of uncertainty and is therefore more complex and will benefit from the attention of a group of people with different ideas, backgrounds and experience. The chapter on working with groups covers the roles that people play in groups or teams, and the same applies to the leaders and leadership skills. See Chapters 6 and 14 for more information.

There are some skills and tools that are particularly useful for project management and these may be found in Chapter 16. They include:

- project definitions/group charters
- managing meetings

- building agendas
- effective meetings
- problem-solving
- structures
- brainstorming
- forcefield analysis
- gantt charts
- communication.

Conclusion

Project management is not only a very useful skill but it also requires more skills and knowledge to manage a complex project than this book is able to address. However, I believe that the overview in this chapter contains enough information with which to manage a small-to-medium-sized project and, combined with the information on the management of change in Chapter 13, and on working with groups and facilitation in Chapter 14, the reader could manage a project with confidence.

Clinical Governance – The Tools for the Job

16

Chapter Contents:

- general skills
- managing meetings
- working with groups or teams
- change management and project management skills.

Various tools, techniques and skills, which have been referred to throughout this book, can be used in the quest for a system of clinical governance and continuous quality improvement.

General Skills

Working with a Flip Chart

- print in large capital letters and concentrate on listening and writing legibly and accurately
- stand facing the flip chart or to the side at all times, except when tearing pages and sticking them on a wall or another chart
- carry tape or some other form of adhesive to attach the sheets of paper to the wall, preferably something that does not leave a mark
- use bold or dark colours such as black, green and blue to make the chart more readable. Never use more than three colours on one page
- stick to basic graphics when you start: for example, use bullets or an arrow for listed items and a border around a page or paragraph that has one block of data. You can also use lighter colours like yellow or pink to highlight a key concept, or a simple symbol to highlight a word or phase
- if possible make sure that there are two flip charts available to maintain the group memory (see below). This allows you to have two people recording

data during brainstorming sessions or to record separately sets of data that will be integrated with each other at a later stage

■ have a supply of stickers that people can use to indicate choices on brainstormed lists. Different coloured dots and other types of stickers are very useful; members of the group can use them, for example, to indicate choices on brainstormed lists.

Managing Meetings

There needs to be effective use of meeting room space. The physical environment is very important as people think and behave better in orderly, arranged surroundings. A good facilitator arrives at the meeting room in good time to do the following:

■ check on the seating arrangements
■ move things around if they do not seem to be positioned correctly
■ make sure that there is a small table to put materials on
■ check that the flip charts have enough paper
■ check markers and make sure that they all work
■ ensure that all audiovisual equipment leads are secure so that no one trips over them
■ ensure that audiovisual equipment is in working order
■ think through each activity which has been planned and make sure the space will accommodate it
■ put out a welcome sign to greet participants or create some last-minute flip charts for the group.

While the meeting or workshop is in progress, keep an eye on the physical conditions in the room. Check that groups are not too close to one another and that they are not distracting each other. Are people too hot or too cold? Respond accordingly to ensure they are comfortable. Unfortunately, it is often the case that the environment is less than perfect and from experience I can say that it is quite possible to facilitate extremely effective meetings in even the most cramped and inhospitable surroundings.

The group memory is critical to group work, so it is important to have enough flip charts, or somewhere to hang up sheets from the flip chart, to cover the whole meeting or workshop.

Whenever there is a significant amount of small-group work, each group should have a record of its work – its own group memory. It is important to find out whether the education centre, organisation or hotel allows the use of temporary adhesives or tape or has certain rules which must be followed, then plan accordingly.

When facilitating large groups there is often a need to break the group down into small groups. Some facilitators advise against using break-out rooms unless it is really necessary. This is mainly because of the management of people returning from break-out rooms is nearly always problematic. The small groups sometimes misinterpret their remit, fail to integrate their ideas and feel isolated from the large group rather than a part of it. On the other hand, using break-out rooms can help a small group concentrate and get its work done better, and if the facilitator divides his/her time between the groups and ensures that small groups return to the main group at the same time, then the break-out room system can work. The best solution is to arrange to use a room large enough for the entire group to stay together throughout the session. The analysis of feedback from groups is that the noise is not seen as a major problem and the 'buzz' of small groups at work together creates a kind of group energy and enthusiasm that is lost when people go off to different locations.

When facilitating large groups, such as at conferences or large workshops where several small groups will be working at the same time, it is a good idea to use a microphone if one is available. The amplification of the facilitator's voice brings a clarity and cohesiveness to managing the group. It also saves the facilitator from having to raise his/her voice in order to be heard. It is also a good idea to have mobile microphones available for small-group leaders to use when they present reports to the larger group. If the location is a hotel, then use small narrow tables or circular tables as these work well for many types of groups.

Building the Agenda

A well-thought-out agenda is an essential foundation for an effective meeting. First, ensure that the purpose and aims of the meeting are made clear and that a carefully thought-out sequence of activities for achieving those purposes and aims is developed. The agenda should be agreed at least three working days before the meeting and preferably fourteen to twenty-one working days before the meeting.

When planning the agenda for a meeting:

- list on a piece of paper the overall purpose/aim of the meeting. If a group of people are doing this, allow enough time for the group to discuss this and be quite clear about the purpose of the meeting
- list any issues or items that need to be dealt with in the meeting to achieve the purpose/aim and any relevant news or information items. If this is a regular meeting of a group or committee, then remember to include the minutes or notes of the previous meeting and any matters arising from them

- sort the issues and information items into what you have to deal with in this meeting and what you can deal with another way: for example, items that must be brought to this meeting; items that can wait until the next meeting; items that can be dealt with outside the meeting, such as a news item that could be include in a newsletter, and so on until you have the items that are essential for this meeting
- list the anticipated outcomes for the meeting: for example, whether the outcome of an item is for approval or agreement by the group or committee; whether it is to be delegated to a member of the group or committee or indeed to another group of people, and so on
- prioritise the outcomes in order of importance with the weighty items at the beginning of the agenda. Leave news and information items to the end of the agenda unless they are critical to the meeting
- transfer all agenda items to a new sheet of chart paper, listing them in order of priority
- for each item, assign a person to be responsible for ensuring that the intended outcome is achieved
- estimate the time slots for each item but allow some extra time rather than planning each moment of it
- if this is a group meeting which is to be facilitated, then the following roles should be assigned:
  - ☐ leader
  - ☐ facilitator (for entire group)
  - ☐ flip chart recorder (if problem-solving group memory to be used)
  - ☐ minute-taker/record-keeper
  - ☐ small-group facilitators
  - ☐ timekeeper
  - ☐ process observer (a person assigned to focus on how the group is doing with specific process skills, which will be monitored during the meeting).
- check out the leader's preferred way of running the meeting. Any of the following may be relevant:
  - ☐ *leader-run using a consultative approach*: here the leader runs the meeting, facilitating discussion and making clear decisions before proceeding from one item to the next. The leader tries not to get involved in the content of decisions but prefers to ask questions and looks for consultative information for the decision that he/she will make
  - ☐ *leader-run and facilitator-assisted*: here the facilitator leads the group through the items, turning to the leader for decisions following consultation with the group
  - ☐ *leader-run with periodic facilitator assistance*: the leader operates as in the consultative approach except for specified items that he/she hands over to the facilitator for discussion and problem-solving using a consensus approach

- [ ] *facilitator-led using team-based decisions*: the leader agrees to accept all decisions agreed on by the group. He/she participates fully as an equal group member, with no greater authority than any other member
- [ ] *leader-run and facilitated*: here the leader functions both as a decision-maker and facilitator, choosing when to play which role.

Whichever approach the leader takes, he/she is responsible for the group and the decisions, not the facilitator.

- identify which method of making decisions will be adopted if this has not already been decided. These include:
  - [ ] *absolute consensus*: everyone must agree to support a decision before a decision is made
  - [ ] *consultative decision*: the leader makes the decision after listening to all advice, points of view, ideas and recommendations made by the group or committee
  - [ ] *consultative consensus*: the leader makes a decision only after listening to the views of the members and striving for consensus
  - [ ] *modified consensus*: the group seeks consensus on all items, agreeing to support the decision even though it may not agree with all of the decision. If this definition of consensus cannot be achieved, there is a fallback on the leader for either a decision or a postponement of the item
  - [ ] *voting*: the members vote on decisions and it is specified as to whether a majority, two-thirds, or other kind of vote determines the decision.

Note any agenda items that will be exceptions to the normal chosen approach for decision-making for this meeting. For example, if the accepted approach is normally one of consultative decision-making, but the leader feels that one item really requires the consensus of the entire group, then this item should be marked as an exception.

- identify any supporting papers that are required and decide which ones should be sent to the group or committee prior to the meeting
- establish the location and start and finish time of the meeting.

Summary of Key Actions that Lead to Effective Meetings

Responsibilities of the chairman, leader or project manager:

- set objectives
- review roles
- establish focused agenda

- set ground rules
- make assignments
- distribute agenda in advance
- start and end meeting on time
- work the agenda
- do not allow interruptions or sidetracking
- encourage creative, proactive participation.

Responsibilities of those attending the meeting:

- be on time
- be attentive
- be prepared
- participate
- be positive
- stick to the agenda
- take notes (for comments or questions).

The process of the meeting:

- clarify objective
- review agenda
- work through each agenda item
- review action items, issues and progress
- assign and document action items
- next steps
- summarise meeting
- follow up on action items.

To be most effective, a meeting should not exceed one hour.

Working with Groups or Teams

Leadership

The decision about who will lead the group is often one that ultimately makes the difference between success and failure in a group. Groups with a leader in place early on in their development usually move through the stages of group development more quickly than those groups who delay the choice of leader. Groups without leaders are more likely to fail in their task than those with a leader. The following are the principal criteria that a group can use to choose its leader and all are valid reasons for doing so:

- *expertise*: the person has the most expertise in the problem to be solved or the group task to be undertaken
- *initiation of work*: the person is most likely to be called upon to initiate work
- *workload expectancy*: the person will be called upon to do the greatest amount of work
- *functional responsibility*: the person has the most 'natural responsibility' for the work in the system
- *hierarchical status*: the person has the highest hierarchical status of all the group members. Many groups fail if the group leader has a lower hierarchical status than other members of the group. However, if the person with the highest hierarchical status has less expertise in a particular area of the project than another member of the group, the option may be to have a joint leadership.

A good practice to adopt early on in the life of a group is to encourage everyone to be a leader, establishing a group culture of shared leadership. This can be done by introducing or reintroducing task maintenance behaviours and asking group members to assert leadership by monitoring the behaviour of the group with regard to those behaviours. If shared leadership is the preferred option, then go through the exercise of monitoring task and maintaining behaviours before the meeting (see Chapter 6 for more information). The group then identifies where it needs to focus attention for this particular meeting and designates leaders to monitor group performance in these areas.

Being an Effective Facilitator

What makes an effective facilitator? There are some key skills that every facilitator should have in his/her portfolio and these include the ability to:

- listen intensely; be a model listener, paraphrase often and 'mirror' what is said
- maintain good eye contact and stay connected to the group and each of its members
- trust in the resources of the group; keep focused on the process of getting things done and remain detached from what the group decides to do
- always address people by their first name
- stay awake and concentrate on every moment of the meeting or session
- organise, connect, and summarise information to conclude and achieve a sense of completion
- protect each and every idea offered by the group and not allow ideas to be attacked until evaluation time

- be a facilitator, not a performer; be interested in the work of the group and not interesting
- encourage everyone to express themselves, and validate varying points of view offered; keep track of who talks and who does not, encouraging balanced participation
- be the guide, not the group leader and support the group leaders
- keep in mind the outcomes that the group are seeking and be flexible in the approach to helping them achieve those outcomes.

Introducing People to Each Other – Ice-Breaking Technique

The most commonly used approach is to ask all the members of the group, in turn, to say something about themselves, their background and what they bring to the group. There is a way of making this a little more fun and a lot more interesting. This technique is designed to introduce people to each other in groups, using an approach that builds an understanding of each person's background. Start the session by inviting each member of the group to draw pictures on a sheet of flip chart paper, depicting:

- his/her working life to date
- his/her family environment
- his/her personal background
- his/her interests outside work
- something that members of the team are unlikely to know about him/her, for example an unusual hobby or a claim to fame.

Then invite each member of the team, in turn, to present and explain his/her pictures.

Using the Group Memory

The group memory is the ongoing record of the group task, which is logged on flip charts and made clearly visible to all group members. Either the facilitator, or someone known as a recorder, writes the comments and ideas of group members on the flip chart and then puts the charts around the meeting room for all to see. After the meeting, the pages are transcribed and serve as the ongoing meeting record for the group. The group memory is an essential part of the work of a group resolving a complex problem. This approach prevents the groups from becoming confused about what happened when, what decisions were made and how they were reached.

At each meeting, in order to establish and maintain the group memory, the facilitator should carry out the following steps:

- identify a member of the group to be responsible for maintaining the group memory and, if the group is to be divided into smaller groups, decide who will continue to record in these groups
- Doyle and Straus (1976), who pioneered the widespread use of the group memory technique, recommend that the group memory be placed directly in front of the group. Use a semi-circle of seats without any tables. The semi-circular seating arrangement is excellent for problem-solving task groups but less useful when the group are reviewing or referring to a number of documents, in which case tables are essential. Use one or more flip charts on stands and keep a supply of adhesive to attach the completed charts on to the walls
- explain to the group about the concept of the group memory and say that everything goes on to the flip chart
- record all information for a specific agenda item on a separate page
- before moving from one agenda item to the next, number each of the flip chart pages. If the data is to be used in subsequent parts of the meeting, then mount the pages on the wall. Some pages may also be mounted to show specific agreements or resolutions which the group has made. During the meeting remove any mounted charts that are no longer required so that the room does not become cluttered with information
- at the end of the meeting collect the charts, number them ready for typing up verbatim as a permanent record prior to being distributed to all group members before the next meeting.

Project Definition/Group Charter

Drawing up a project charter or defining the project is essential to a group as it sets out the purpose of the group's work. Groups that have been set up to work over a long period of time, groups working on complex tasks and special project teams need to take the time necessary to clarify the work of the group if they are to be successful. A group charter statement is an excellent way to clarify the work of the group.

Every group needs to have a clearly worded statement, which is known as a project definition or charter. The following steps are useful in the process of developing the project definition or charter:

- carry out a brainstorming exercise to establish the purposes of the group and list them on a flip chart or piece of paper

- list all the purposes of the group in order of priority, starting with the primary purpose of the group. If this is not fulfilled, it will mean that the group has failed
- discuss what the group sees as the potential outcome of its work and the desired future state in measurable terms. Review the outcomes and highlight any that the group can agree will definitely be needed for a successful outcome
- elicit the expected barriers to achieving the desired outcomes and identify problems related to the accomplishment of these outcomes
- take similar problems and group them together to create a smaller list of groups of problems
- put the list of problems in order of priority then highlight the top 20 per cent. These become the group's key problems
- establish the estimated length of time for the group to meet the targets that they set previously
- the group now decides which of the following choices they will make in the event of three key scenarios:
  - □ to disband when it has completed its tasks
  - □ to continue as a monitoring and problem-solving group until its tasks are completed
  - □ to review the decision to continue as a group at a later date.
- identify the person who will make the decisions and to whom the group's recommendations will be submitted. Also identify any regular meeting to be led by the appointed decision-maker where recommendations will be reviewed prior to decisions being approved
- schedule the first meeting, when the person responsible for approving the recommendations will review the group's recommendations
- write a brief group mission statement of fewer than fifty words that clearly sets out the task of the group
- set a date to review the charter statement and make revisions.

Reflective Listening

Reflective listening is a very valuable skill; it can be used to initiate reflective conversations and to encourage members of a group to listen carefully to one another's points of view and the various experiences each brings to the group. The members of the group take turns reflecting upon a question asked by another group member, sharing their thoughts, and then asking the next person a question.

The facilitator gives the group an overview of the session and sets out the ground rules which are:

- only one person speaks at a time
- there should be no interrupting, correcting, or helping
- there should be no judgements, especially of oneself.

One group member is given the talking stick (this can be anything from a stick to a ruler) and is asked to generate a broad question related to a topic area. The group member holding the stick reflects and then directs the question to the person sitting beside him/her. This person takes the stick, responds to the question, taking as long as is needed, poses another question to the person sitting next to him/her, and passes the talking stick to that person. The process continues until everyone has had a turn.

The group is asked to discuss what the experience was like for them and what they noticed about the activity.

The facilitator follows the same ground rules as participants and should not try to help anyone in the group. Sometimes a person will misunderstand the question but the exercise should continue nonetheless.

Giving and Receiving Feedback

Feedback is essentially for the benefit of the receiver rather than the giver. The process should be seen as a positive experience for all involved. This includes negative feedback which, if given for the right reasons, can also be a positive experience. There is an opportunity to learn from mistakes when these are fed back to the receiver in an honest and open way. The facilitator has a role in both the giving and receiving of feedback:

Giving feedback: be 'other-centred', honest, own the feedback and use 'I' statements. When giving feedback focus on behaviour and not on the person. Base the feedback on observation and not inference. Feedback should be descriptive and not judgemental. It is about sharing information and ideas and not about giving advice or direction. Feedback is specific and given immediately, not generalised and given after a delay. It is important to focus on items that can be changed and not on those outside the control of the receiver. Mix and balance positive and negative feedback; try not use the positive without the negative, and vice versa.

Receiving feedback: be open and avoid filtering and interpreting. The receiver of feedback should be receptive and not defensive. Listen carefully and resist the temptation to interrupt or challenge the giver of the feedback. The receiver must acknowledge and not ignore the feedback, and he/she must check his/her understanding of the information rather than assume what the giver of the feedback means. The receiver may discuss the feedback if required to do so but should not sulk or refuse to respond to negative feedback; remember, it is about learning and moving on.

Intervention Skills

There are times when the facilitator must make the decision to intervene if there are problems with the processes within the group. For example, if there is hostility between two members of the group, the group is being destructive to itself, an individual is withdrawing from the group, there is competition for the leadership or there is poor communication. Some suggestions for dealing with problems within a group are given below.

Encouraging all Members of the Group to be Actively Involved

Some people enjoy the dynamics of a group and readily contribute but there are also those who hold back and just watch. Being part of a group is not a spectator sport and it is the responsibility of the facilitator or the leader to ensure that everyone contributes so that the group works effectively. The following suggestions may help:

- divide the group into pairs, or groups of three or four; the smaller group will encourage people to join in
- divide the group into pairs to work on a specific aspect of a problem or a project, for example a name for the group. After the groups of pairs have met to generate their recommendations, then combine two of the pairs together to make a larger group of four. This group then discusses the same issue, compares lists and adds more recommendations. Join two groups of four together and repeat the process. As the groups grow larger, the quieter members of the group tend to grow in confidence as they receive recognition for their recommendations
- move to 'round robin' participation; ask everyone to take a turn offering his/ her thoughts or ideas. This has to be carefully handled as sometimes this has the negative effect of putting people on the spot and they withdraw further
- call on those who have not been participating. If a member of the group has not been contributing, address him/her by name and say, 'I notice that you have been doing a lot more thinking than talking. Is there anything you would like to contribute at this stage?'
- introduce another ice-breaking technique, as set out earlier in this section. This will help to build the participative atmosphere

- acknowledge the problem that members of the group are not joining in by saying, 'I notice that we seem to be having some problems working as a group. Can someone help us explore these issues?'
- ask group members to pause and reflect upon their participation within the group. Ask them to remain silent and think about the role they are playing in the group. For example, have they all been joining in and sharing their thoughts and ideas? Have they been talking too much, too little, or about the right amount? Which members of the group need to be heard from more? What group task and group maintenance behaviours have they been practising? What adjustments, if any, do they want to make to maximise the success of the group? After the moment of silence, either discuss people's thoughts or simply move on. Alternatively, use this activity prior to a break and start again with the group after the break
- ask each member of the group to select a partner for interview. On a flip chart, write a list of questions that represent aspects of the task that members are working on. These questions form the interview and the answers to the questions should be written down, so that each member of the group is ready to share his/her findings with the whole group
- review the agenda and change it. If the lack of participation is being caused by a problem with the process and the agenda needs to be revised, then either discuss this with the whole group or the leader and make any modifications as necessary to get the group working effectively on the task
- stop the meeting or session, talk to the leader and have a brief look at what is not going right, why, and what to do about it.

The Individual who Does not Join in with the Group

Some people remain silent in group meetings; they seem unable or unwilling to speak in a group setting. They may be shy, frightened of looking stupid or unsure of themselves and what they have to offer to the group. If unchecked they are likely to withdraw from the group, so the facilitator needs to take action which may include:

- outside the group activity take the person to one side and talk to him/her privately to find out what the problem is
- within the group ask the individual to contribute, for example, 'John, we have not heard from you on this. What are your views about ... ? Choose your time carefully and do not ask him about his views unless you are sure he has something to contribute with confidence and conviction, or it is an area where he has some expertise. Then thank him for his contribution
- early in the life of the group make sure that everyone contributes during ice-breakers and 'getting to know you' sessions.

The Group does not Keep to the Agenda

Some groups have trouble staying on the subject or following the agenda of a meeting. This may be because individuals in the group are distracted by their own personal agenda, because they disagree with the agenda or task, or because they simply want to avoid tackling the task. The following options may help to resolve the problem:

- take the group back and revisit the agenda
- ask the group if it feels that the current discussion is helpful or necessary
- ask the group why it is not sticking to the agenda
- offer to change or reschedule the task or the agenda
- ask the group if the present discussions are important to everyone or if they can be postponed until after the meeting and then handled by a few members of the group
- ask the group what is going on
- take a break before continuing.

When an Individual Member of the Group Does not Keep to the Agenda

Sometimes one or more of the group are clearly not working to the same agenda as the rest of the group. This becomes obvious as they talk about things that are irrelevant to the group's task. To put a stop to this, some of the following ideas may help:

- ask these members of the group to relate what they are saying to the current agenda
- ask if the group may come back to their point at a later stage in the group's task and write their issues on the flip chart
- ask others in the group if they have anything to add to what the other members of the group have said
- stop them and explain that it is not appropriate at this stage of the group's work; ask them to bring it up later at a different stage of the group's task.

Problem-Solving

When most groups are set up they have a broad picture of the problem they have to resolve. It is often said that in order to agree upon a solution, you must first agree on the problem. Problem-solving techniques help to clarify the problem. One such technique is detailed below:

- ask each member of the group to write down what he/she thinks the problem is. Then list all their responses on a flip chart
- lead the group through a series of questions designed to elaborate accurately on the problem. Select no more than eight questions from the following list:
  - [ ] what happens?
  - [ ] then what happens? (Repeat several times until all scenarios are identified.)
  - [ ] where does the problem occur?
  - [ ] when does the problem occur?
  - [ ] how frequently does the problem occur?
  - [ ] how long has the problem been going on?
  - [ ] what resources are involved in the problem?
  - [ ] what systems, processes or procedures are involved in the problem?
  - [ ] who is most affected by the problem?
  - [ ] who or what type of person gets hurt most by the problem?
  - [ ] who has the authority and control to correct the problem?
  - [ ] what other processes or procedures does the problem have an impact on?
  - [ ] when was the problem first identified as being significant?
  - [ ] what happened that the problem became so important that this group is working on it?
  - [ ] is this problem like many other problems that have occurred in the past? If the answer is yes, does there appear to be a pattern emerging?
  - [ ] where could this problem be occurring but at present is not? (for example, other departments or trusts)
  - [ ] when could this problem be occurring but at present is not?
  - [ ] who might have this problem but does not?
  - [ ] how did things work before this problem occurred?
- write the selected questions on flip charts, with one question at the top of each chart page
- lead the group through the process of generating the information in answer to the questions. Encourage them to be objective when putting forward their answers to the questions. Record all the information on the flip chart without comment or disagreement. Go through all the questions
- go back to each question and ask, 'Does anyone have a concern related to any of this recorded information? Do you feel it is inaccurate or unclear?' Then either change the statements so that they are acceptable to both the person who had the concern and the person who originally generated the information, or eliminate the statements. Alternatively, allow some additional discussion related to the problem, noting any relevant comments on the appropriate chart page
- ask the group to write the problem in statement form in fewer than one hundred words. The statement should end with the sentence, 'The primary

causes of the problem appear to be ...' Once the group have clarified the problem, then the solution is on the horizon

■ feed the statement back to the group and check that it is satisfied that it has described the problem.

Disruptive Behaviour in Groups

Difficult people

Sometimes there are people in the group who cause problems through inappropriate or unhelpful behaviours. While each situation will be different, there are some approaches that the facilitator or the leader can use:

■ if possible, talk to the individual on his/her own, state the problem and help him/her towards more acceptable behaviour
■ do not judge a person's behaviour to be right or wrong
■ approach the individual as a friend and not as someone in authority
■ keep a balance between protecting the group from the unhelpful behaviour while protecting the individual from attack by the rest of the group
■ accept what the individual is doing; at the same time, describe it and ask about it
■ legitimise his/her feelings, perceptions or rights
■ work with the individual and the disruptive behaviour when it will be productive for the group, or defer this to a time when the group is likely to perform well, despite the distraction
■ use the group's ground rules for participation, so that it can self-monitor and enforce these rules when someone disrupts the group.

Conflict resolution

Covey (Covey 1989; Covey et al., 1994), offers a simple approach for resolving conflict between two members of a group who are not listening to each other. He suggests that nearly every two-person conflict can be resolved by invoking a communication rule that says, 'You cannot make your point until you restate the point of the other person to his or her satisfaction.'

When two members of the group become entrenched in their conflicting positions, the facilitator or the group leader stops the discussion and points out the need for the two members of the group to listen to one another in order for the group to succeed. If they agree, then the next steps are:

■ ask the two members to undertake an exercise that requires them to use their listening skills. Emphasise that they will be working to improve the performance of the entire group

- when the two members agree to participate, then write up the 'seek first to understand' rule on a flip chart. This rule is that you cannot make your point until you have restated the point of the other person to his/her satisfaction. Ask both members if they understand the rule
- ask them to proceed with the discussion. Ask member one to start making his/her point. If member two interrupts, remind him/her of the rule and allow member one to finish. Then ask member two, who has been listening, to state member one's viewpoint
- ask member one if he/she is satisfied that member two has grasped the essence of his/her point. If member one is not satisfied, then ask him/her to repeat the point until he/she is satisfied that member two understands the point
- once member one feels that he/she has been heard, then member two makes a point and the process is repeated. The discussion proceeds in this way until both parties feel that they have fully expressed their standpoint and have been heard
- the facilitator or the group leader monitors the discussion, making sure that neither member proceeds to make a point until the other is satisfied that he/she has been 'heard'.

The unresponsive, silent or complaining group

Sometimes a particular activity or task leaves the group unresponsive, silent or complaining. There may be many reasons behind this behaviour, from a feeling that the task is too difficult to fears about the impact of the outcome. Therere are a number of ways to get the group back on track:

- ask the group what is going on
- provide feedback on what you see and ask why
- try a different approach to start the activity or discussion
- take a short break. During the break ask some of the group why they are reluctant to complete the task or why they are silent
- ask the group if they have any suggestions as to how to do it differently
- ask the group if this approach is helpful
- ask the group how they would like to take things forward
- ask individuals to respond.

A member of the group dominates the discussion

It may happen that someone in the group talks too long, too loud or too often, making it difficult if not impossible for others in the group to participate. Here are a few suggestions to curb this sort of behaviour in a group:

- very politely stop the person, thank him/her, and say that you would like to hear from someone else
- refer to the agenda and timeframes
- break eye contact, move away from the person and stop focusing your attention on the individual
- move closer and closer to the person, maintaining eye contact. Place yourself in front of him/her with the result that the problematic behaviour will start to stand out
- summarise what the person has said and move to someone else
- set a time limit before the discussion starts of, for example, no more than two minutes each for comments. Keep everyone who contributes to the time limit. Alternatively, if one of the group has a reputation for 'hogging' the floor, then at the start of the meeting say that the intention is for the group to monitor the time people spend talking, which will mean talking more for some and less for others
- introduce an inclusion activity to get everyone participating.

People who interrupt while others are speaking

Some people cut in when others are speaking or jump into a conversation too soon. When they do this they disrupt the group and in particular the person speaking, who is prevented from finishing what he/she was saying or stopped from completing his/her argument or point of view. These interruptions are usually verbal but a group member can equally be interrupted by non-verbal negative expressions. The problem is most marked in large groups where people are keen to be heard and become frustrated while waiting to get into the discussion. One solution is to ask people to raise their hand when they have something to say; the facilitator acknowledges each person and verbally puts the names of the people who want to speak in an order, and then directs the group to hear from each person in turn.

The ground rules of the group will include the need for group members to respect each individual's contribution and not interrupt, but this still seems to happen. To resolve the problem of the constant interrupter, it is necessary to start by reinforcing the ground rules, and if that does not work:

- stop the person who is interrupting and ask him/her to wait while the speaker completes what he/she is saying
- some members of the group may become impatient when listening to someone making a point so suggest that they write down their thoughts and wait their turn
- be neutral and consistent. It is important to be seen to be consistent so do not let some people get away with it and not others.

People with their own personal agenda

It can be very disruptive when someone in the group continually inserts a concern, a disagreement or an alternative or additional agenda item. This is annoying if it is repetitive and distracts from the group task. The following suggestions may help to contain and resolve this type of behaviour:

- very politely ask the group member to explain how what he/she is saying relates to the current agenda item
- make a note of the point on the flip chart, thank the person, and move on
- ask the person what he/she wants the group to do with the information
- give the person a time limit for his/her point of view.

The person who repeats the same point over and over again

Sometimes people get caught up in something they care passionately about and they just cannot let go. If they repeat themselves over and over again, this will annoy and disrupt the group. The solution is similar to that for the problem when a member of the group has his/her own personal agenda: acknowledge the point and somehow put it away so that the group can move on. The following may be helpful:

- acknowledge the importance of the point and the person's beliefs, passion and determination
- write the point on the flip chart to demonstrate that his/her point has been heard
- explain how and when the point will be dealt with
- ask the group member if it is all right to move on and to leave the point for the moment
- give the group member a definite time when the point will be made.

People in a group who make private comments to others during a meeting

In any group in any meeting there may be people who insist on making private comments to one another. This distracts the group and undermines the people who are speaking at the time. Here are some suggestions to resolve this problem:

- invite the people concerned to share what is being said
- stop the conversation, look at the people talking and ask them to stop
- request that they join the group

■ move closer to the people having the side conversation and repeat the topic under discussion, asking if everyone can focus on having just one conversation at a time.

The person who is negative or hostile

There may be some people in the group who are always sceptical, negative and cynical, and they can be very distracting because they distort the work of the group. They are often heard to say, 'We have tried that and it didn't work' or 'That won't work!' Alternatively, they huff, puff, tut and make disapproving faces, and the body language says it all. The following suggestions should help to curb this behaviour:

■ first get them to express their point of view and acknowledge it
■ then feed back to them exactly what was said, paraphrasing their view the first couple of times they speak. Use their exact words if you can, or at least keep very close to what was said and how it was said
■ point out to them the negative pattern
■ ask them if there is any aspect of the group's task that they feel good about
■ ask them to say what they believe is required to complete the task. Write down their ideas on the flip chart and ask the group to respond.

The person who attacks, criticises or picks arguments

Some people enjoy 'having a go at' other members of the group and indeed the facilitator is often seen as fair game. These attacks can be personal or more general, and an attempt to discredit or change what the group is doing. Whatever the reason, the individual must be stopped as this sort of behaviour will disrupt and could ultimately destroy the group as members withdraw, fearful of becoming a target for the attacks. There are some approaches that the facilitator can employ:

■ describe to the person what he/she is doing but be sure to be non-judgemental in the way you express yourself
■ ask the person if something that has occurred during the meeting has caused him/her to launch the personal attack or argue the point so aggressively
■ stop the argument or personal attack. Ask the group member for a statement about his/her position at the centre of the argument or personal attack and write all the points on the flip chart. Then ask the rest of the group to discuss and record their position on each of the statements. Discuss the problem together
■ ask the individual what the group can do to respond to his/her concerns.

The clown

Humour is essential in any group as part of the dynamics of working together. However, sometimes a member of the group may overuse humour by acting the clown and joking about everything. This overdose of humour can distract the group from the task in hand. Some tactics to control the clown include:

- ignoring the behaviour and the individual
- asking him/her to stop it
- pointing out to the individual that what he/she is doing is distracting the group from its task
- having a quiet word with the individual outside the meeting and explaining the effect that his/her behaviour is having on the group. Discuss the agenda and the timescales and get him/her to focus on the agenda and the task.

Poor attendance

Some people have a tendency to arrive late or leave early, miss meetings, or leave meetings to take a phone call or answer a bleep. This behaviour is selfish and disrupts the group by delaying its start or progress. There is an element of 'my time is more important than the group's time', which indicates a lack of commitment to the group's task. There are a few ways to deal with this, for example:

- at the start of the group's life discuss all issues concerning attendance, including arriving on time, not leaving meetings, not taking calls or answering bleeps during a meeting, and not leaving before the end of the meeting. Agree dates and times for all meetings for the duration of the group's life and make sure that these dates are in everyone's diary. Get commitment from the group and enforce it
- speak to those concerned outside the meeting
- get the group to agree that if members are absent when a decision is made, then they must abide by the decision of the group. Also get the group to agree that there will be no reviews for people who were absent at the time.
- do not review anything or stop the meeting for such people
- ask group members to tell the group when and why they have to leave, arrive late or miss a meeting
- ask one of the group to update the latecomer on a break
- if an individual is missing meetings on a regular basis, then the leader of the group should replace him/her. Avoid the use of temporary replacements to fill in for another member; the group is a dynamic body and constant change of membership will destroy this.

Change Management and Project Management Skills

All the skills and attributes previously mentioned support effective change management and project management. However, I have included a few skills which are specifically relevant to change management and project management.

The Structured Interview

This is a technique to get answers to a series of questions from specific people. A number of interviewees are asked the same questions and the answers are compared.

- work out what questions need to be asked and write them down in a checklist format
- test the questions to ensure that they cover all areas that are required to be tested and will result in the data that you require. Check that the questions are clear and unambiguous
- validate the interviewees' responses by taking a selection of the first interviews and making sure that the data collected is what was required and anticipated. If this is not the case, revise the questions
- structured interviews have the advantage of only getting answers to the questions listed and a set of responses from one interviewee can therefore be compared to those from another. Also, the structured interview provides objectivity, whereas unstructured interviews result in unstructured data and are difficult to analyse and therefore subjective.

Techniques for Generating Solutions

Brainstorming

This is a technique for generating a large number of ideas from a group of people in a short space of time.

- get a group of people together who are involved in finding a solution to a problem, are involved in the proposed area for change, and have a vested interest in the proposed change or will be affected by the change
- make sure that all members of the group have a clear understanding of the purpose of the brainstorming session

■ make sure that the group understands that the session is about gathering and generating as many ideas as possible. When an idea is put forward, it will be written on the flip chart for everyone to see. Any contribution must be valued and not ridiculed, however outrageous it may seem

■ invite the group to call out its ideas as to how the change may be implemented or the problem solved. The ideas are written on the flip chart as stated, succinct statements are encouraged and it is made clear that no discussion or criticism is allowed.

Brainstorming is a simple but versatile and powerful technique that stimulates and generates lots of ideas. It can be applied to any problem or change issue and is of most benefit at the start of the change process. However, these sessions require skilled facilitation.

Activity diagrams

This is a useful technique to apply to a list of ideas already generated by brainstorming or other techniques:

■ write each idea on a separate 'post-it'

■ stick all the 'post-its' on a wall

■ move the 'post-its' into groups of similar ideas or themes

■ work out titles to capture the clusters of 'post-its' and write these on a flip chart. Then stick the groups of 'post-its' under the correct titles

■ if appropriate, prioritise the titles into a sequence.

A group or an individual may suggest these sets of random ideas through the brainstorming process. The process of establishing an affinity between ideas and groups of ideas may also be a group or individual activity.

Forcefield analysis

A forcefield analysis is a technique with which to identify the forces which assist or obstruct the implementation of change. To undertake a forcefield analysis, take a piece of paper and describe the planned change in a simple sentence, and then list the driving forces which support the change on the left-hand side of the paper and the restraining forces on the right-hand side. Establish which of the restraining forces pose the greatest threat to change and highlight them for specific action in the change plan. Then determine which of the driving forces represent the best levers for implementing change and highlight them for action. It is important to maximise the driving forces, but breaking down the barriers to change of the restraining forces is generally more effective than promoting the favourable ones.

Block schedule

This is a technique (see Table 15.2) to help the planning process by putting the planning activities into a visual implementation plan.

A visual implementation plan gives a picture of the change plan, helps to organise the project and can also be used to identify who is responsible for the action by putting his/her initials in the appropriate shaded box:

- using squared paper or a spreadsheet, create a matrix across the top for the timescales in the form of days, dates or months. Then enter the activities vertically down the side of the table
- make a list of the milestones or set target dates and a separate list of those activities still to be planned
- insert the list of activities in chronological order into activity slots on the left-hand side of the table
- take the milestones or key target dates and block shade the appropriate box or cell
- take the remaining activities and fit them in between the milestones and block shade the appropriate box or cell.

Conclusion: Making a Difference

When the NHS was created in 1948, national standards of care were not thought to be necessary. It was generally believed that standards of care for patients would rise automatically all over the country and so it was left to individual health authorities to set the required standard to be achieved (DoH, 2000). However, in reality many professional groups carried out their own evaluations of treatment and care, which over time has lead to a healthcare system often described as a 'postcode lottery'. Different values of care and access to treatment have multiplied, often dependent on the preferences of key individuals rather than on the most efficacious care and treatments. The Government, through the NHS Plan (DoH, 2000), identified this approach to care as being unacceptable in the twenty-first century and planned to 'reduce the unjustified variations and achieve a truly National health service'.

Achieving demonstrable improvements in the areas of healthcare that matter most to patients is the challenge we all face under clinical governance (DoH, 1999). Yet this now goes beyond being just a vision and has become an absolute expectation of NHS staff, patients, carers and the Healthcare Commission, to name just a few. If we understand that engaging front-line staff is essential to achieve this, then we must enable their involvement by giving them the tools and knowledge to make a difference, and I hope that the information within the pages of this book has contributed to some of that knowledge. However, resources, both human and monetary, in our modern health service are stretched to the limit, despite the Government's recent efforts substantially to increase funding. We need, therefore, to utilise the best, latest and most advanced technology available in order to provide smarter solutions. We need to look to new software to improve efficiency in capturing and reporting on quality improvement data to support ongoing monitoring of the care that is provided for our patients. As part of multidisciplinary and multi-agency teams, we need to work together as we follow the pathway of the key elements of clinical governance, as set out in Figure 1. 7, to ensure that our trust or healthcare organisation has all the processes in place that demonstrate evidence of an effective system of clinical governance through:

- good leadership at all levels
- good systems of education, training, supervision and appraisal
- mechanisms for quality improvement
- evidence-based practice
- patient-focused care
- patient and public involvement in service planning
- collaborative care
- good communication
- effective team working/collaborative care
- an effective system of risk management
- effective management of high-quality information
- evidence of learning from mistakes
- an open learning culture
- an open 'no blame' culture.

This will lead to improved patient care, a culture that values patients and staff, and an organisation that demonstrates continuous quality improvement.

Appendix: An Overview of the History of Quality Assurance

This appendix has been designed to give a quick overview of quality assurance and bring together the key events, people, legislation, publications and systems that make up the signposts on the quality assurance journey from the first century to the present day.

Date	Event	Comments
1st century AD	Romans	The earliest studies of quality assurance were probably undertaken by the Romans, who reported on the efficiency of their military hospitals.
1780–1845	Elizabeth Fry	Described the quality of patient care in the hospitals she visited.
1860, 1874	Florence Nightingale	Evaluated the care delivered to the sick. She kept notes on her observations and used the information to establish the level of care being provided to improve care in areas that were below standard (Nightingale, 1860; 1874).
1863	Louisa M. Alcott	During the American Civil War she wrote about the quality of nursing care in *Hospital Sketches*. In this publication, she described the contrast between the chaos of the 'Hurly-Burly House' and that of the organised and compassionate care at the Armoury Hospital (Alcott, 1960).
1910	Ernest Codman MD, 'End Result System of Standardisation', USA	Under this system a hospital would track every patient it treated long enough to determine whether the treatment was effective. If the treatment was not effective, the hospital would then attempt to determine why, so that similar cases could be treated successfully in the future (JCAHO, 2002).
1913	First accreditation in the USA	Established to ensure 'that those institutions having the highest ideals may have proper recognition before the profession' (Roberts et al., 1987).

1917	American College of Surgeons USA	The American College of Surgeons financed a compilation of minimum standards published. Franklin Martin and John Bowman drafted the five-point minimum standard, which became the basis of the American College of Surgeon's programme in hospital standardisation and the foundation for all subsequent standards (JCAHO, 2002).
1918	The American College of Surgeons	The American College of Surgeons began on-site inspections of hospitals (JCAHO, 2002).
1919	Isabel Stewart	Stewart looked at ways of measuring the quality of nursing care and the effective use of resources. She developed an eight-point list known as 'Stewart Standards', using professional opinion rather than a rating scale. The eight-point list included: ▪ safety ▪ therapeutic effect ▪ economy of time ▪ economy of energy and effort ▪ economy of material and costs ▪ finished workmanship ▪ simplicity and adaptability (Stewart, 1919).
1930s before World War II	Quality Control	Inspection processes used in industry gave way to quality control. Quality control is the process of measuring actual quality performance, comparing it with a standard, and acting on the difference (Juran and Gryna, 1980).
1936	Miss G. B. Carter and Dr H. Balme	Published a book on the importance of evaluating care. They recommended that a multidisciplinary team, consisting of the ward sister, the doctor and the administrator, should discuss the progress and evaluate the care of all patients, by reviewing the medical and nursing records, at the end of every month (Carter and Balme, 1936).
1938–45	Total Quality Management (TQM), USA	The concept of TQM originated in the USA during World War II from work by Deming (1982) and Juran (Deming, 1982; Juran and Gryna, 1980), employees of the armaments industry.
1945	Quality assurance	After World War II, quality control was superseded by quality assurance, where the emphasis is on assuring quality rather than the use of controlling systems once things have gone wrong. The British Standards Institution (1987),

		defined quality assurance as a management system designed to give the maximum confidence that a given acceptable level of quality of service is being achieved with a minimum of total expenditure.
1946	NHS Services Act	The act committed the government at the time to fund the health service, which rested on the principles of collectivism, comprehensiveness, equality and universality (Allsop 1986). The NHS was established in 1948.
1950	A survey of general practice by Collings	Collings established that there was poor quality of care, and his survey contributed to the formation in 1952 of the College of General Practitioners. Collings's study observed current practice and found it to be lacking but his findings did not directly change the delivery of care (Collings, 1950).
1950s	Japan	It is said that the quality revolution in industry started in Japan in the 1950s inspired by the writings of Deming and Juran (Macdonald and Piggott 1990).
1950s	Dr Joseph M. Juran	Juran came from the USA and had an engineering background. In the early 1950s he was invited to Japan where he lectured on quality. He is best known for the broad management aspects of quality, the important role of communication, the co-ordination of functions and the 'human' element. He also stated that an understanding of the human element associated with the job will help to solve technical problems and that such an understanding may be the prerequisite of a solution. He focused on quality management from the top of an organisation and identified eight success factors which would indicate that an organisation had improved quality (Juran, 1988). In these organisations top managers had:

■ personally led the quality process
■ adopted quality improvement plans and clearly identified roles and responsibilities
■ included all those affected
■ trained management staff in quality planning, control and improvement
■ trained the workforce to participate in quality improvement
■ included quality improvement in strategic planning

- applied quality improvement to business planning and operational processes
- used modern quality methodology instead of empiricism quality planning.

Juran organised quality management into three parts called a quality trilogy:

- *quality planning*: Determining who the customers are and their needs and developing processes, which result in products, which respond to these needs
- *quality control*: Evaluation of the product performance and comparing this to product goals and then acting on the difference
- *quality improvement*: Identification of improvement projects and establishing the project teams with resources, training and motivation to diagnose the cause of the problems, identify solutions and establish mechanisms to monitor and maintain progress (Juran, 1988).

1952	The American College of Surgeons officially transferred its Hospital Standardisation Programme to the Joint Commission on Accreditation of Hospitals (JCAH)	JCAH published *Standards for Hospital Accreditation* in 1953. In the USA, accreditation is linked with funding. If standards fall below predetermined levels, then the hospital organisation is in jeopardy of losing federal or state funding. The hospital accreditation programmes demand evidence that a hospital has some system of quality assurance. Medical audits have developed into medical record audits, which examine in detail the records post-discharge. Today, these systems are often computerised. Some of these hospitals employ a team of people to examine the records and report their findings to a Quality Assurance Committee (JCAHO, 2002).
1952	Canadian Council on Hospital Accreditation founded	Evidence of standards-setting at a national level in Canada (Wilson, 1983).
1953	Reiter and Kakosh	Developed a system based on the classification of patients into three categories. This classification looked at the way in which nurses plan to work with patients:

- type 1 was professional, where the nurse worked with the patient as in rehabilitation

■ type 2 was curative, where the nurse 'did things' for the patient, such as dressing, treatments and specific tasks

■ type 3 was elementary, custodial or palliative care; that is, nursing care given to a comatose or unresponsive patient.

Reiter and Kakosh developed a series of questions to assess the effectiveness of each type. Their work was published and led to a study of communications as a focal point of quality in nursing (Reiter and Kakosh, 1953).

1958	Dr Faye Abdellah, USA	Developed a method of matching staffing levels to the measurement of quality of care for patients in a large hospital. She chose to measure the level of dissatisfaction observed by patients, nurses and other individuals. Over a period of time, she established 50 of the most common causes for dissatisfaction and developed a weighting value for each one. The area of dissatisfaction was rated from five to zero; for example, an unconscious patient who was left unattended, and therefore at risk, would have scored five, whereas a minor dissatisfaction would have scored zero. The scores were then totalled: a high score indicated poor nursing, whereas a zero score meant that the ward was excellent. Measuring what goes wrong is, however, rather a negative approach to evaluating a ward, as it does not measure the positive qualities. This method did not establish if the staffing level equated with quality of care; in fact, it proved that there was little correlation between the number of staff members and the quality of care. Neither did this system offer solutions to resolve dissatisfaction and improve the quality of care (Abdellah, 1958).
1961	Dr Faye Abdellah	Identified three types of criterion measures in nursing: physiological, sociological and psychological, all of which had to meet certain requirements in terms of validity, reliability, discrimination, relevancy and appropriateness (Abdellah, 1961).
1962	Quality Circles	Launched in Japan as part of an overall quality assurance system. Lochkeed Missiles and Space Company of California sent a team to Japan in 1973

		who concluded that Quality Circles were not culturally based and it was vital to retain as much of the Japanese model as possible.
1964	J. Drew, California	Undertook a survey of 21 hospitals to establish what quality assurance techniques were being used. It was established that 42 different techniques were being used and that they fell into the following categories:

■ comments from patients and others
■ special rounds of patient units
■ checks and tests of procedures
■ patient and other records
■ others, for example inspection teams of outside agencies, nurses, consultants, infection control nurses and so on.

The survey highlighted that each hospital was using at least one quality assurance tool, but that there was a lack of co-ordination and information-sharing between hospitals in the same area. Drew stressed the need for the sharing of techniques in order to establish a uniform and complete system of quality control. Since then, nurses all over the world have evaluated the care given to their patients to a greater or lesser degree (Drew, 1964).

1966	Salmon Report, UK	The implementation of this report introduced industrial management techniques and the idea of improving efficiency and saving money in the National Health Service (DoH, 1966).
1967	Philip B. Crosby	One of America's quality gurus, with a background in quality control. He combines the preventative focus of quality assurance with the Deming and Juran systematic and disciplined approach, while taking account of prevailing staff attitudes. A significant contributor to quality, although his work has been developed in industry many of the principles he proposed have relevance to and influence over health care.

Crosby (1979) defined quality management as a 'systematic way of guaranteeing that organised activities happen the way they are planned. It is a management discipline concerned with preventing problems from occurring by creating the attitudes and controls that make prevention possible.' Crosby also

		highlights 'customer requirements' as the cornerstone of quality. He maintains that quality is 'no more and no less than conformance to customer requirements'. His best-selling book, *Quality is Free*, was first published in 1979. His approach is known as the Quality Improvement Process (QIP). Crosby (1988) sets out three questions which are essential to answer: ■ what is the definition of quality? ■ how is it achieved? ■ how can it be measured?
1967	The Cogwheel Report	In this report, audit was described as a proper function for practising clinicians, but there was still a distinct dearth of mechanisms for monitoring the effectiveness of patient care.
1969	Hospital Advisory Service established	This service was established to monitor the care of people with mental illness and elderly care groups, and the National Development Team/Group for those with learning disabilities. Both these bodies are responsible for inspecting clinical areas and establishing the level of clinical practice. They report on good practice and criticise bad practice.
1969	Avedis Donabedian	Donabedian's approach to describing an organisation is based on the systems theory of input, throughput and output. When applied to healthcare, he divided the evaluation of quality of care into the evaluation of the structure in which care is delivered (input), the process of care (throughput) and the outcome (output) (Donabedian, 1969).
1970s	Criticism of General Medical Council	In the 1970s the General Medical Council was criticised for its inability to stop doctors overprescribing heroin and other addictive drugs to patients, and there were concerns that Britain's doctors had not become involved in medical audit.
1970s	The introduction of the Nursing Process	The Nursing Process, which had been used widely across the USA, was first used in the UK in the 1970s where it has been adapted and implemented, to a greater or lesser extent, throughout the country.
1971	Joint Commission on Accreditation, Standards of Nursing Care, USA	This is about implementing a more objective and systematic review of patient care and performance (Palmer, 1978).

1972	Phaneuf's Nursing Audit	This is a retrospective appraisal of the nursing process as reflected in the patient's records. There are 50 items in the audit, which was devised around the seven functions of nursing, as described by Lesnik and Anderson, in 1955, in their book, *Nursing Practice and the Law*.
1972	Rush Medicus	In 1972 the Rush Medicus instrument (Hegyvary and Hausman, 1975), was developed by the Rush Presbyterian St Luke's Medical Centre and the Medicus Systems Corporation of Chicago from 1972 and was completed in 1975. This system evolved from research in two main areas:

■ the development of a 'conceptual framework', stating what is being measured – as this constitutes a patient-centred approach, the Nursing Process and patient needs were the identified components

■ the identification of criteria for evaluating the quality of care within this framework.

Within the system, there are a series of objectives and subobjectives, which represent the structure of the Nursing Process. At the same time as the development of this system, criteria were developed and tested to measure each of the subobjectives within the six main objectives. These criteria were written so that a 'yes' or 'no' response indicates the quality of care and, where appropriate, 'not applicable' was applied. Each item was written in such a way as to minimise ambiguity, and to ensure reliable interpretation and response from the observers carrying out the study. The system is computerised and involves a simple dependency rating system, which enables the computer to select 30 to 50 criteria at random for each patient according to his/her dependency rating. Monitor is the UK version of this system.

1973	NHS Reorganisation Act, 1973	This reorganisation was implemented in 1974. The new structure created three tiers of Health Service management below the Department of Health and Social Security at regional, area and district level. New health authorities, responsible for planning and developing services, were established at regional

		and area levels. They were accountable to and appointed by ministerial authority. The Family Practitioner Committees replaced the executive councils and the NHS became responsible for community health services, transferred from local government (Baggott, 1994; DHSS, 1981).
1973	Community Health Councils	Set up as part of the 1974 reorganisation of the Health Service to represent the patients' viewpoint.
1974	Qualpacs, Wandelt and Ager, USA	Developed at Wayne State University College of Nursing, many of the items were derived from the Slater Nursing Performance Rating Scale. Qualpacs uses a method of concurrent review that is designed to evaluate the process of care at the time it is being provided, including a review of the patient's records, patient interview, asking the patient to comment on certain aspects of his/her care, and direct observation of the patient's behaviours related to predetermined criteria (Wandelt and Ager, 1974).
1975	The Slater Nursing Competencies Rating Scale USA	This is an 84-item scale, which is arranged into six subsections that identify nurse–patient interventions or interactions on behalf of the patient. The scale can be used concurrently or retrospectively and evaluates the competence of the nurse while he/she is delivering patient care by observing and measuring his/her performance against predetermined standards within the scale (Wandelt and Stewart, 1975).
1976	Royal Commission – the Alment Report, 1976	The Government established a Royal Commission to consider 'the best use and management of financial and manpower resources of the NHS' (DHSS, 1979). It outlined seven key objectives:

It outlined seven key objectives:
- to encourage and assist individuals to remain healthy
- to provide equality of entitlement to health services
- to provide a broad range of services to a high standard
- to provide equality of access to these services
- to provide a service free at the time of use
- to satisfy the reasonable expectations of its users
- to remain a national service responsive to local needs

(DHSS, 1979b).

1976	The Confidential Enquiry into Maternal Deaths	This enquiry focused on the reasons for inadequate care and the results of this led to changes in practice and a reduction in the number of maternal deaths (Godber, 1976).
1976	Lang's model of conceptual evaluation	Eleven steps to Lang's model for nursing quality assurance: 1. identify and agree values; 2. review literature, known quality assurance programmes; 3. analyse available programmes; 4. determine most appropriate quality assurance programme; 5. establish structure, process, outcome criteria and standards; 6. ratify standards and criteria; 7. evaluate current levels of nursing practice against ratified structures; 8. identify and analyse factors contributing to results; 9. select appropriate action to maintain or improve care; 10. implement selected actions; 11. evaluate quality assurance programme (Lang, 1976).
1977	Medical Service Group founded	The Royal College of Physicians founded the Medical Service Group (Clarke and Whitehead, 1981).
1979	Royal Commission on the National Health Service – the Merrison Report	This report related the problems of declining standards to untrained staff left in charge of wards, unsupervised learners and increased workload, all of which suggest a neglect of students' preparation (DHSS, 1979b).
1979	National Organisation for Quality Assurance in Hospitals in the Netherlands	This organisation was formed (Reerink, 1987).
1979	Australian Council of Hospital Standards	This organisation was founded in 1979.
1979	Patients First	Consultative paper on the structure and management of the NHS, which came into force in 1982 (DHSS, 1979a).
1980	Dr John Øvretveit	Dr John Øvretveit has carried out consultancy research into health and commercial service organisation in the UK and abroad. He is an expert in Total Quality Management (Øvretveit, 1992).
1980	Royal College of Nursing	Published *Standards of Nursing Care*, the start of the setting of standards for the nursing profession in the UK (RCN, 1980).

1981	Royal College of Nursing	Published *Towards Standards* (RCN, 1981).
1982	NHS reorganisation	Area Health Authorities abolished and District Health Authorities created, each with its own Community Health Council (DHSS, 1981).
1982	W. Edwards Deming	One of quality assurance's gurus from the USA. In his early work, Deming recommended uniformity as the path to quality, arguing that the cause of variation in production processes should be identified and systematically reduced to 'a predictable degree of uniformity and dependability, at a low cost and suited to the market' (Deming, 1982). Deming promoted the idea of a 'quality culture' through motivating and developing people (Deming, 1986).
1982	Peters and Waterman published *In Search of Excellence: Lessons from America's Best-Run Companies*	Creating quality requires an organisation to continually strive for excellence. Seven key variables in the organisation to focus on (the Mckinsey 7-S Framework): strategy, structure, staff, systems, shared values, style and skills (Peters and Waterman, 1982).
1982–84	The Korner Report	These reports were produced in order to improve information management in the NHS. They resulted in minimum data sets. These were intended to improve the standardisation of definitions of the data across the UK. There were problems with the collection of data and lack of feedback to the clinical staff who collected the data (Greenhalgh & Co. Ltd, 1993).
1983	Griffiths Management Report	The Griffiths Recommendations and General Management of Health Care were introduced. Quality assurance and the establishment of standards and review mechanisms became the responsibility of all General Managers at Regional, District and Unit level (DHSS 1983).
1984	Government set up the Office of the Health Service Commissioner	Set up to investigate complaints of maladministration. This did not include 'clinical judgement' but the ombudsman was able to comment on the way complaints were handled and the quality of patient care management (DHSS, 1983; 1985).
1984	Monitor, UK	Ball et al. successfully adapted the Rush Medicus methodology, resulting in the development of the monitoring tool called Monitor. The original version was designed for use on acute surgical

		and medical wards. However, more recent versions have been developed for use in care of the elderly wards, district nursing, mental health, paediatric wards, midwifery and health visiting (Ball et al. 1983; Goldstone, 1985a).
1984	Government declaration	The Government signed a declaration that effective mechanisms for quality of health care would be in place by 1990 (WHO, 1985a).
1984	Maxwell's Six Dimensions of Quality	Six Dimensions of Quality (Maxwell, 1984): ▪ acceptability ▪ effectiveness ▪ efficiency ▪ economy ▪ access ▪ equity ▪ relevance.
1985	World Health Organisation	WHO supports the need for quality assurance in health care and develops programmes to increase the knowledge and skills required (WHO, 1985a). Target 31 in the document 'Targets for Health for All' encourages all member states to have by 1990 'built effective mechanisms for ensuring quality of patient care within their health care systems' (WHO, 1985b).
1985	The Royal College of General Practitioners (RCGP)	Issued a policy statement 'Quality in General Practice' (RCGP, 1985).
1985	The Royal College of Nursing Standards of Care Project, led by Professor Alison Kitson	This project was set up with the intention of establishing the academic background to quality of care and encouraging the nursing profession to set and monitor standards (RCN, 1987).
1986	Resource Management Initiative (RMI)	The main objectives of the RMI were to involve clinicians in the decision-making process, and to improve the use of resources. The initiative saw the introduction of Clinical Directorates, headed by Clinical Directors who were, more often than not, doctors. The evaluation of the RMI focused on the improvement of IT systems. For clinical staff the main implications of these initiatives were the devolution of responsibility for budgets and activity levels (DHSS, 1986).
1987	*Promoting Better Health*	Government White Paper set out the government's policies for the future of primary care, which included improving the quality of life through improved

		health promotion, illness prevention and promoting consumer choice, information and complaints about the GP service (DoH, 1987).
1987	The Joint Commission on Accreditation of Hospitals (USA) changed its name to the Joint Commission on Accreditation of Healthcare Organisations (JCAHO)	The change reflected an expanded scope of activities. The Agenda for Change was launched with a set of initiatives designed to place the primary emphasis of the accreditation process on actual organisation performance.
1987	New Zealand set up their Joint Commission on Accreditation for Hospitals	(Darby and Cane, 1987).
1987	The Royal College of Nursing	Published a position statement on nursing, *In Pursuit of Excellence*. The steering group which produced this statement set down three main principles: equity, respect for persons, and caring. The group then provided nine statements to enable nurses to move to the provision of a quality service based on core concepts (RCN, 1987).
1989	King's Fund Centre – Organisational Audit established	A project steering group looked critically at existing systems for setting and monitoring national standards, principally those models of accreditation used in the USA, Canada and Australia. The Australian system was considered to be the most appropriate on which to build its own model, with reference to the Canadian system as appropriate. The King's Fund Organisational Audit was established, with the development of national standards for acute hospitals (Sale, 2000).
1989	*Working for Patients*	This White Paper, published by the Department of Health, covered a wide range of issues and initiatives, including the implementation of the internal market based on a system of contracting for services between purchasers and providers, the extension of the RMI and the formal introduction of medical audit (DoH, 1985).
1989	The formal introduction of medical audit	As part of the NHS reforms the government facilitated the development of programmes intended to measure and improve the quality of care within the NHS (DoH, 1985).

1989	J. S. Oakland	Oakland is a British guru of quality assurance and the author of *Total Quality Management* (1989). He stresses the importance of the customer/supplier interface, which he describes as a 'quality chain', with the customer and the supplier forming the vital links. He concludes that the chain can be broken at any point if an individual or other essential piece of equipment does not meet requirements. He examines the management of quality through two central concepts:

- quality of design – 'a measure of how well the product or service is designed to meet its purpose'
- conformance to design – the extent to which the product or service actually achieves the quality of design. The need to build statistical process control into the production process (Oakland, 1986).

1989	*Caring for People*	The White Paper that preceded the NHS Community Care Act 1990. This paper upheld the central ideas put forward by the Griffiths Report that the lead responsibility for community care should be given to local authorities and supported the principle of case management (DoH, 1989; Baggott, 1994).
1990	*NHS and Community Care Act*	This legislation facilitated the development of the process of contracting between the purchaser and the provider units. The provider units in the form of NHS Trusts and Directly Managed Units were responsible for meeting specifications for services as laid down in the contract with the purchaser (commissioner). The purchaser (commissioner) was looking for value for money and quality care from the providers. Other changes included performance appraisal, league tables, the growth of managerialism, customer orientation, quality assurance systems, installation of comprehensive resource management systems, the creation of trusts and GP fundholding, mergers and acquisitions. The act also gave local authorities the power to inspect premises used for the provision of community care services, excluding those premises registered under the Registered Homes Act in England and Wales (DoH, 1990).

1990	The Audit Commission	The Audit Commission was created to enhance the efficiency and financial probity in local government. As a result of the 1989 White Paper, its remit was extended to the NHS. Since October 1990 the Audit Commission has been responsible for the external audit of the National Health Service in England and Wales. The Audit Commission has responsibility for reviewing the financial accounts of all health service bodies and examining the health authorities' use of resources for economy, efficiency and effectiveness. Each year the Commission publishes around six detailed audits.
1990	*Working Paper 10 – Education and Training: Further Guidance*	This paper addressed the issue of pre-registration education and training for health professionals. The paper excluded doctors and dentists (NHSME, 1990).
1991	*The Patient's Charter*	The charter sets out a number of national rights and service standards that every patient could expect. Seven out of the ten rights in the charter were already in existence, for example the right to be treated on the basis of need, regardless of ability to pay; the right to be registered with a GP. The three new rights concerned not being on a waiting list for treatment for more than two years, and receiving detailed information about local health services, including waiting times and quality standards. Patients also had a right to full and prompt investigation of any complaints. The rights in the charter are not legal rights (DoH, 1991).
1991–97	King's Fund Organisational Audit	King's Fund Organisational Audit launched the programme on a fee-paying basis with clients recruited from the NHS and independent sector; developed and revised programmes for primary care, health authorities, community, mental health and learning disabilities services, and developed standards for nursing and residential care homes.
1991	*Health of the Nation*	*Health of the Nation* set targets for reducing morbidity by concentrating on health promotion and disease prevention (DoH, 1991).
1991	*Framework of Audit of Nursing Services*	A framework for auditing nursing services was published by the NHS Executive (NHSME, 1991).

1992	*An Information Management and Technology Strategy for the NHS in England*	Key principles within the strategy: Non-repetitiveness of data (all individuals should have one NHS number); operational data to be utilised so that information can be collected where care is delivered; security and confidentiality of information a priority; standards in place to ensures that these principles were maintained even though information is accessible and shared across the NHS (NHSME, 1992).
1993	*Risk Management in the NHS*	In 1992 the Department of Health commissioned risk management consultants to develop a manual training guide on risk management for the NHS – published in 1993. This publication resulted in trusts implementing comprehensive systems for reporting of adverse outcomes and serious incidents. The reports are used to develop a database of information to enable the trust to identify common patterns and prevent incidents in the future. Risk may be defined as 'the reduction of harm to an organisation, by identifying and, as far as possible, eliminating risk' (NHSME, 1993).
1994	*Corporate Governance in the NHS, Code of Conduct, Code of Accountability*	The development of a framework of corporate governance was outlined in this document and the focus directed at NHS Trust boards in ensuring and demonstrating that the conduct of the board was exemplary (DoH, 1994).
1995	*The Patient's Charter and You*	A revised updated Patient's Charter which included specific standards for GP services, hospital services, community services, ambulance services, dental, optical and pharmaceutical services, maternity services (DoH, 1995).
1996	Clinical Negligence Scheme for Trusts (CNST)	In England the National Health Service Litigation Authority set up by statute in 1996 has implemented risk management standards, which all member trusts of the CNST must work towards achieving set standards by a given date (Mayatt, 1995).
1996	The process of complaints in the NHS was changed	The aim of these changes was to reduce inconsistency to responding and investigating complaints and to introduce more openness with the participation of laypeople.
1997	*The New NHS. Modern, Dependable*	The Government set out its plans to modernise the NHS by abolishing the internal market and enabling health professionals to focus on patients.

		It stressed that 'local doctors and nurses, who best understand patients' needs, will shape local services'. Patients will be guaranteed national standards of excellence so that they will have confidence in the quality of the services they receive (DoH, 1997).
1997	*Designed to Care in Scotland*	Modernising healthcare in Scotland (secretary of state for Scotland, 1997).
1997	Caldicott Report	*The Caldicott Committee. Report on the Review of Patient-Identifiable Information* (DoH, 1997).
1997 and 1998	Locality commissioning pilot projects were set up	The aim was to develop more locally sensitive services. This paper was an endorsement of the strengths and potential developments in primary care and the establishment of Primary Care Groups (PCGs).
1998	White Paper *NHS Wales: Putting Patients First*	Modernising healthcare in Wales (secretary of state for Wales, 1998).
1998	White Paper *Fit for the Future*	Modernising healthcare in Northern Ireland (DoH for Northern Ireland, 1988).
1998	King's Fund Organisational Audit relaunched as the Health Quality Service	The concept of performance indicators is piloted, and standards and an assessment programme for primary care groups initiated.
1998	Publication of a consultation paper outlining a National Performance Framework	The consultation paper consisted of six areas: 1. Health improvement, which covered overall health of populations, reflecting social and environmental factors, individual behaviour, NHS care. 2. Fair access to provision of services in relation to need, including geographical, socio-economic, demographic and care groups. 3. Effective delivery of appropriate healthcare including clinical effectiveness and evidence-based practice which is appropriate to need, timely, in line with agreed standards, provided according to best practice and delivered by appropriately trained and educated staff. 4. Efficiency, for example cost per unit of care or outcome and productivity of labour and capital. 5. Patient/carer experience, which included being responsive to individual needs and preferences; assuring patients of skill, care and continuity of service; involving the

		patient in making informed choices and decisions; patients being treated within an acceptable length of time and easy access to care within an acceptable environment. Health outcomes of NHS Care, which refers to reduced levels in risk factors, reduced levels of disease, impairment and complications of treatment.
		6. Improved quality of life for patients and carers and a reduction in the number of premature deaths.
		This performance framework was created with the aim of monitoring the performance of the NHS and improving quality (DoH, 1998).
1998	White Paper *A First Class Service: Quality in the New NHS*	The main elements of this document are:
		▪ clear national standards for services and treatments through National Service Frameworks and a National Institute for Clinical Excellence
		▪ local delivery of high quality healthcare, through clinical governance underpinned by modernised professional self regulation and life long learning
		▪ monitoring progress through a commission of health improvement, a framework for assessing performance and a national survey of patient and service user experience (DoH, 1998).
1998	Clinical Governance	'A framework through which NHS organisations are accountable for continuously improving the quality of their services and safeguarding high standards of care by creating an environment in which excellence in clinical care will flourish' (DoH, 1998a).
1998	*Reducing Junior Doctors' Hours*	Continuing action to meet new deal standards, rest periods and working arrangements, improving catering and accommodation for junior doctors (DoH, 1998c).
1998	European Working Time Directives	The Working Time Directives restricted working hours to 48 per week which specifically excluded junior doctors. However, it was recognised that junior doctors working long hours would affect the quality of patient care, and trusts were advised to recognise this fact (Working Time Regulations 1998).

1999	Primary Care Groups	Primary Care Groups (PCGs) were set up with a requirement to identify a lead person for clinical governance (DoH, 1997b).
1999	The Health Quality Service (HQS) – accreditation for the UK	The Health Quality Service (HQS) gained accreditation from the UK Accreditation Service as an ISO9002 certification body allowing an organisation to pursue ISO9002 in addition to HQS accreditation by working with the same programme. A new accreditation programme was introduced for acute hospitals, community mental health, learning disability and specialist palliative care services; a new programme for hospice care was launched, and a revised programme developed for primary care teams (www.hqs.org.uk).
1999	The National Institute for Clinical Excellence (NICE) was formed	NICE was formed as part of the Government's framework for improving the NHS as set out in *A First Class Service: Quality in the New NHS* (DoH, 1998). NICE was established to provide guidance to health professionals and patients in England and Wales on the clinical and cost effectiveness of select technologies and other health interventions. The Institute is a Special Health Authority, which appraises health technologies and commissions clinical guidelines. It also funds clinical audit at national level and provides funds for effective practice publications.
1999	Controls assurance	Controls assurance is part of governance and has been described as 'a holistic concept based on best governance practice' (NHSME, 1999). 'A process, built on best governance practice, by which NHS organisations demonstrate that they are doing their reasonable best to manage themselves so as to meet their objectives and protect patients, staff, visitors and other stakeholders against risks of all kinds' (Emslie, 2001).
1999	The NHS Performance Assessment Framework	This is a mechanism by which NHS organisations monitor the delivery of health services against the government's plans for improvement.
1999–2002	National Service Frameworks	A set of National Service Frameworks have been developed with nationally agreed standards which cover major care areas and disease groups and include National Service Frameworks for: ■ Mental Health 1999 ■ Coronary Heart Disease 2000

- National Cancer Plan 2000
- Older People 2001
- Diabetes 2001
- Renal Services 2002
- Children Services
- Long-term conditions focusing on neurological conditions (under development).

2000	Commission for Health Improvement (CHI)	The CHI was set up to monitor the quality of clinical services at local level and intervene if necessary to deal with problems (DoH, 1998a). CHI started its first round of evaluations in 2001.
2000	Care Standards Act, 2000	<ul><li>national minimum standards for care homes for older people, monitored by the National Care Standards Commission from April 2002</li><li>national minimum standards for Care Homes for Younger Adults and National Minimum Standards for Adult Placements (December 2001) (DoH, 2001b).</li></ul>
2000	NHS Plan	The Government has taken the concepts of quality management set out in *A First Class Service. Quality in the New NHS* and developed the NHS Plan. The NHS Plan is 'a radical action plan for the next ten years setting out measures to put patients and people at the heart of the health service and promising a 6.3 per cent increase in funding over five years to 2004'. The NHS Plan promises:

- more power and information for patients
- more hospitals and beds
- more doctors and nurses
- much shorter waiting times for hospitals and doctor appointments
- cleaner wards, better food and facilities in hospitals
- improved care for older people
- tougher standards for NHS organisations and better rewards for the best.

Priorities are to:

- target diseases which are the biggest killers, such as cancer and heart disease
- pinpoint the changes that are most urgently needed to improve people's health and wellbeing and deliver the modern, fair and convenient services which people want.

The Modernisation Board will lead the changes, headed by the health secretary, it will have an advisory role and comprise leading figures from healthcare institutions such as the Royal Colleges, together with clinical staff and managers from within the NHS and patient representatives.

Ten task-forces have been put in place to drive the improvements outlined in the NHS Plan. Six of these focus on improving services for coronary heart disease, cancer, mental health, older people, children, waiting times and access to services. The remaining four concentrate on how these improvements are to be made, and focus on the NHS workforce, quality, reducing inequalities and promoting public health, and investment in facilities and information technology.

A new Modernisation Agency plays a crucial role in ensuring that the commitments in the plan are translated into reality. The new agency works with NHS Executive regional offices and with all NHS trusts to help them redesign their services around the needs and convenience of patients. The Modernisation Action Team was formed in March 2000, the five teams represented: patient access, performance and productivity, partnership, professional and the workforce, and prevention. The NHS Plan (DoH, 2000b).

2001	The Patient Advice and Liaison Service (PALS)	The role of PALS is to provide information to patients about health and local health services both NHS and voluntary services and support groups. PALS are in a position to alert Trusts and PCTs to gaps in service provision and possible or potential problems. They also support patients with concerns, problems and complaints, helping them through the process to resolve issues as quickly as possible (DoH 2001a).
2001	The National Clinical Assessment Authority (NCCA)	The NCCA was established as a Special Health Authority in April 2001 with a remit to provide support to the NHS when the performance of an individual doctor is giving cause for concern. The NCCA works closely with the General Medical Council and the Healthcare

Commission as part of a framework to protect patients and improve the quality of care. The publication of the report *An Organisation with a Memory* (DoH, 2000a) drew attention to the absence of a systematic approach to identifying serious lapses in standards of care and analysing the events, learning from them and putting in systems of introducing change to prevent them recurring (DoH, 2000).

2001	The National Patient Safety Agency	This agency was set up in July 2001 following the publication of *Building a Safer NHS* (NHS Confederation, 2001). The role of the National Patient Safety Agency is to run a national reporting system for the recording of adverse healthcare events (DoH, 2001).
2001	The Modernisation Agency	The Modernisation Agency was created in April 2001 and it is part of the Department of Health and was set up to help healthcare staff redesign local health services in line with good practice (DoH, 2000b).

The Agency provides a problem-solving service to the NHS which:

- helps to diagnose problems and support possible solutions. The agency has a key role in conjunction with the Strategic Health Authorities in the assessment of an NHS organisation for eligibility to access the NHS Plan Performance Fund and how the fund may be used
- provides practical tools and training skills
- secures patient and carer involvement
- co-creates solutions, which means that the Agency adapts and modifies innovation and best practice from one trust so it can be used by another trust
- identifies good practice, for example the NHS Beacons Learning Handbook which lists services that have been innovative in meeting specific heathcare needs across all sectors. The Beacons Learning Handbook can be obtained through the Beacon website, www.nhs.uk/beacon.

2002	The Commission for Health Improvement (CHI) became the Commission for Healthcare Audit and Inspection (CHAI)	The Government announced in 2002, subject to primary legislation, that a new single commission was to be set up to inspect both the public and private healthcare sectors. The CHI has been succeeded by the CHAI, with more responsibilities (see under Healthcare Commission). It has incorporated the Office for Information on Healthcare Performance and manages the national patient and NHS staff surveys (DoH, 2002).
2003	Commission for Patient and Public Involvement in Health (CPPIH)	Community Health Councils were abolished in 2003 and the CPPIH was set up with responsibility to make appointments to Patient Forums. This organisation sets national standards and provides training and monitoring of the Patient's Advice and Liaison Service (PALS), Patient Forums and the Independent Complaints Advocacy Services (ICAS).
2004	*Standards for Better Health* – healthcare standards for services under the NHS	A consultation document published in February 2004. The consultation period ended May 2004. This document proposed the establishment of two sets of standards covering NHS healthcare in England: ▪ a set of 24 core standards establishing a level of quality of care which can be expected by all NHS patients, regardless of where they are treated. The standards come into effect from the end of 2004 ▪ the second set of standards proposed are ten developmental standards, designed to enable the overall quality of healthcare to rise to a higher standard in the long term as additional resources invested in the NHS take effect. Criteria with which to measure the standards to be developed and subsequently monitored by CHAI (Healthcare Commission). The standards have been divided into the following domains: ▪ safety ▪ clinical and cost effectiveness ▪ governance ▪ Patient Focus ▪ Accessible and Responsive Care ▪ Care Environment and Amenities ▪ Public Health (DoH, 2004).

| 2004 | The Healthcare Commission | The Healthcare Commission is a new organisation established in April 2004 and is the public name of the CHAI. This new organisation covers England and Wales and brings together the CHI, the National Care Standards Commission (NCSC) (inspection and licensing of private and voluntary healthcare) and the Audit Commission who undertake national 'Value for Money' studies in healthcare. In future it is expected that the Mental Health Act Commission will merge into the Healthcare Commission once further legislation has been completed. The Healthcare Commission pilot for mental health reviews with the Commission for Social Care Inspection is planned for 2005 (DoH, 2004). |

References

Chapter 1

BSI (British Standards Institution) (1990) *Quality Management and Quality Systems Elements – Draft Guidelines for Services*. Milton Keynes: British Standards Institution.

CHI (Commission for Health Improvement) (2002) *A Guide to Clinical Governance Reviews – Primary Care Trusts.*

Crosby, P. B. (1979) *Quality is Free*. New York: McGraw-Hill.

Crosby, P. B. (1988) *The Eternally Successful Organization: The Art of Corporate Wellness*. New York: McGraw-Hill.

Deming, W. (1986) *Out of Crisis*. Cambridge, MA: Massachusetts Institute of Technology.

Deming, W. E. (1982) *Quality, Productivity and Competitive Position*. Cambridge, MA: Massachusetts Institute of Technology.

DoH (Department of Health) (1997) *The New NHS, Modern, Dependable*. London: HMSO.

DoH (Department of Health) (1998) *A First Class Service: Quality in the New NHS*. London: HMSO.

DoH (Department of Health) (1999) *Clinical Governance: Quality in the New NHS*. London: HMSO.

DoH (Department of Health) (2000a) *An Organisation With a Memory*. London: HMSO.

DoH (Department of Health), (2000b) *The NHS Plan, A Plan for Investment, A Plan for Reform*. Norwich: HMSO.

DoH (Department of Health) (2001a) *Assuring the Quality of Medical Practice: Implementing Supporting Doctors, Protecting Patients*. London: HMSO.

DoH (Department of Health) (2001b) *Involving Patients and the Public in Healthcare: A Discussion Document*. London: HMSO.

DoH (Department of Health) (2003) *The NHS Complaints Reforms: Making it Right*. London: HMSO.

DoH (Department of Health) (2004) *Standards for Better Health – Health Care Standards for Services under the NHS, a Consultation Document in February 2004*. London: HSMO.

Donabedian, A. (1990) 'The Seven Pillars of Quality', *Archives of Pathology and Laboratory Medicine*, 114: 14–16.

Drew, J. (1964) 'Determining Quality of Nursing Care', *American Journal of Nursing*, 64(10): 82–5.

Ishikawa, K. (1976) *Guide to Quality Control*. Tokyo: Asian Productivity Organisation.

Ishikawa, K. (1985) *Total Quality Control – The Japanese Way*. Englewood Cliffs, IL: Dorsey Press.

Juran, J. M. (1988) *Juran on Planning for Quality*. New York: Free Press.

Juran, J. M. (1989) *Juran on Leadership for Quality*. New York: Free Press.

Lang, N. (1976) *Issues in Quality Assurance in Nursing, ANA Issues in Evaluation Research*. Kansas City: American Nursing Association.

Lugon M. and Secker-Walker J. (eds) (2001) *Advancing Clinical Governance*. London: Royal Society of Medicine Press Ltd.

Macdonald, J. and Piggott, J. (1990) *Global Quality – The New Management Culture*. London: Mercury Books.

Maxwell, R. (1984) 'Quality Assessment in Health', *British Medical Journal*, 288: 1470–2.

NHS Confederation (2001) *Building a Safer NHS*. London: HMSO.

NHS Executive (2002) *Delivering the NHS Plan, Next Steps on Investment, Next Steps on Reform*. London: HMSO.

NICE (National Institute for Clinical Excellence) (2000) www.nice.org.co.uk

Oakland, J. S. (1986) *Statistical Process Control*. London: Heinemann.

Oakland, J. S. (1989) *Total Quality Management*. London: Heinemann.

Øvretveit, J. (1992) *Health Service Quality: An Introduction to Quality Methods for Health Services*. Oxford: Blackwell Scientific Publications.

Peters, T.J. and Waterman, R. H. (1982) *In Search of Excellence: Lessons From*

America's Best-Run Companies. New York: Harper and Row.

Shewhart, W. A. (1931) *The Economic Control of Quality Manufactured Products.* New York: Van Nostrand Reinhold.

Williamson, J. W. (1979) 'Formulating Priorities for Quality Assurance Activity: Description of Method and its Application', *Journal of the American Medical Association,* 239: 631–7.

Chapter 2

Bristol Royal Infirmary Inquiry (2001) *Learning from Bristol: The Report of the Public Inquiry into Children's Heart Surgery at the Bristol Royal Infirmary 1984–1995.* London: HMSO.

Cadbury Report: *Report of the Committee on the Financial Aspects of Corporate Governance* (1992) London: Gee.

DoH (Department of Health) (1994) *Corporate Governance in the NHS, Code of Conduct, Code of Accountability.* London: HMSO.

DoH (Department of Health) (1998) *A First Class Service – Improving Quality in the New NHS.* London: HMSO.

DoH (Department of Health) (1999) *Governance in the New NHS. Controls Assurance Statements 1999/2000 Risk Management and Organisational Controls HSC 1000/123.* London: HMSO.

DoH (Department of Health) (2000), *The NHS Plan: A Plan for Investment, a Plan for Reform.* London: HMSO.

NHS Executive (1999) *Clinical Governance: Quality in the New NHS.* London: Department of Health.

Nolan Report (1995) *Report on Standards in Public Life,* chaired by Lord Nolan. London: HMSO.

Chapter 3

DoH (Department of Health) (1997) *The New NHS, Modern, Dependable.* London: HMSO.

DoH (Department of Health) (1998) *A First Class Service – Improving Quality in the New NHS.* London: HMSO.

DoH (Department of Health) (2000), *The NHS Plan: A Plan for Investment, a Plan for Reform.* London: HMSO.

DoH (Department of Health) (2001) *Essence of Care – Patient-Focused Benchmarking for Healthcare Practitioners.* HMSO: London.

Gordon, R. I. (1969) *Interviewing Strategy: Techniques and Tactics.* Homewood, IL: Dorsey Press.

Kelson, M. (1996) 'User Involvement in Clinical Audit: A Review of Developments and Issues of Good Practice', *Journal of Evaluation in Clinical Practice,* 2, 96–109.

Maccoby, E. et al. (1968) 'The Interview: A Tool of Social Science', in G. Lundzey (ed.), *Handbook of Social Psychology,* vol. 1, *Theory and Method.* Reading, MA: Addison-Wesley.

NHS Executive (1999) *Clinical Governance: Quality in the New NHS.* London: Department of Health.

Nehring, V. and Geach, B. (1973) 'Patients' Evaluation of their Care: Why They Don't Complain', *Nursing Outlook,* 21(5), 317–21.

Oppenheim, A. N. (1979) *Questionnaire Design and Attitude Measurement.* London: Heinemann.

Payne, S. I. (1951) *The Art of Asking Questions.* Princeton, NJ: Princeton University Press.

Wilson, J. (1999) 'Acknowledging the Expertise of Patients and their Organisations', *British Medical Journal,* 319, 771–4.

Chapter 4

Clinical Negligence Scheme for Trusts (1997) *Risk Management Standards and Procedures: Manual of Guidance*. Bristol: CNST.

Clothier Report (1992) *Report of the Independent Inquiry Relating to Deaths and Injuries on the Children's Ward at Grantham and Kestevan General Hospital during the Period February to April 1991*, chaired by Sir Cecil Clothier. London: HMSO.

CNST (Clinical Negligence Scheme for Trusts) (2002) *Clinical Risk Management Standards for Maternity Services, Draft 4*. London: NHS Litigation Authority and Clinical Negligence Scheme for Trusts.

DoH (Department of Health) (1994) *Corporate Governance in the NHS, Code of Conduct, Code of Accountability*. London: HMSO.

DoH (Department of Health) (1999) *Governance in the New NHS. Controls Assurance Statements 1999/2000 Risk Management and Organisational Controls HSC 1000/123*. London: HMSO.

DoH (Department of Health) (2000) *An Organisation with a Memory: Report of an Expert Group on Learning from Adverse Incidents in the NHS Chaired by the Chief Medical Officer*. London: HMSO.

DoH (Department of Health) (2001) *Building a Safer NHS for Patients*. London: HMSO.

Griffiths, N. (2000) 'Controls Assurance: The Shape of Things to Come', *The Healthcare Risk Resource*, vol. 3 no. 1. London: Healthcare Risk Resources International Ltd.

NHS Executive (1999) *Guidelines for Implementing Controls Assurance in the NHS*. London: Department of Health.

NHS Litigation Authority (2002) *Clinical Risk Management Standards*. London: NHS Litigation Authority.

Standards Australia (1999) *Risk Management AS/NZS 4360:1999*. Strathford, NSW: Standards Association of Australia.

Williams, C. A. and Heins, R. M. (1976) *Risk Management and Insurance*. New York: McGraw-Hill.

Wilson, J. H. (1994) 'Quality in Clinical Care Healthcare Risk Modification', Health Business Summary, April.

Wilson J. and Tingle, J. (1999) (eds) *Clinical Risk Modification: A Route to Clinical Governance*. Oxford: Butterworth Heinemann.

Chapter 5

Casley, S., Allsopp, D., Page S. and Turner, A. (1998) *The Practice Development Unit: An Experiment in Multidisciplinary Innovation (The Contribution of the Seacroft PDU)*. London: Whurr Publishers Ltd.

Donabedian, A. (1990) 'The Seven Pillars of quality', *Archives of Pathology and Laboratory Medicine*, 114: 14–16.

Kelson, M. (1996) 'User Involvement in Clinical Audit: A Review of Developments and Issues of Good Practice', *Journal of Evaluation in Clinical Practice*, 2, 96–109.

Lang, N. M (1976) 'Quality Assurance – The Idea and its Development in the United States', in M. Willis and M. Linwood (eds), *Measuring the Quality of Care*. Edinburgh: Churchill Livingston.

Maxwell, R. J. (1984) 'Quality Assessment in Health', *British Medical Journal*, 12, May, 1470–2.

NHS Executive (1996) *Complaints, Listening, Acting, Improving*. London: Department of Health.

Chapter 6

DoH (Department of Health) (1994) *Being Heard: Report of the Review Committee on NHS Complaint Procedures*, chaired by Professor Alan Wilson. London: HMSO.

DoH (Department of Health) (1995) *Acting on Complaints: The Government's Proposals*. London: HMSO.

DoH (Department of Health) (2000) *The NHS Plan, a Plan for Investment, a Plan for Reform*. London: HMSO.

DoH (Department of Health) (2001) *Working together – Learning Together: A Framework for Lifelong Learning for the NHS*. London: HMSO.

DoH (Department of Health) (2002) *Primary Care Workforce Planning Framework. www. doh.gov.uk/pricare/pcwpf.htm*

DoH (Department of Health) (2003) *NHS Complaints Reform: Making Things Right.* London: HMSO.

DoH (Department of Health) (2004) *Standards for Better Health. Health Care Standards for Services under the NHS, a Consultation Document.* London: HMSO.

Hagerty, B. (1986) 'A Second Look at Mentors: Do You Really Need One to Succeed in Nursing?', *Nursing Outlook*, 34 (1), 16–19, 24.

Levinson, D. J., Darrow, C. N., Klein, D. B., Levinson, M. H. and McKee, B. (1978) *The Seasons of a Man's Life.* New York:

Marquis, B. L and Hutson, C. J. (2000) *Leadership Roles and Management Function in Nursing: Theory and Application* (3rd edn). Philadelphia, PA: Lippincott.

McSherry, R. and Simmons, M. (2001) 'The Importance of Research Dissemination and the Barriers to Implementation', in R. McSherry, M. Summons and P. Abbot, *Evidence – Informed Nursing: A Guide for Clinical Nurses* London: Routledge.

Morton-Cooper A. and Palmer, A. (2000) *Mentoring, Preceptorship and Clinical Supervision – A Guide to Professional Roles in Clinical Practice* (2nd edn). Oxford: Blackwell Science.

NHS Executive (1996) *Complaints, Listening, Acting, Improving.* London: Department of Health.

Palmer, E. A. (1987) *The Nature of the Mentor.* Unpublished thesis, South Bank Polytechnic.

RCN (Royal College of Nursing) (2000) *Clinical Governance: How Nurses get Involved.* London: Royal College of Nursing.

Stewart, R. (1996) *Leading in the NHS: A Practical Guide* (2nd edn). London: Macmillan Business.

Chapter 7

American Academy of Family Physicians (1999) *Family Practice Management*

Binnie, A. and Titchen, A. (1999) *Freedom to Practice: The Development of Patient-Centred Nursing.* Oxford: Butterworth-Heinemann.

Chief Medical Officer (1995) *Maintaining Medical Excellence.* London: HMSO.

Cutcliffe, J., Jackson, A., Ward, M., Cannon, B. and Titchen, A. (1998) 'Practice Development in Mental Health Nursing', *Mental Health Practice*, 2(4), 27–31.

DoH (Department of Health) (1992) *Health of the Nation.* London: HMSO.

DoH (Department of Health) (1993) *A Vision for the Future.* London: HMSO.

DoH (Department of Health) (1997) *The New NHS, Modern, Dependable.* London: HMSO.

DoH (Department of Health) (1998a) *Clinical Governance: Quality in the New NHS.* London: HMSO.

DoH (Department of Health) (1998b) *A First Class Service: Quality in the NHS.* London: HMSO.

DoH (Department of Health) (1998c) *Quality in the New NHS.* London: HMSO

DoH (Department of Health) (2000) *The NHS Plan: A Plan for Investment, a Plan for Reform.* London: HMSO.

DoH (Department of Health) (2001) *Learning from Bristol: The Report of the Public Inquiry into Children's Heart Surgery at the Bristol Royal Infirmary, 1984–1995.* London: HMSO.

Donaldson, L., Gray, J. and Muir, J. (1998) 'Clinical Governance: A Quality Duty for Health Care', *Quality in Health Care*, 7.

Draper, J. (1996) 'Nursing Development Units: An Opportunity for Evaluation', *Journal of Advanced Nursing*, 23(2), 267–71.

Dunning, M. (1998) 'Securing Change: Lessons from the PACE Programme', *Nursing Times*, 94(34), 51–2.

Garbett, R. and McCormack, B. (2001) 'The Experience of Practice Development: An Exploratory Telephone Interview Study', *Journal of Clinical Nursing*, 10(1), 94–102.

Garbett, R. and McCormack, B. (2002a) 'A Concept Analysis of Practice Development', *NT Research*, 7(2), 87–100.

Garbett, R. and McCormack, B. (2002b) 'The Qualities and Skills of Practice Developers', *Nursing Standard*, 16(50), 33–6.

Gerrish, K. (2001) 'A Pluralistic Evaluation of Nursing/Practice Development Units', *Journal of Clinical Nursing*, 10(1), 109–18.

Graham, I. (1996) 'A Presentation of a Conceptual Framework and its use in the Definition of Nursing Development within a Number of Nursing Development Units', *Journal of Advanced Nursing*, 23(2), 260–6.

Harvey, G., Loftus-Hills, A., Rycroft-Malone, J., Titchen, A., Kitson, A., McCormack, B. and Seers, K. (2002) 'Getting Evidence into Practice: The Role and Function of Facilitation', *Journal of Advanced Nursing*, 37(6), 577–88.

Kitson, A., Ahmed, L. B., Harvey, G., Seers, K., Thompson, D. R. (1996) 'From Research to Practice: One Organizational Model for Promoting Research-Based Practice', *Journal of Advanced Nursing*, 23(3), 430–40.

Kitson, A. and Currie, L. (1996) 'Clinical Practice Development and Research Activities in Four District Health Authorities', *Journal of Clinical Nursing*, 5(1), 41–51.

Luker, K. (1997) 'Research and the Configuration of Nursing Services', *Journal of Clinical Nursing*, 6, 259–67.

Manley, K. (2000) 'Organisational Culture and Consultant Nurse Outcomes: Part 2 – Consultant Nurse Outcomes', *Nursing in Critical Care*, 5(5), 240–8.

Marsh, S. and MacAlpine, S. (1995) *Our Own Capabilities*. London: King's Fund.

McCormack, B. (1998) 'Caring for Older People – Enabling Change in the "Messy" World of Practice', *Journal of Nursing Care* (Winter), 8–11.

McCormack, B., Kitson, A, Harvey, G, Rycroft-Malone, J, Titchen, A. and Seers, K. (2002) 'Getting Evidence into Practice: the Meaning of "Context"', *Journal of Advanced Nursing*, 38(1), 94–104.

McCormack, B., Manley, K., Titchen, A., Kitson, A. and Harvey, G. (1999) 'Towards Practice Development – A Vision in Reality or a Reality without Vision', *Journal of Nursing Management*, 7, 255–64.

McCormack, B. and Wright, J. (1999) 'Achieving Dignified Care through Practice Development – A Systematic Approach', *Nursing Times Research*, 4(5), 340–52.

McMahon, A. (1998) 'Developing Practice through Research', in B. Roe and C. Webb (eds), *Research and Development in Clinical Nursing*. London, Whur Publishing Ltd.

Thomas, S. and Ingham, A. (1995) 'The Unit-Based Clinical Practice Development Role: A Practitioner's and a Manager's Perspective', in K. Kendrick, P. Weir and E. Rosser (eds), *Innovations in Nursing Practice*. London: Arnold.

Titchen, A. (1998) *Critical Companionship: A Conceptual Framework for Supporting Practice Development*. Oxford: RCN Institute.

Unsworth, J. (2000) 'Practice Development: A Concept Analysis', *Journal of Nursing Management*, 8, 317–26.

Vaughan, B. (1996) 'Developing Nursing', *Nursing Standard*, 10(15), 31–5.

Vaughan, B. and Edwards, M. (1995) *Interface Between Research and Practice*. London: King's Fund.

Ward, M. J. et al. (1998) *Instruments for Measuring Practice and Other Healthcare Variables*, vols 1 and 2. Boulder City, CO: Western Interstate Commission for Higher Education.

Williams, C., Lee, D. and Lowry, M. (1993) 'Practice Development Units: The Next Step?', *Nursing Standard*, 8(11), 25–9.

Chapter 8

Appleby, J., Walshe, K. and Ham, C. (1995) *Acting on the Evidence. A Review of Clinical Effectiveness: Sources of Information, Dissemination and Implementation*. Birmingham: NAHA.

Bassett, M. (1993) 'Nurse Teachers' Attitudes to Research; a Phenomenological Study', *Journal of Advanced Nursing*, 19, 1–8.

Belsey J. and Snell, T. (2001) *What is Evidence-Based-Medicine?* www.evidence-based-medicine.co.uk

Berwick, D. M. (1989) 'Continuous Quality Improvement: An Ideal in Healthcare', *New England Journal of Medicine*, 320, 53–6.

Crombie, I. (1997) *The Pocket Guide to Critical Appraisal*. London: BMJ Publishing.

DoH (Department of Health) (1993) *Improving Clinical Effectiveness*. London: HMSO.

DoH (Department of Health) (1996a) *Clinical Guidelines: Using Clinical Guidelines to Improve Patient Care within the NHS*. London: HMSO.

DoH (Department of Health) (1996b) *Promoting Clinical Effectiveness – A Framework for Action in and Through the NHS* (Culyer Report). London: NHSE.

Grimshaw, J. and Russell, I. (1993) 'Achieving Health Gain Through Clinical Guidelines. 1: Developing Scientifically Valid Guidelines', *Quality in Health Care*, 2: 243–8.

Hill, A. and Spittlehouse, C. (2001) *What is Critical Appraisal?* www.evidence-based-medicine.co.uk

Kongstvedt (ed.) (1995) *Essentials of Managed Care*. Gaithersburg, MD: Aspen.

Long, A. and Harrison, S. (1996) 'Evidence-Based Decision Making', *Health Service Journal*, 106: 1–11.

May, A., Alexander C. and Mulhall, A. (1998) 'Research Utilisation in Nursing: Barriers and Opportunities', *Journal of Clinical Effectiveness*, 3(2) 59–63.

McSherry, R. (1997) 'What do Registered Nurses and Midwives Feel and Know about Research?', *Journal of Advanced Nursing*, 25, 985–8.

Milne, R. and Chambers, L. (1993) 'Addressing the Scientific Quality of Review Articles', *Journal of Epidemiology and Community Health*, 47(3): 169–70.

RCN (Royal College of Nursing) (1995) *Clinical Guidelines: What You Need to Know*. London: RCN.

Sackett, D. L., Rosenburg, W. and Haynes, R. B. (1997) *Evidence Based Medicine: How to Use Practice and Teach EBP*. London: Churchill Livingstone.

Swage, T. (1998) 'Clinical Care Takes Centre Stage', *Nursing Times*, 94(14): 40–1.

Zander, K. and McGill, R. (1994) 'Critical and Anticipated Recovery Paths: Only the Beginning', *Nursing Management*, 25 (8): 34–40.

Chapters 9

DoH (Department of Health) (2001) *Building on the Information Core: Implementing the NHS Plan*. London: HMSO.

DoH (Department of Health) (2002) *Developing 21st Century IT Support for the NHS*. London: HMSO.

Secretary of State for Health (1998) *Information for Health*. London: NHS Executive.

Welsh Office, 1999. *Better Information – Better Health. Information Management and Technology for Health Care and Health Improvement in Wales*. Cardiff: The Welsh Office.

Chapter 10

DoH (Department of Health) (1997) *The New NHS, Modern Dependable*. London: HMSO.

Donabedian, A. (1990) 'The Seven Pillars of Quality', *Archives of Pathology and Laboratory Medicine*, 114: 14–16.

Morton-Cooper, A. and Bamford, M. (1997) *Excellence in Health Care Management*. Oxford: Blackwell Science.

Rowntree, D. (1987) *Assessing Students: How Shall We Know Them?*, revised edn. London: Kogan Page Ltd.

Towell, D. and Harries, C. (1979) *Innovation in Patient Care*. London: Croom Helm.

Chapter 11

Audit Commission (2000) *Getting Better all the Time: Making Benchmarking Work*. London: Audit Commission

Caddow, P. (1986) 'Questions on Quality', *Nursing Times*, September 10, 44-8.

CHI (Commission for Health Improvement) (2002) *A Guide to Clinical Governance Reviews Primary Care Trusts*. London: CHI.

Crosby, P. B. (1979) *Quality is Free*. New York: McGraw-Hill.

Crosby, P. B. (1984) *Quality without Tears*. New York: McGraw-Hill.

Deming, W. E. (1982) *Quality, Productivity and Competitive Positions*. Cambridge, MA: Massachusetts Institute of Technology.

Deming, W. E. (1986) *Out of the Crisis.* Cambridge, MA: MIT Centre for Advanced Engineering Study.

DoH (Department of Health) (1998) *A First Class Service: Quality in the New NHS.* London: HMSO.

DoH (Department of Health) (1999) *Making a Difference: Strengthening the Nursing, Midwifery and Health Visiting Contribution to Health and Healthcare.* London: HMSO.

DoH (Department of Health) (2000) *The NHS Plan: A Plan for Investment, A Plan for Reform.* London: HMSO.

DoH (Department of Health) (2001a) *Essence of Care – Patient-Focused Benchmarking for Healthcare Pracitioners.* London: HMSO.

DoH (Department of Health) (2001b) *NHS Performance Ratings. Acute Trust, Specialist Trusts, Ambulance Trusts, Mental Health Trusts 2001/02.* London: HMSO.

DoH (Department of Health) (2001c) *NHS Performance Ratings. Acute Trusts, Specialist Trusts, Ambulance Trusts, Mental Health Trusts 2002/02.* London: HMSO.

DoH (Department of Health) (2003) *Essence of Care Benchmarking Framework.* London: HMSO.

DoH (Department of Health) (2004) *Standards for Better Health – Health Care Standards for Services under the NHS, a Consultation Document in February 2004.* London: HMSO.

Handy, C. (1985) *Understanding Organisations* (3rd edn). London: Penguin.

Ishikawa, K. (1985) *Total Quality Control – The Japanese Way.* Englewood Cliffs, NJ: Prentice-Hall.

JCAH (Joint Commission on Accreditation of Hospitals) (1953) *Standards for Hospital Accreditation.* Chicago: JCAH.

JCAHO (Joint Commission on Accreditation of Healthcare Organisations) (2002) *A Journey through the History of the Joint Commission.* Chicago: JCAHO.

JCAHO (Joint Commission on Accreditation of Healthcare Organisations) (1990) *Primer on Indicator Development and Application.* Chicago: JCAHO.

Juran, J. M. (1980) *Quality, Planning and Analysis.* New York: McGraw-Hill.

Koch, H. C. H. (1991) *Total Quality Management in Healthcare.* Harlow: Longman.

NHS Executive (1994) *Networking: A Guide for Nurses, Midwives Health Visitors and the Professions Allied to Medicine.* Leeds: NHSE.

NHS Executive (2000) *Improving Quality and Performance in the New NHS, NHS performance indicators.* Health Service Circular 200/2003. London: NHS Executive.

Oakland, J. (1993) *Total Quality Management* (2nd edn). Oxford: Butterworth Heinemann.

Reid, E (1986) 'Performance Indicators', *Nursing Times*, September 10, 44–8.

Roberts, C. J., Coale, J. G and Redman, R. (1987) 'A History of the Joint Commission on Accreditation of Hospitals', *Journal of the American Association*, 258(7), 936-40.

Robson, M. (1984) *Quality Circles – A Practical Guide.* Aldershot: Gower.

Sale, D. N. (2000) *Quality Assurance: A Pathway to Excellence.* Basingstoke: Macmillan.

Scrivens. E. (1995) *Accreditation: Protecting the Professional or the Consumer?* Buckingham: Open University Press.

Vetter, N. (1986) 'Performance Indicators in Care of the Elderly', *Nursing Times*, April 1, 30–2.

Zairi, M. (1999) *Benchmarking for Best Practice: Continuous Learning through Sustainable Innovation.* Oxford: Butterworth Heinemann.

Chapter 12

Donabedian, A (1969) 'Evaluating the Quality of Medical Care', *Hilbank Memorial Fund Quarterly*, 44(2), 166–206.

Goldstone, L. A., Ball, J. A. and Collier, M. (1983) *Monitor: An Index of the Quality of Nursing Care for Acute Medical and Surgical Wards.* Newcastle-upon-Tyne: Newcastle-upon-Tyne Polytechnic Products.

Hegyvary, S. T. and Haussman, R. K. D. (1975) 'Monitoring Nursing Care Quality', *Journal of Nursing Administration*, 15(55), 17–20.

Jelinek, R. C., Haussman, R. K. D., Hegyvary, S. T. and Newmann, T. F. A. (1976) Monitoring Quality of Nursing Care, part 2: Assessment and Study of Correlates. Bethesda, MD: Department of Education, Health and Welfare.

Lesnik, M. J and Anderson, B. E. (1955) *Nursing Practice and the Law* (2nd edn). Philadelphia, PA: Lippincott.

Phaneuf, M. C. (1972) *The Nursing Audit*: Detroit: Appleton-Century-Crofts.

RCN (Royal College of Nursing) (1980) *Standards of Nursing Care*. London: RCN.

RCN (Royal College of Nursing) (1981) *Towards Standards*. London: RCN.

Wandelt, M. A. and Ager, J. W. (1974) *Quality Patient Care Scale*. New York: Appleton-Century-Crofts.

Wandelt, M. A. and Stewart S. D. (1975) *Slater Nursing Competencies Rating Scale*. Detroit: Appleton-Century-Crofts.

Phaneuf, M. C. (1976) *Nursing Audit. Self-Regulation in Nursing Practice* (2nd edn). New York: Appleton-Century-Crofts.

NHS Executive (1996) *Promoting Clinical Effectiveness: A Framework for Action in and through the NHS*. London: NHS Executive.

Chapter 13

Beckhard, R. and Harris, R. (1987) *Organisational Transitions* (2nd edn). Reading, MA: Addison-Wesley.

Bennis, W., Benne, K. D. and Chin, R. (eds) (1988) *The Planning of Change*. New York: Holt, Reinhart and Winston.

Bowman, M. P. (1986) *Nursing Management and Education; A Conceptual Approach to Change*. London: Croom Helm.

Broome, A. (1998) *Managing Change, Essentials of Nursing Management* (2nd edn). Basingstoke: Macmillan.

Burns, J. M. (1978) *Leadership*. London: Harper and Row.

Fretwell, J. E. (1985) *Freedom to Change. The Creation of a Ward Learning Environment*. London: Royal College of Nursing Publications.

Gillies, D. A. (1988) *Nursing Management, A Systems Approach* (2nd edn). New York: W. B. Saunders/Harcourt Brace Jovanovich.

Hinings, R. (1983) *Planning, Organising and Managing Change*. Luton: Local Government Training Board.

Kanter, R. M. (1984) *The Change Masters*. London: Allen and Unwin.

King's Fund (1999) *Promoting Action on Clinical Effectiveness (PACE) Experience,* *Evidence and Everyday practice*. London: King's Fund.

Lewin, K. (1953) 'Studies in Group Decisions', in D. Cartwright and A. Zander (eds), *Group Dynamics: Research and Theory*. Evanstone, IL: Row Peterson.

Mintzberg, H. (1973) *The Nature of Managerial Work*. Prentice-Hall.

NHS Executive (1999) Health Service Circular 1999/065 *Clinical Governance: Quality in the New NHS*. London: Department of Health.

Plant, R. (1987) *Managing Change and Making it Stick*. London: Fontana.

Rogers, B. cited in Welch, L. B. (1979) 'Planned Care in Nursing', *Nursing Clinics in North America*, 14 (2), 311.

Rogers, B. (1983) *Diffusion of Innovation* (3rd edn). New York: Free Press.

Rogers, E. and Shoemaker, F. (1971) *Communication of Innovations: A Cross Cultural Report*. New York: Free Press.

Towell, D. and Harries, C. (1979) *Innovation in Patient Care*. London: Croom Helm.

Turrell, E. A. (1986) *Change and Innovation: A Challenge for the NHS*. London: Institute of Health Services Management.

Chapter 14

Belbin, R. M. (1981) *Management Teams – Why They Succeed or Fail*. Oxford: Heinemann.

Drucker, P. F. (1977) *Management: Tasks, Responsibilities, Practices*. Basingstoke: Pan Books.

Handy, C. B. (1985) *Understanding Organizations*. Harmondsworth: Penguin Books.

Justice, T., and Jamieson, D. W. (1999) *The Facilitator's Fieldbook*. New York: American Management Association.

Marquis, B. L. and Hutson, C. J (2000) *Leadership Roles and Management Function in Nursing: Theory and Application* (3rd edn). Philadelphia, PA: Lippincott.

Schein, E. (1969) *Process Consultation*. London: Addison-Wesley.

Stewart, J. (1996) *Managing Change Through Training and Development*. London: Kogan Page Ltd.

Tuckman, B. W. (1965) 'Developmental Sequences in Small Groups', *Psychological Bulletin*, 63(6), 384–99.

Chapter 15

Bentley, C. (2002) *Practical PRINCE2*. London: HMSO.

Collins (1988) *Collins Modern English Dictionary*. Glasgow: William Collins.

Critchley, B. and Casey, D. (1984) 'Second Thoughts on Team Building', *Management Education and Development*, 15(2), 163–75.

Harrington, H. J., Conner, D. R. and Horney, N. L. (2000) *Project Change Management*. New York: McGraw-Hill.

Project Management Institute, Standards Committee (1996) *A Guide to the Project Management Body of Knowledge*. Upper Darby, PA: Project Management Institute.

Chapter 16

Covey, S. R. (1989) *The Seven Habits of Effective People*. New York: Simon and Schuster.

Covey, S. R., Merrill, A. R. and Merrill, R. R. (1994). *First Things First*. New York: Simon and Schuster.

DoH (Department of Health) (1999) *Making a Difference: Strengthening the Nursing, Midwifery and Health Visiting Contribution to Health and Healthcare*. London: HMSO.

DoH (Department of Health) (2000) *The NHS Plan, A Plan for Investment, a Plan for Reform*. London: HMSO.

Doyle, M. and Straus, D. (1976) *How to Make Meetings Work: The New Interaction Method*. New York: Jove Books.

Appendix

Abdellah, F. (1958) *Effects of Nursing Staffing on Satisfactions with Nursing Care*. Chicago: American Hospital Association Monograph.

Alcott, L. M. (1960) *Hospital Sketches*, ed. B. Z. Jones. Cambridge, MA: Belknap Press.

Allsop, J. (1986) *Health Policy and the National Health Service*. London: Longman.

Alment Report (1976) *Competence to Practice. Committee of Enquiry into Competence to Practice*. London: HMSO.

Baker, A. (1976) 'The Hospital Advisory Service', in G. McLachlan (ed.), *A Question of Quality*. London: Oxford University Press, 203–16.

Baggott, R. (1994) *Health and Health Care in Britain*. Basingstoke: Palgrave Macmillan.

Ball, J. A. Goldstone, L. A. and Collier, M. M. (1983) *Monitor: An Index of the Quality of Nursing Care for Acute Medical and Surgical Wards*. Newcastle-upon-Tyne: Newcastle-upon-Tyne Polytechnic Products.

BSI (British Standards Institution) (1987) *Quality Systems Part 1: Specification for Design/ Development, Production, Installation and Servicing*. Milton Keynes: BSI.

Carter, G. B. and Balme, H. (1936) *Importance of Evaluating Care*.

Clarke, C. and Whitehead, A. G. W. (1981) *The Collaboration of the Medical Services Group to the Royal College of Physicians to Improvement in Care*, in G. McLachlan (ed.), *Reviewing Practice in Medical Care: Steps to Quality Assurance*. London: Nuffield Provincial Hospital Trust, 33–40.

Collings, J. S. (1950) 'General Practice in England Today: A Reconnaissance', *The Lancet*, 535–85.

Crosby, P. B. (1979) *Quality is Free*. New York: McGraw-Hill.

Crosby, P. B. (1988) *The Eternally Successful Organization. The Art of Corporate Wellness*. New York: McGraw-Hill.

Deming, W. E. (1982) *Quality, Productivity and Competitive Position*. Cambridge, MA: Massachusetts Institute of Technology.

Deming, W. (1986) *Out of Crisis*. Cambridge, MA: Massachusetts Institute of Technology.

Department of Health for Northern Ireland (1998) *Fit for the Future*. Belfast: Department of Health.

DHSS (Department of Health and Social Security) (1979a) *Patients First*. London: HMSO.

DHSS (Department of Health and Social Security) (1979b) *Report of the Royal Commission on the National Health Service (the Merrison Commission)*. London: HMSO.

DHSS (Department of Health and Social Security) (1981) *The NHS (Constitution of District Health Authorities)*. London: HMSO.

DHSS (Department of Health and Social Security) (1983) *NHS Management Inquiry (The Griffiths Management Report)*. London: HMSO.

DHSS (Department of Health and Social Security) (1985) *Report of the Committee on Hospital Complaints Procedure*. London: HMSO.

DHSS (Department of Health and Social Security) (1986) *Health Services Management: Resource Management In Health Authorities (Management Budgeting). HN(86)34*. London: HMSO.

DoH (Department of Health) (1966) *Report of the Committee on Senior Nursing Staff Structure (Salmon Report)*. London: HMSO.

DoH (Department of Health) (1987) *Promoting Better Health*. London: HMSO.

DoH (Department of Health) (1989a) *Caring for People*, London: HMSO.

DoH (Department of Health) (1989b) *Working for Patients*. London: HMSO.

DoH (Department of Health) (1990) *NHS and Community Care Act*. London: HMSO

DoH (Department of Health) (1991a) *Health of the Nation*. London: HMSO.

DoH (Department of Health) (1991b) *The Patient's Charter*. London: HMSO.

DoH (Department of Health) (1994) *Corporate Governance in the NHS, Code of Conduct, Code of Accountability*. London: HMSO.

DoH (Department of Health) (1995) *The Patient's Charter and You*. London: HMSO.

DoH (Department of Health) (1997a) *The Caldicott Committee. Report on the Review of Patient-Identifiable Information*. London: HMSO.

DoH (Department of Health) (1997b) *The New NHS, Modern, Dependable*. London: HMSO.

DoH (Department of Health) (1998a) *A First Class Service: Quality in the New NHS*. London: HMSO.

DoH (Department of Health) (1998b) *National Performance Frameworks*. London: HMSO.

DoH (Department of Health) (1998c) *Reducing Junior Doctors' Hours. Continuing Action to Meet New Deal Standards Rest Periods and Working Arrangements, Improving Catering and Accommodation for Juniors, Other Health Points*. Health Circular 240. London: HMSO.

DoH (Department of Health) (2000a) *An Organisation With a Memory*. London: HMSO.

DoH (Department of Health) (2000b) *The NHS Plan, a Plan for Investment, a Plan for Reform*. London: HMSO.

DoH (Department of Health) (2001a) *Involving Patients and the Public in Healthcare: A Discussion Document*. London: HMSO.

DoH (Department of Health) (2001b) *National Minimum Standards For Care Homes For Older People*. London: HMSO.

DoH (Department of Health) (2002) *Delivering the NHS Plan, Next Steps on Investment, Next Steps on Reform*. London: HSMO.

DoH (Department of Health) (2004) *Standards for Better Health*. London: HMSO.

Donabedian, A. (1969) 'Medical Care Appraisal – Quality and Utilization', *Guide to Medical Care Administration*, vol. II. New York: American Public Health Association.

Drew, J. (1964) 'Determining Quality of Nursing Care', *American Journal of Nursing*, 64 (10), 82–5.

Emslie, S. (2001) 'Controls Assurance in the National Health Service in England – The Final Piece of the Corporate Governance Jigsaw', *Corporate Governance*, 12, March, Abg Professional Information, London.

Godber, G. (1976) 'The Confidential Enquiry into Maternal Deaths', in G. McLachlan (ed.), *A Question of Quality*. London: Oxford University Press, 24–33.

Goldstone, L. and Ball, J. (1984) 'The Quality of Nursing Services', *Nursing Times*, 29(8), 56–9.

Greenhalgh & Co. Ltd in conjunction with a five regional consortium (1993) *Using Information in Contracting – Setting the Context*. London: HMSO.

Hegyvary, S. T. and Hausman, R. K. D. (1975) 'Monitoring Nursing Care Quality', *Journal of Nursing Administration*, 15(55), 17–26.

JCAHO (Joint Commission on Accreditation of Healthcare Organizations) (2002) *A Journey through the History of the Joint Commission*. Chicago: JCAHO.

Juran, J. M. (1988) *Juran on Planning for Quality*. New York: Free Press.

Juran, J. M. (1989) *Juran on Leadership for Quality*. New York: Free Press.

Juran, J. M. and Gryna, F. M. (1980) *Quality Planning and Analysis*. New Delhi: McGraw-Hill.

Lang, N. (1976) *Issues in Quality Assurance Nursing, ANA Issues in Evaluative Research*. Kansas City: American Nursing Association.

Lesnik, M. J. and Anderson, B. E. (1955) *Nursing Practice and the Law* (2nd edn). Philadelphia, PA: Lippincott.

Macdonald, J. and Piggott, J. (1990) *Global Quality – The New Management Culture*. London: Mercury Books.

Mayatt, V. L. (1995) *The CNST – How to meet the Risk Management Standards and Reduce Financial Losses*. HRRI Conference, Edinburgh: Paper Sedgwick UK Ltd.

Maxwell, R. (1984) 'Quality Assessment in Health', *British Medical Journal*, 288, 1470–2.

NHSME (1990) *Working Paper 10 – Education and Training: Further Guidance*. EL (90)/119.29 June 1990. London: HMSO.

NHSME (1991) *Framework of Audit for Nursing Services*. London: HMSO.

NHSME (1992) *An Information Management and Technology Strategy for the NHS in England*. London: HMSO.

NHSME (1993) *Risk Management in the NHS*. London: HMSO.

NHSME (1999) *Governance in the New NHS; Controls Assurance Statements*. London: HMSO.

Nightingale, F. (1860) *Notes on Nursing*. London: Harrison and Sons.

Nightingale, F. (1874) *Address from Florence Nightingale to the Probationer Nurses in the Nightingale Fund School at St Thomas's Hospital who were Formerly Trained There*. Printed for private use 23 July 1874. Nut-

ting Collection, Teachers College, Columbia University.

Oakland, J. S. (1986) *Statistical Process Control*. London: Heinemann.

Oakland, J. S. (1989) *Total Quality Management*. London: Heinemann.

Øvretveit, J. (1992) *Health Service Quality*. Oxford: Blackwell Scientific Publications.

Palmer, R. E. (1978) 'The March of History: Growing Regulations and Growing Costs', *Hospital Progress*, 59(9), 58–61.

Peters, T. J and Waterman, R. H. (1982) *In Search of Excellence: Lessons From America's Best-Run Companies*. New York: Harper and Row.

Reerink, E. (1987) 'Quality Assurance in the Health Care System in the Netherlands', *Australian Clinical Review*, 7(24), 11–15.

Reiter, F. and Kakosh, M. (1953) *Quality of Nursing Care: A Report of a Field Study To Establish Criteria 1950–1953*. New York: Graduate School of Nursing, New York Medical College.

Roberts C. J., Coale, J. G. and Redman, R. (1987) 'A History of the Joint Commission on Accreditation of Hospitals', *Journal of the American Medical Association*, 258(7), 936–40.

RCGP (Royal College of General Practitioners) (1985) *Quality in General Practice*. London: RCN.

RCN (Royal College of Nursing) (1980) *Standards of Nursing Care*. London: RCN.

RCN (Royal College of Nursing) (1981) *Towards Standards*. London: RCN.

RCN (Royal College of Nursing) (1987) *In Pursuit of Excellence. Position Statement on Nursing*. London: RCN.

Sale, D. N. (2000) *Quality Assurance: A Pathway to Excellence*. Basingstoke: Macmillan.

Secretary of State for Scotland (1997) *Designed to Care in Scotland: Renewing the National Health in Scotland*. Edinburgh: HMSO.

Stewart, I. (1919) 'Possibilities of Standardisation of Nursing Techniques', *Modern Hospital*, 12(6), 451–4.

Wandelt, M. A. and Ager J. W. (1974) *Quality Patient Care Scale*. New York: Appleton-Century-Crofts.

Wandelt, M. A. and Stewart, D. S. (1975) *Slater Nursing Competencies Rating Scale*. New York: Appleton-Century-Crofts.

Wilson, J. (1983) 'The Canadian Hospital Accreditation Program', *Canadian Nurse*, 79, 48–9.

Working Time Regulations (1998) London: HMSO.

WHO (World Health Organisation) (1985a) *Targets For Health For All*. Geneva: WHO Regional Office for Europe.

WHO (World Health Organisation) (1985b) *The Principles of Quality Assurance Report on WHO Meeting. Euro Report and Studies 94*. Copenhagen: WHO.

Index